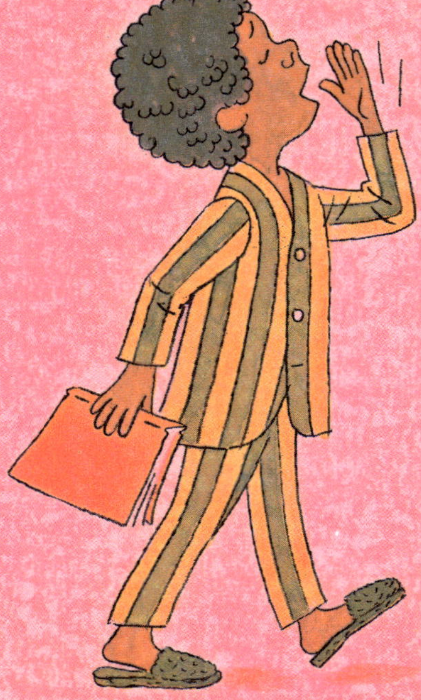

What makes you **YAWN**
when you get sleepy?
(See page 62)

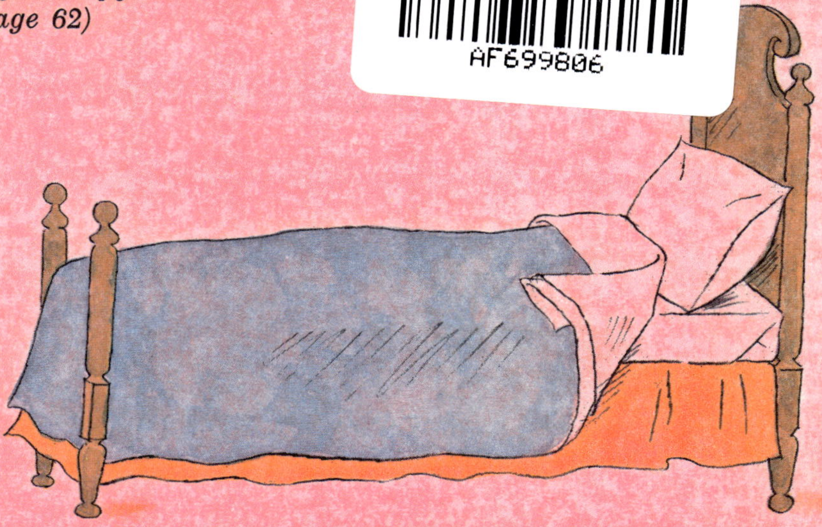

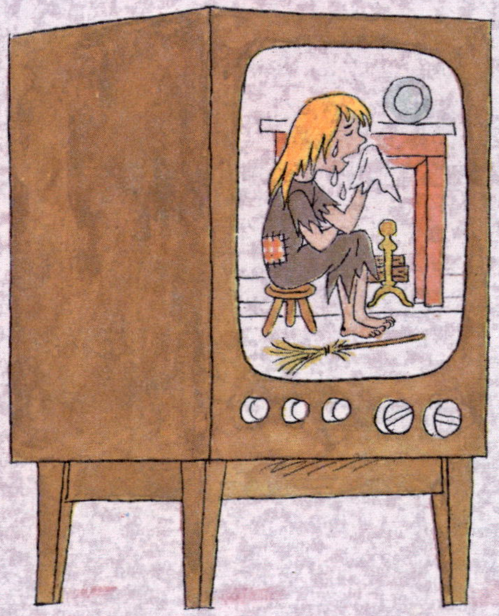

Where do your tears come from
when you **CRY?**
(See page 67)

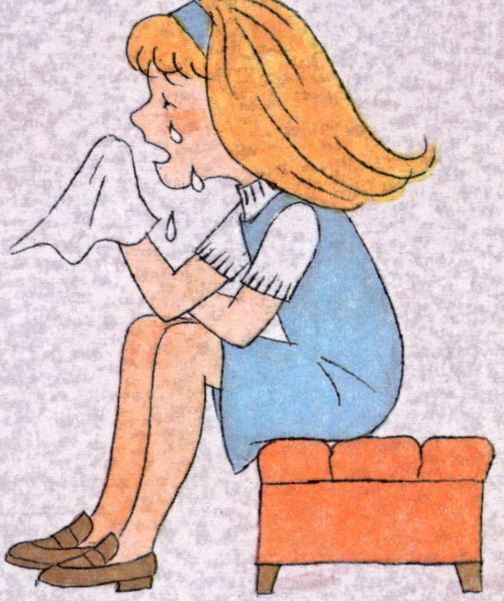

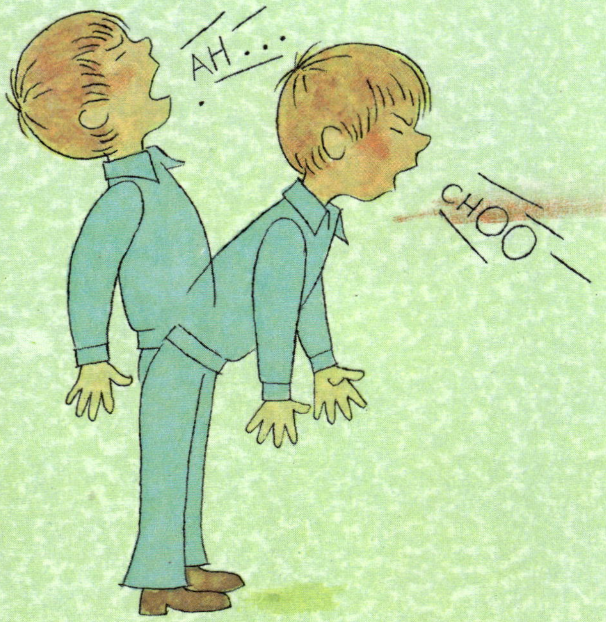

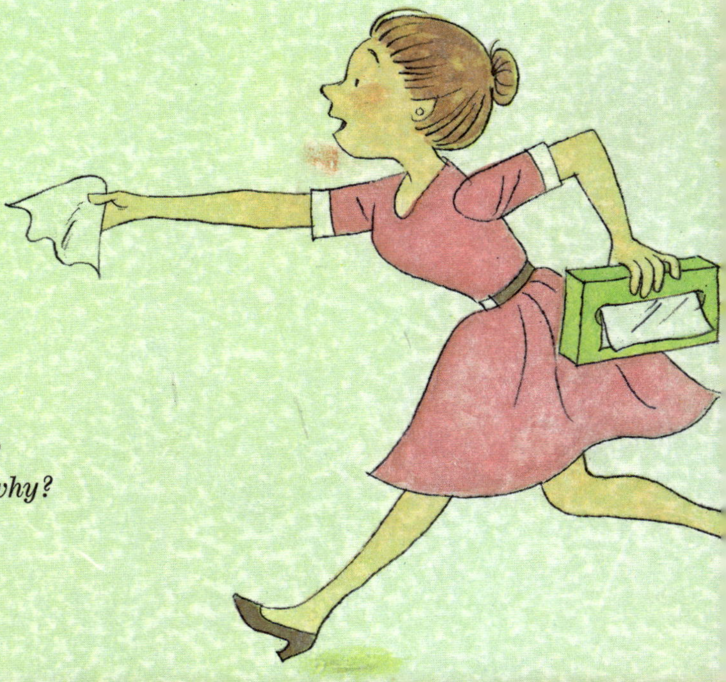

Your nose feels irritated,
then you **SNEEZE**... why?
(See page 43)

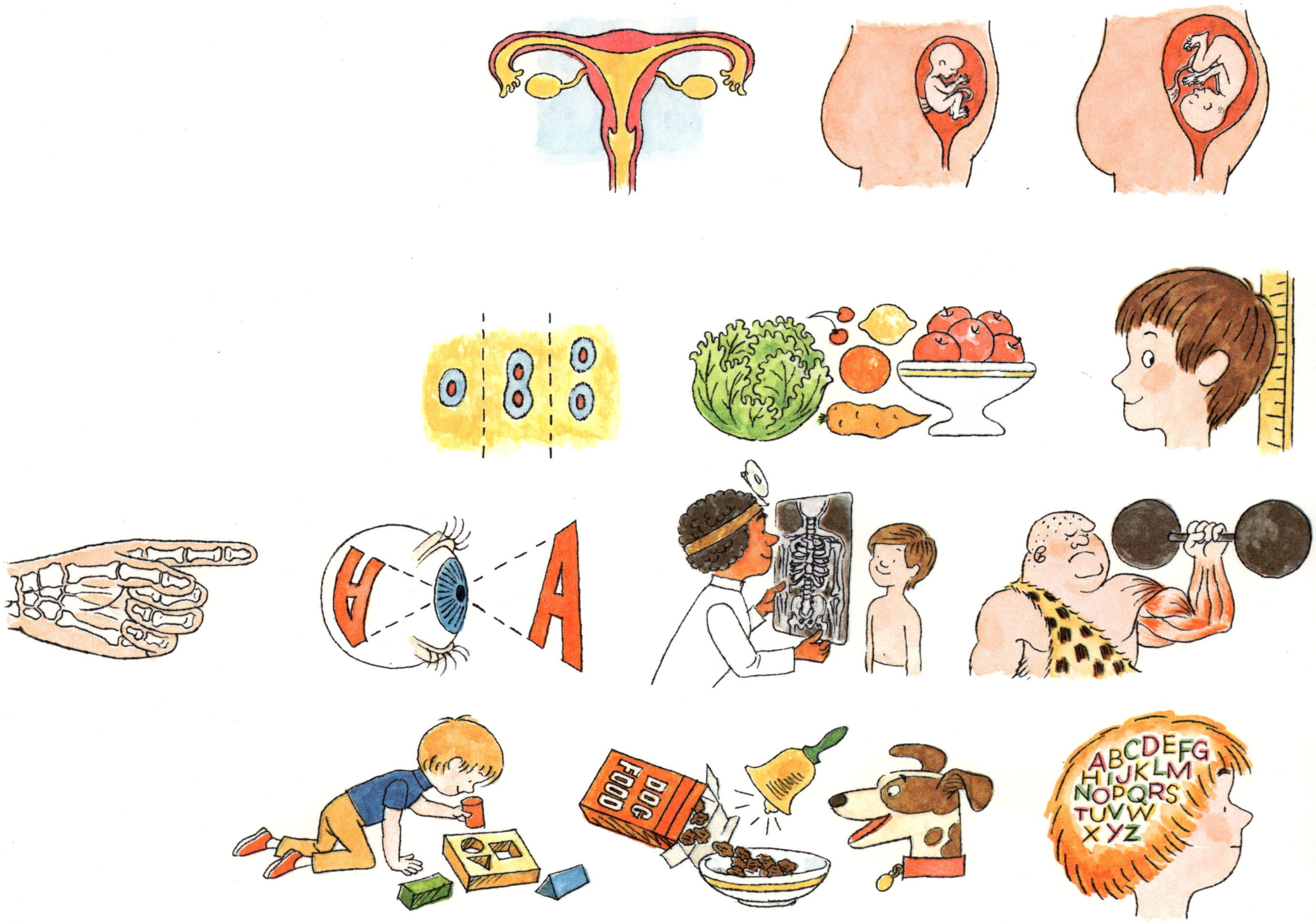

to HOLLY

Joe Kaufman's

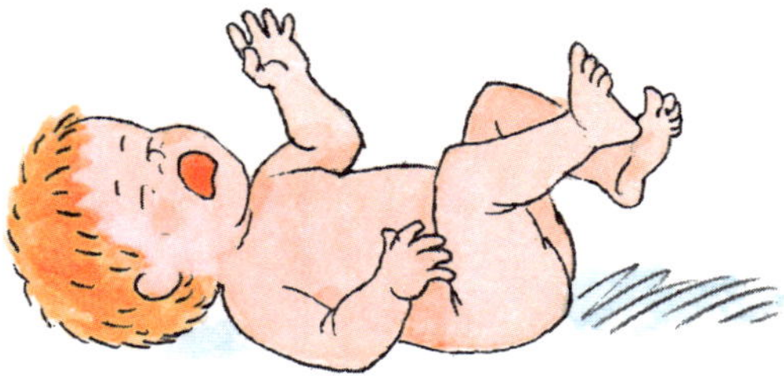

HOW WE ARE BORN

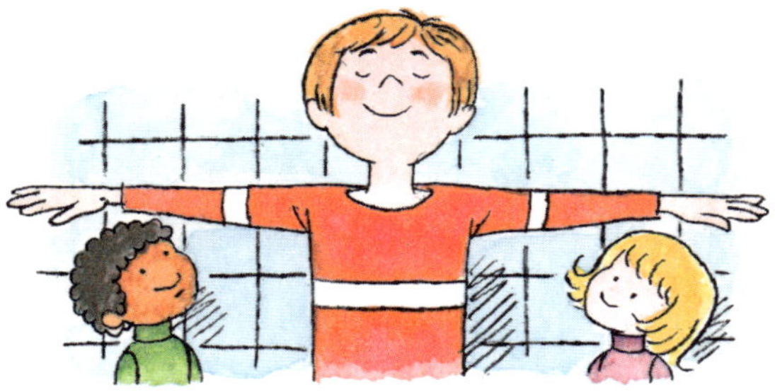

HOW WE GROW

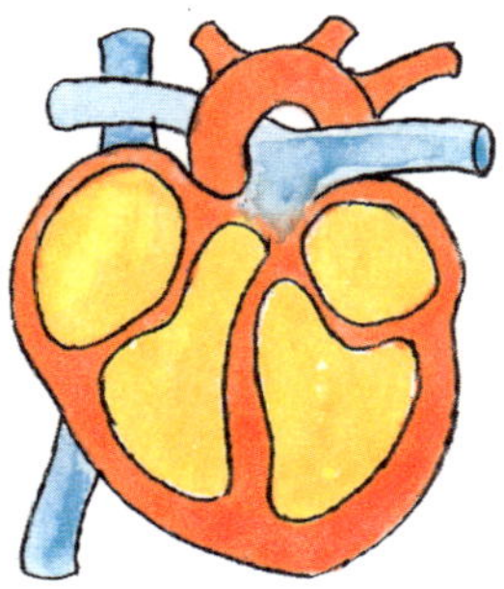

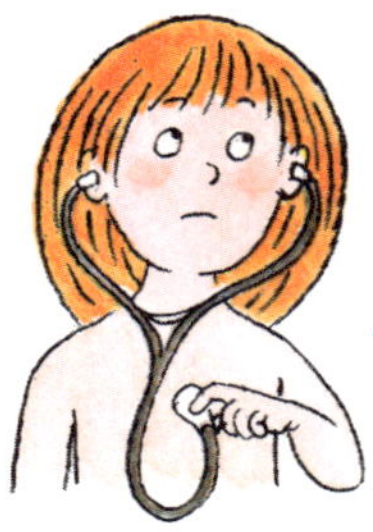

HOW OUR BODIES WORK

...AND HOW WE LEARN

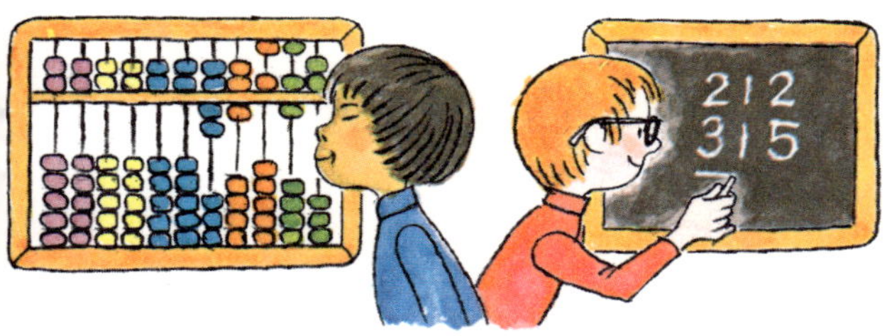

Written and Illustrated by JOE KAUFMAN

In consultation with MARSHALL KAUFMAN, B.M.E.
New York University Medical Center

ELLEN KAUFMAN, M.D. *and* ARTHUR KAUFMAN, M.D.
University of New Mexico School of Medicine Faculty

Golden Press · New York
Western Publishing Company, Inc.
Racine, Wisconsin

Printed in the U.S.A.

Library of Congress Catalog Card Number: 75-11069

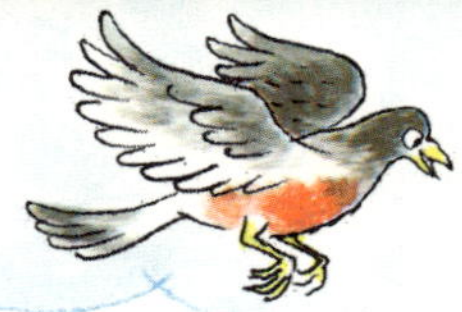

CONTENTS

A NOTE TO PARENTS: This book has been designed to give children an understanding of their bodies—and to help parents answer the many questions they ask. It provides a basic introduction to all the body structures and their functions, and also covers a variety of related topics. The book is primarily for young readers from six to twelve, who will find ideas and concepts to fascinate them at every stage of their growth. The whole family, in fact, will enjoy reading and sharing the information offered here.

The exercises on pages 32-33 are from the book *Youth Physical Fitness*, published by The President's Council on Physical Fitness. The tooth-cleaning method on page 80 is from the pamphlet "Cleaning Your Teeth and Gums," published by The American Dental Association, Chicago, Illinois.

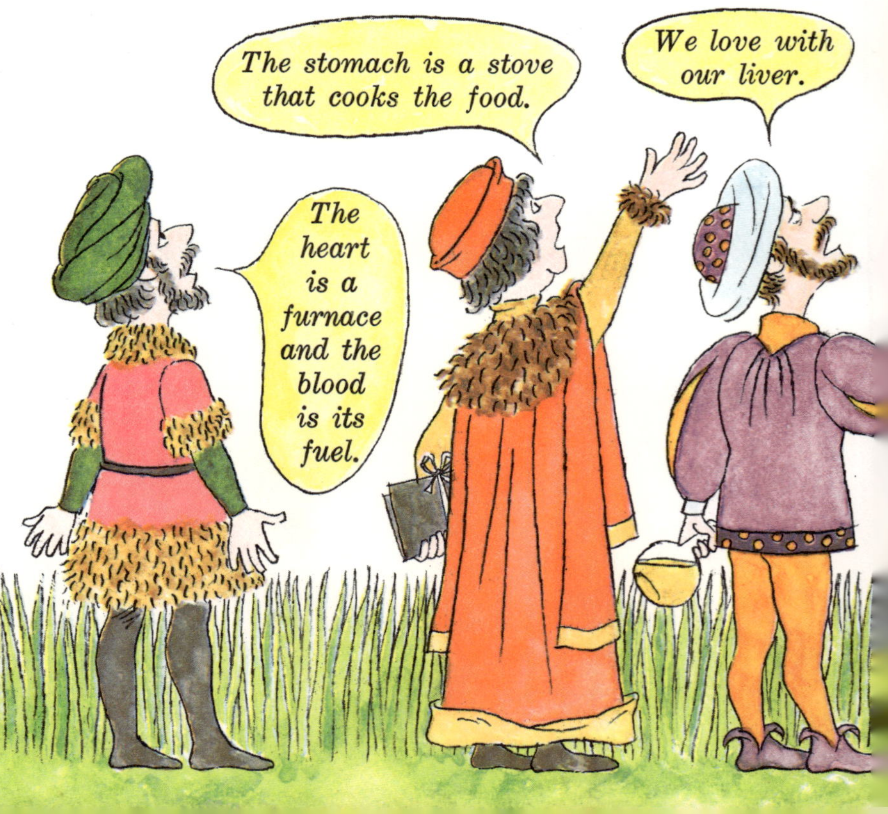

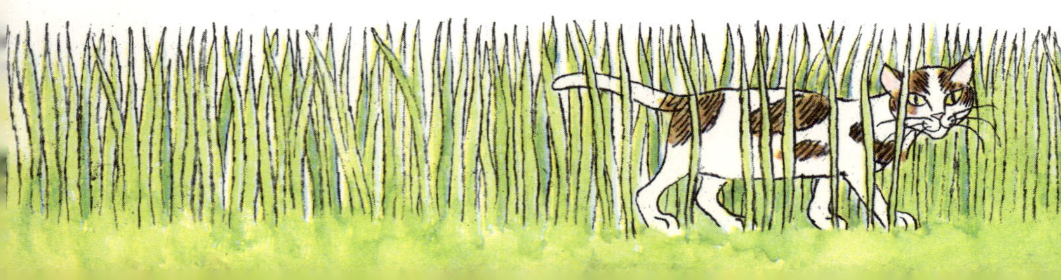

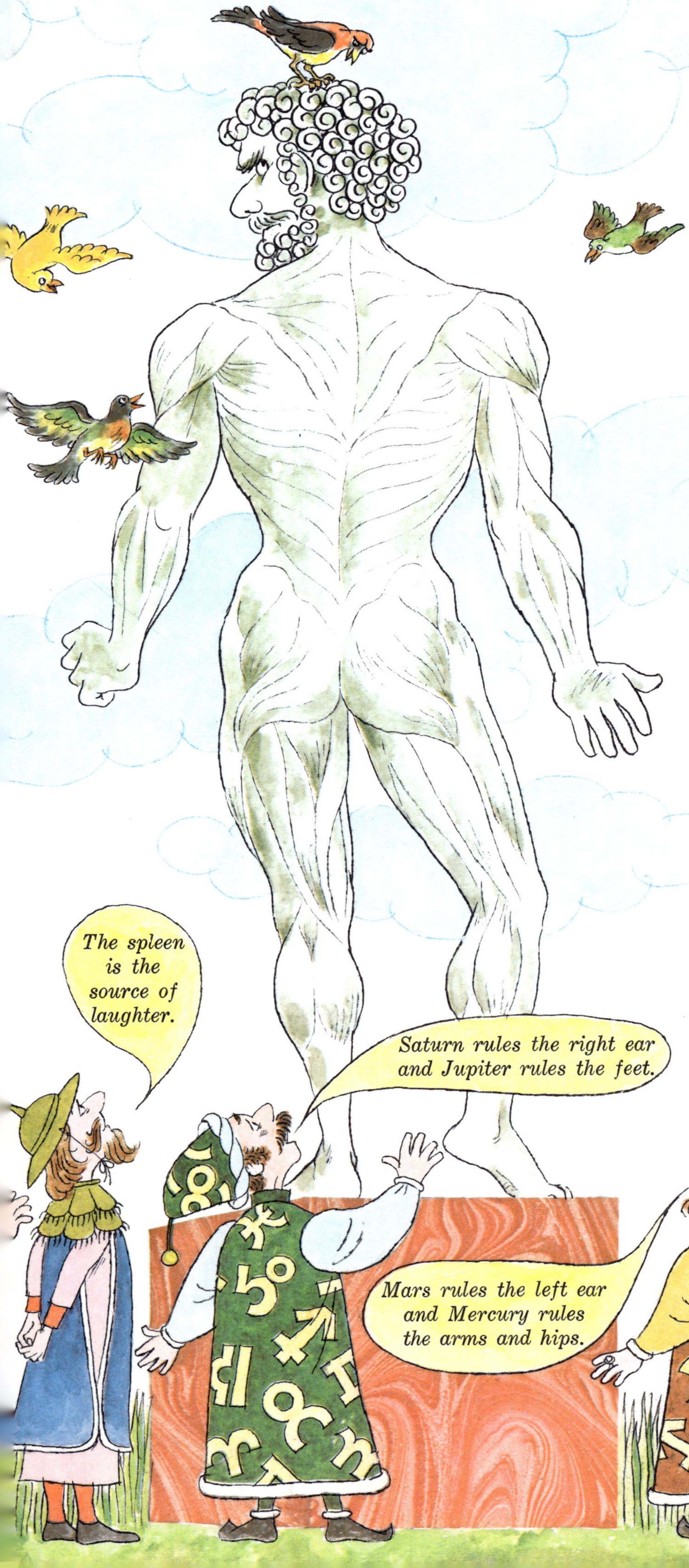

EARLY IDEAS about how the body worked, and what the functions of the different organs inside the body were, seem strange to us now. Where did the ancient astrologers get the funny idea that Saturn rules the right ear and Mars rules the left ear? And how did the doctors of the old Orient decide that the gall bladder is the seat of courage?

The answer is that these people had very little scientific knowledge to help them make better judgments. As a matter of fact, they had superstitions and fears that prevented them from carrying out scientific investigation. So the people wondered and guessed at how babies began and how they grew to be adults. And they guessed at which foods helped the body grow and which foods kept it from getting sick. They made many other guesses about how the body works—this was all they could do with their limited knowledge.

Only in the last three centuries did people learn that blood circulates—that the heart pumps it through the arteries, and that it returns through the veins to start its trip again. Before that there were other ideas about the blood. One idea was that the blood flowed endlessly from the liver to the heart, which people thought was a sort of furnace that burned the blood as fuel.

Today, after centuries of studying the human body, its muscles and bones, its brain and all its other organs, doctors and scientists know quite a lot about it, and are learning more all the time. Some of that knowledge is in this book. We hope it will help you begin to understand that fascinating subject—your own body.

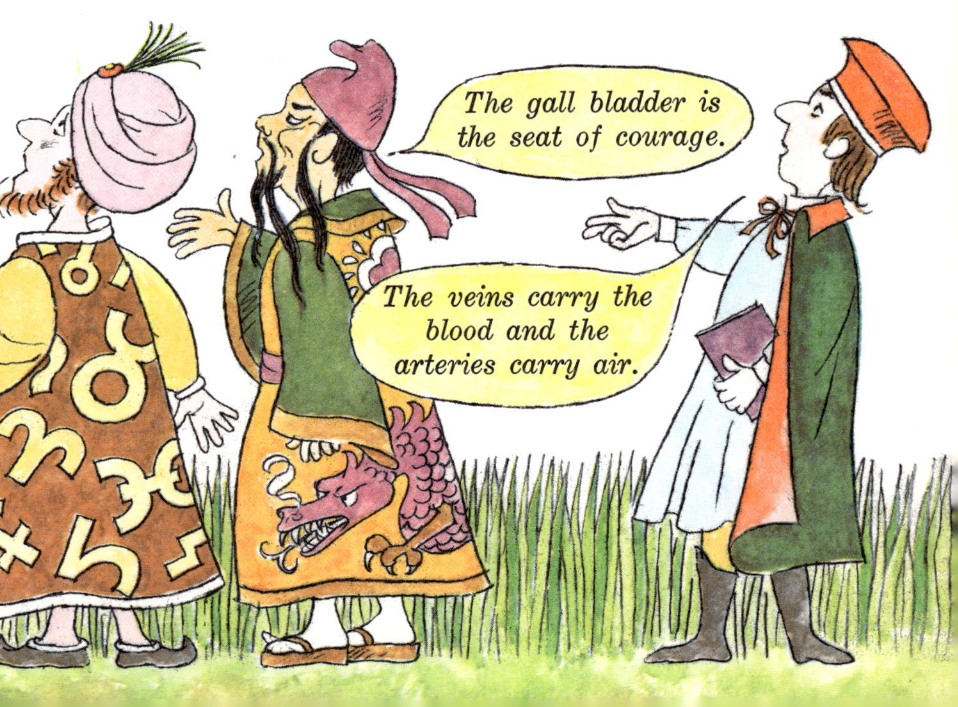

When a baby turtle hatches, it heads for the water for its first swim.

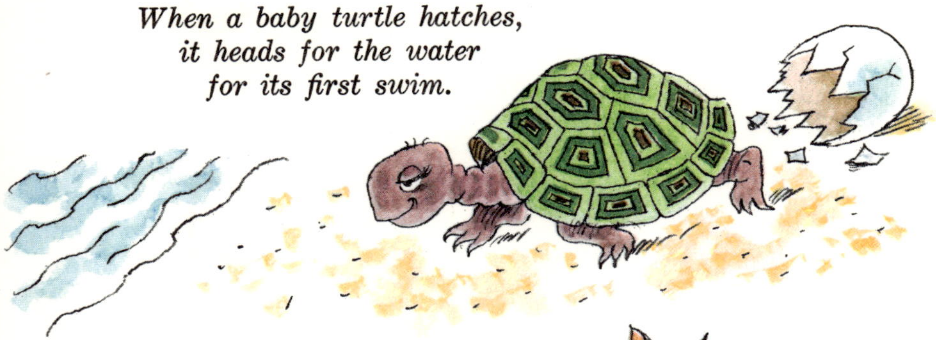

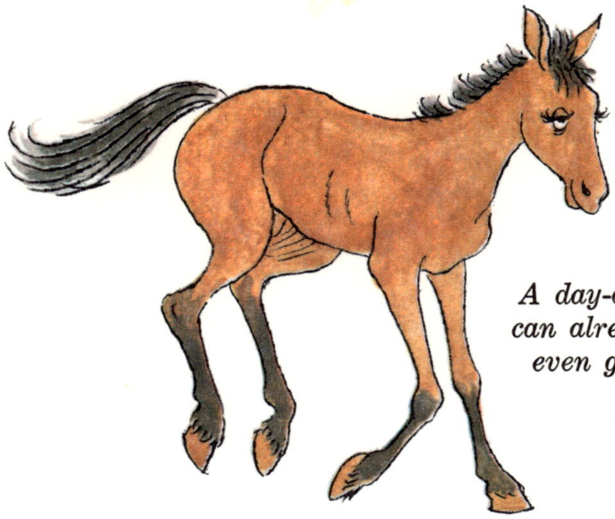

A day-old baby horse can already walk, and even gallop a little.

The NEWBORN BABY is usually about twenty inches long, and probably weighs about seven pounds. Of course, some babies may be bigger and some may be smaller. The baby's face may be red and wrinkled, and its head probably looks very big. The baby's skin color is lighter than it will be later, because the pigments that color the skin won't be working for several days or even weeks.

Before being born, the baby got all its oxygen from its mother. Now the baby must use its lungs for the first time, and begin to breathe on its own.

Before being born, the baby lived in a warm, dark comfortable place inside its mother. The newborn baby's first cry tells you that now it is hungry or cold or maybe bothered by bright lights. There are no tears when the baby cries because its tear ducts won't

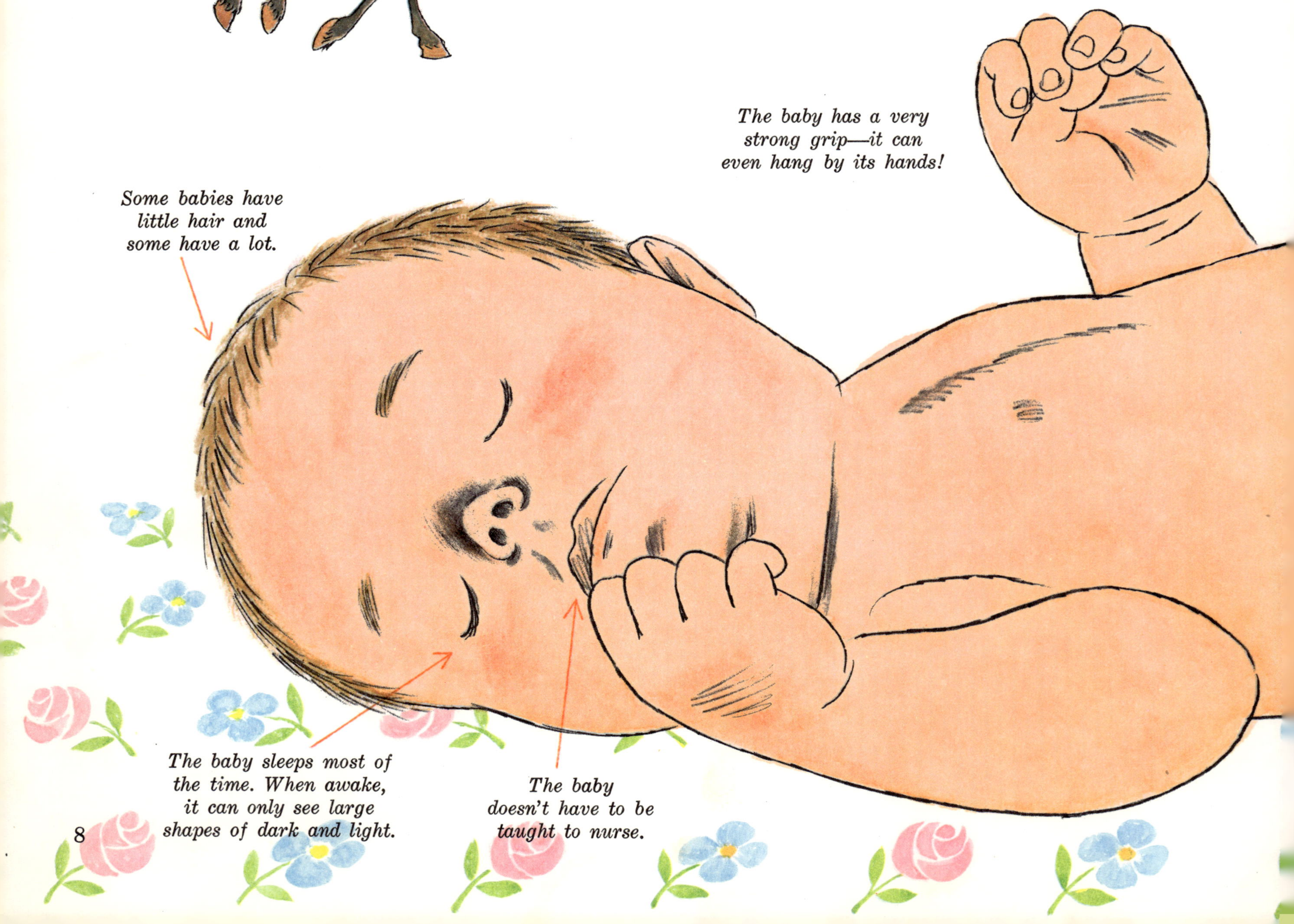

The baby has a very strong grip—it can even hang by its hands!

Some babies have little hair and some have a lot.

The baby sleeps most of the time. When awake, it can only see large shapes of dark and light.

The baby doesn't have to be taught to nurse.

be working for a week or two. The baby's ears are clogged and won't hear well for a day or so. Its eyes wander and may sometimes seem to be a little crossed. The baby needs time to learn to use its eyes, as well as the rest of its body.

But the baby is born knowing how to eat. If the mother's breast or a bottle is put to its mouth the baby is soon sucking away. The baby is also born with a very strong grip, strong enough to support its own weight. If you put the baby on its stomach, it will move as though trying to swim. And if you hold the baby so that its feet just touch the ground, the baby moves them in a walking motion.

But what the baby does most of all is sleep, about 18 hours out of every 24. A newborn baby needs lots of sleep to grow.

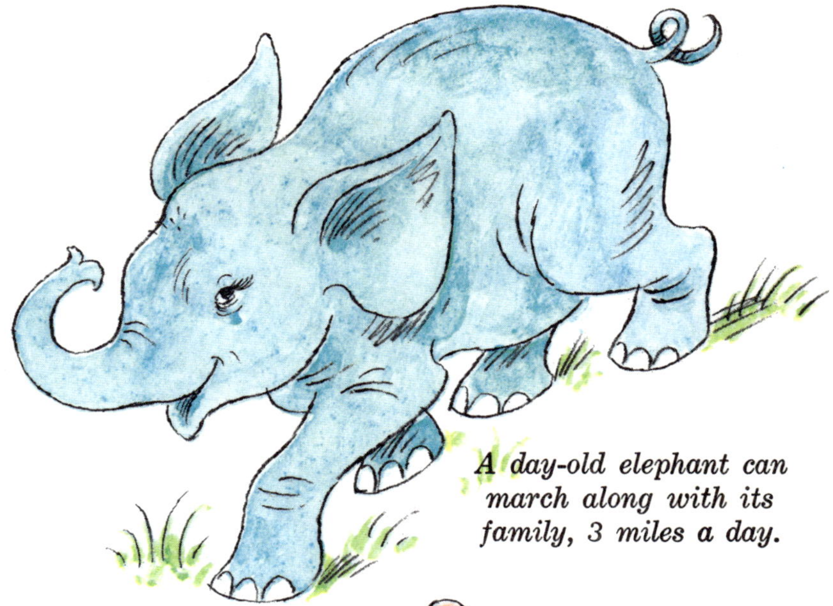

A day-old elephant can march along with its family, 3 miles a day.

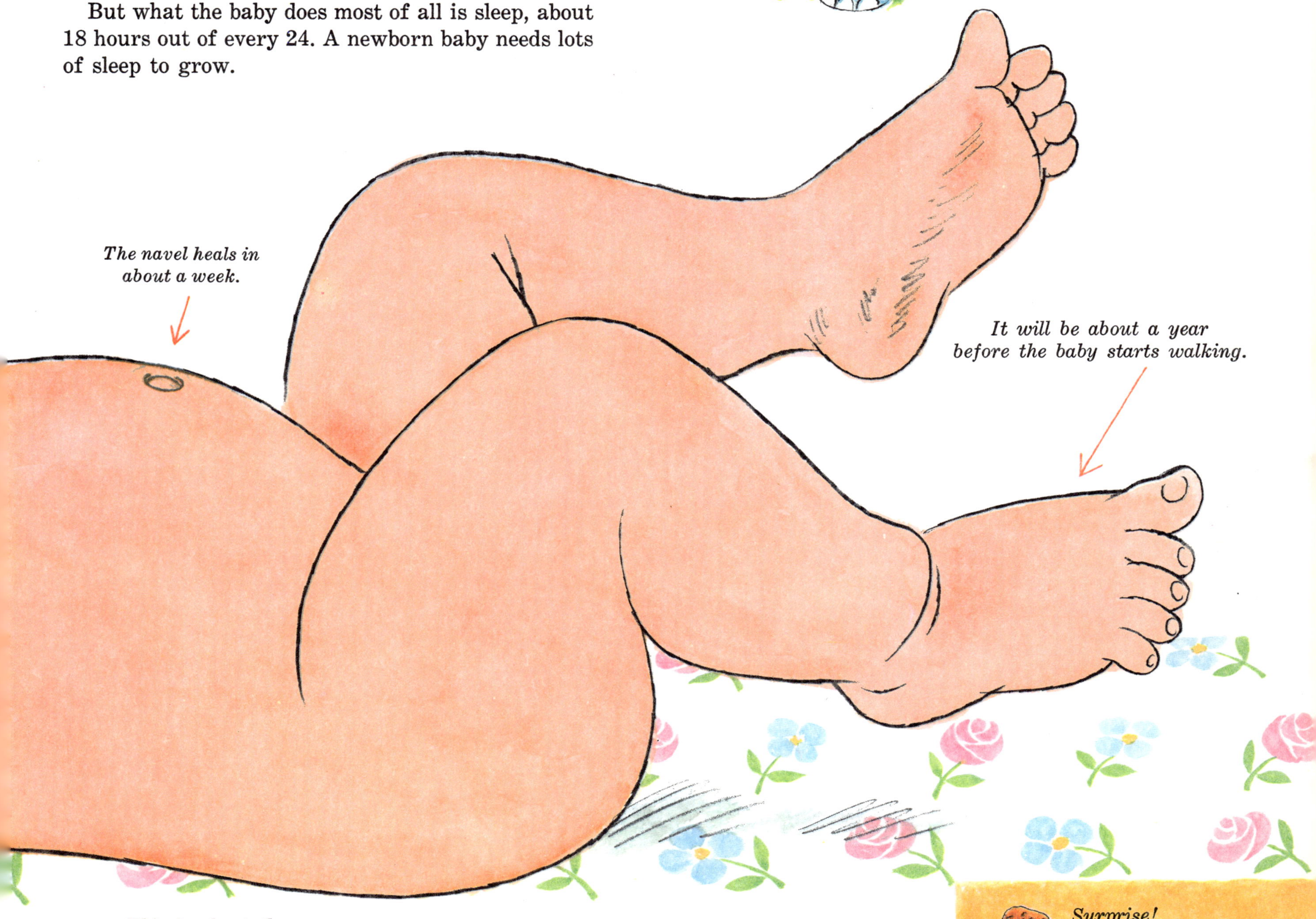

The navel heals in about a week.

It will be about a year before the baby starts walking.

This is about the real size of a newborn baby.

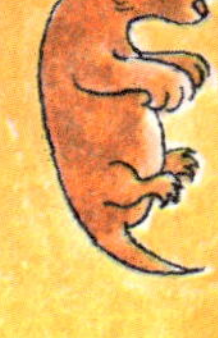

Surprise! A newborn kangaroo is only an inch long. It nurses in its mother's pouch for four months.

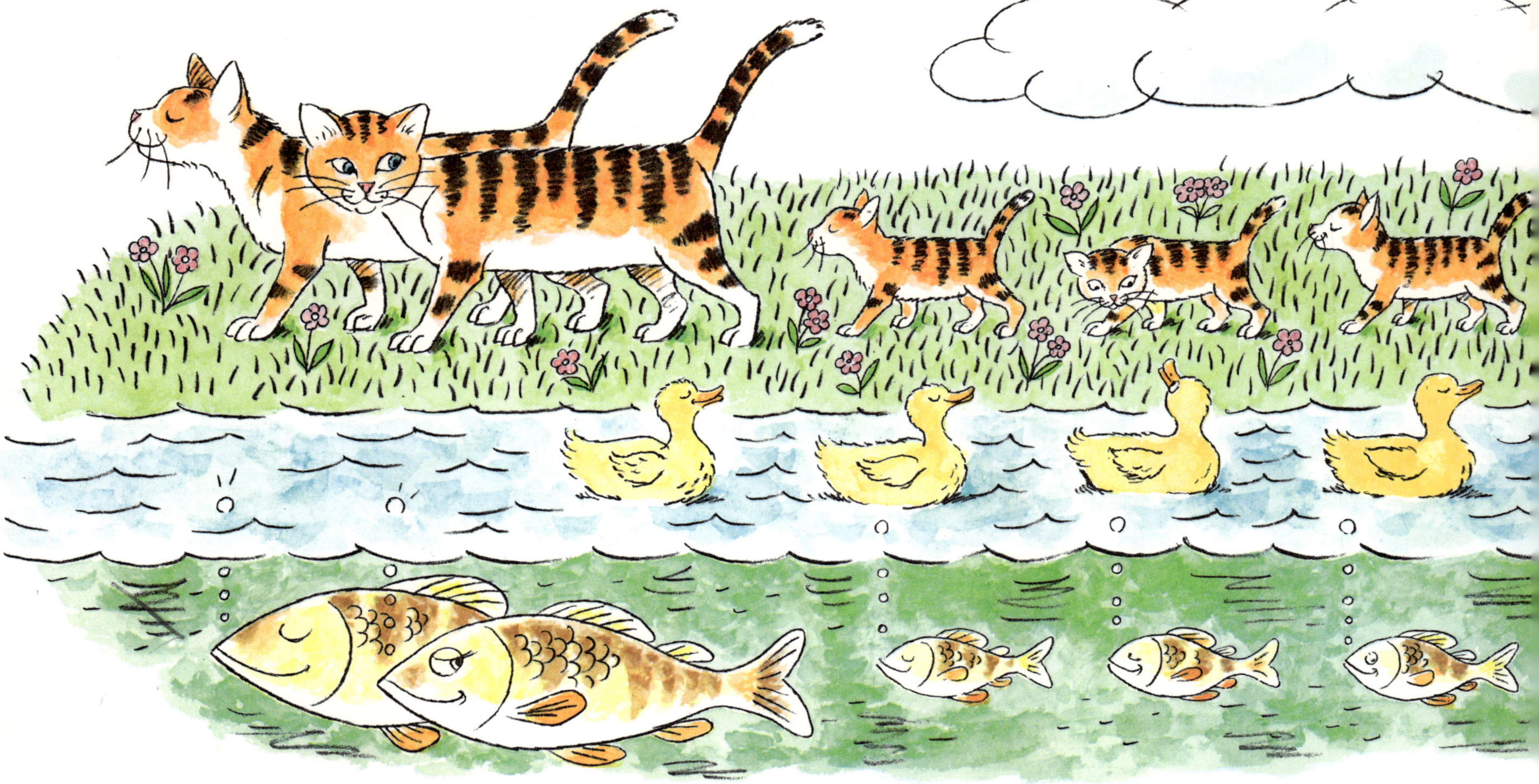

A BABY BEGINS when a sperm cell from the father meets an egg cell from the mother. The sperm gets inside the egg cell, and together they become a new and different cell, part like the mother's and part like the father's. This is a fertilized cell, a cell which is ready to begin growing into a baby. An egg cell from any animal can only be fertilized by a sperm cell from the same kind of animal.

A baby fish begins when the female fish finds a safe spot under the water and lays many eggs. The male fish swims over the eggs, and spreads sperm over them from an opening near his tail. The tiny sperm cells swim to the eggs, and push inside them. The fertilized eggs will develop into baby fish.

In many animals, the egg cell needs to stay inside the mother, because it must be protected after fertilization. The sperm cells from the father must go into the mother's body to find the egg cell to fertilize.

A baby duck begins when the male duck gets on the female duck's back, so that his sperm can come out of an opening under his tail and go into an opening under the female's tail. The sperm cells wiggle their way to the female's egg cells. A fertilized egg cell develops inside the mother into a large duck egg with a tiny duckling inside. The mother lays the egg, then sits on it to keep it warm while the duckling grows inside it. In a few weeks, the egg hatches and out comes the duckling.

For the sperm of a male cat to get to the egg cells of the female, the male cat stretches his body over the female's back and his penis gets hard so it can go into her vagina. The sperm cells come out of the male's penis, go into the female's vagina and find their way to the egg cells. The fertilized egg cells grow inside the mother for about two months—developing into kittens, ready to be born.

Sperm cells as seen through a microscope—they move by wiggling their tails.

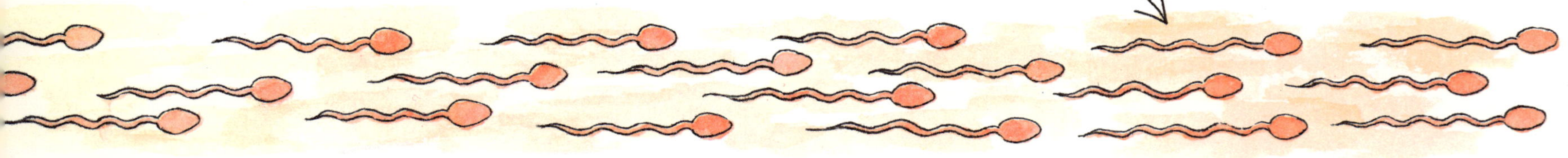

A human baby begins very much like all other babies—the father's sperm cell must fertilize the mother's egg cell. Hundreds of tiny egg cells are stored in the mother's two ovaries. Once a month, one egg cell leaves an ovary and travels through a tube to the uterus. If it isn't fertilized during this trip, it passes out of the mother's body.

The sperm cells are made in the father's testicles. After the father puts his penis into the mother's vagina, the sperm cells travel through a tube from his testicles to his penis, then go into the mother's vagina. There they begin their trip in search of the egg cell. Millions of sperm cells meet the egg cell in the tube leading from the ovary to the uterus. But it takes only one sperm cell to fertilize the egg cell. Once the egg cell is fertilized, it moves to the uterus, where it will spend nine months growing into a human baby ready to be born.

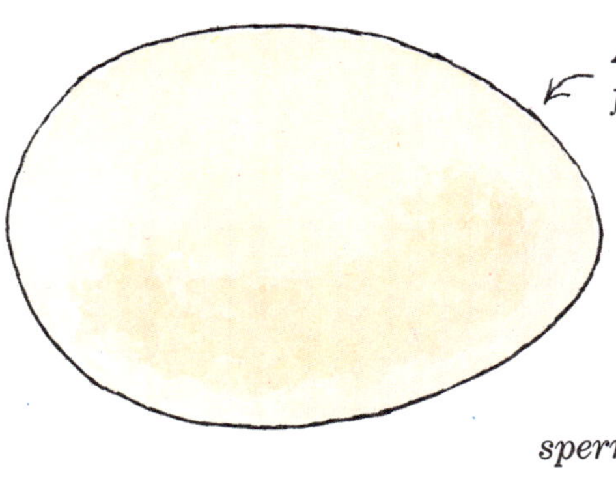

A baby chick will hatch from this fertilized egg.

This is the actual size of a human egg cell.

You can't see a sperm cell without a microscope.

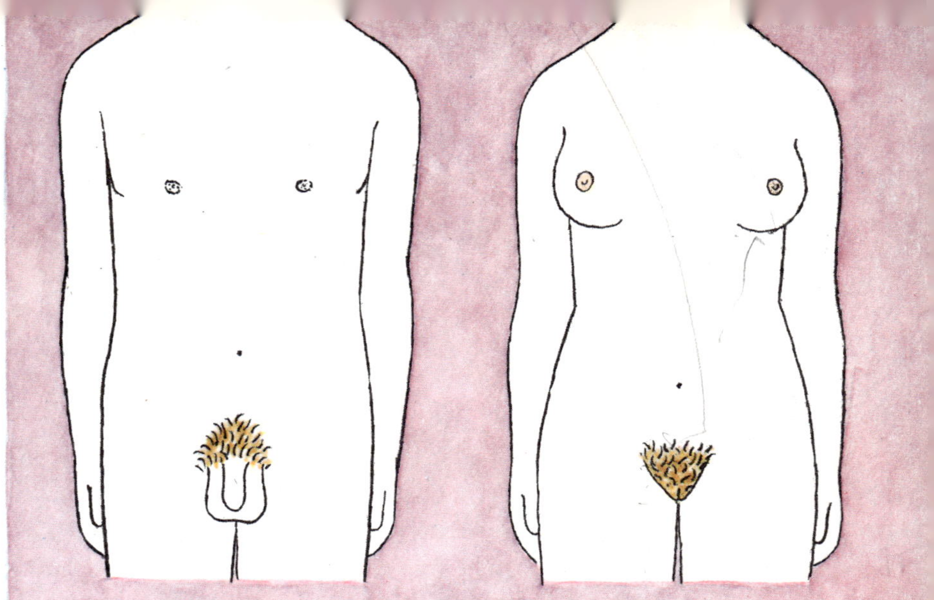

A man's penis and testicles hang outside his body.

A woman's vagina, uterus, and ovaries are tucked inside her body.

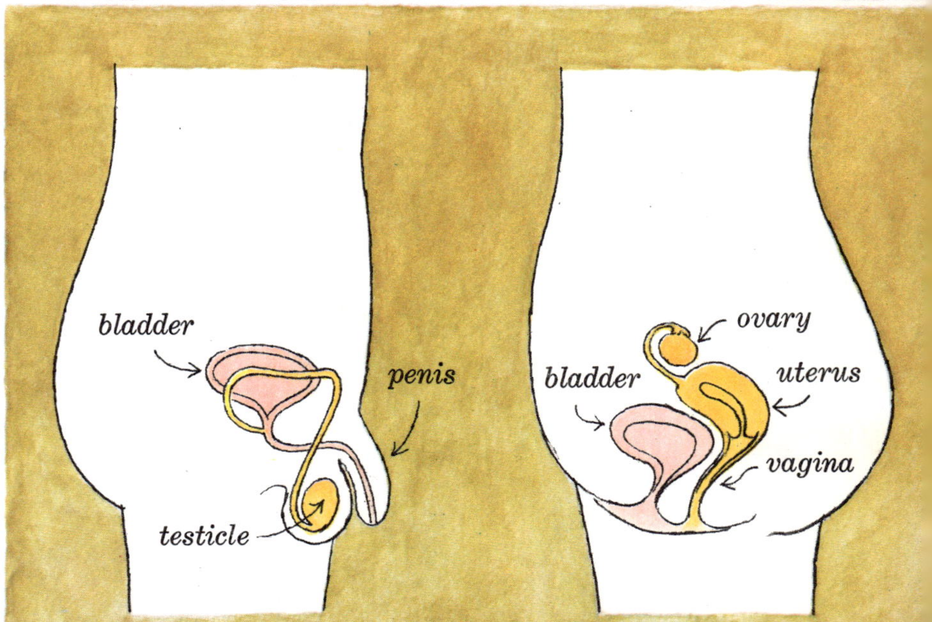

Inside view—a man's penis and testicles

Inside view—a woman's vagina, uterus, and ovaries

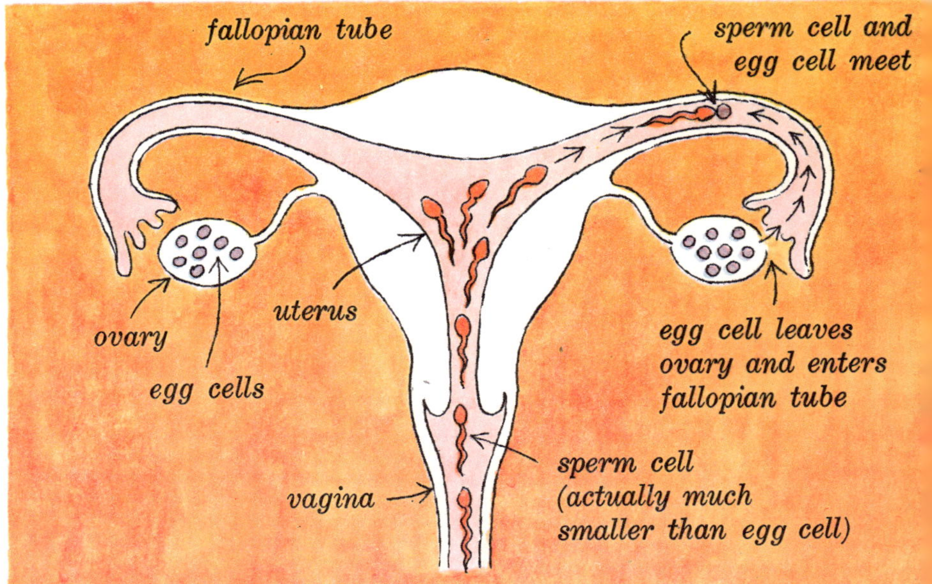

Sperm cells enter vagina, then uterus, then fallopian tubes, where one sperm cell meets an egg cell coming from the ovary.

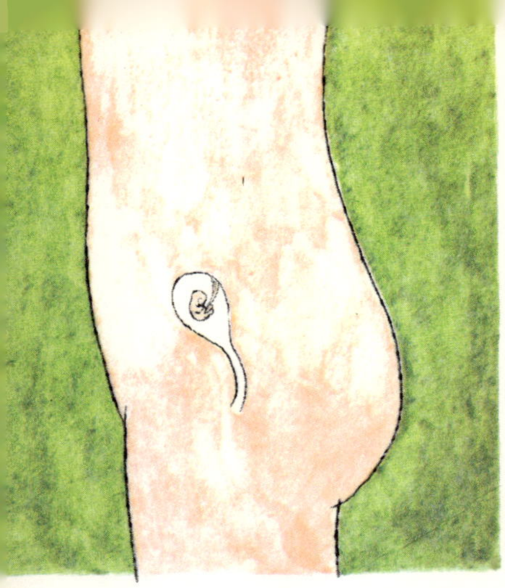

First month—a quarter of an inch long, but growing nicely.

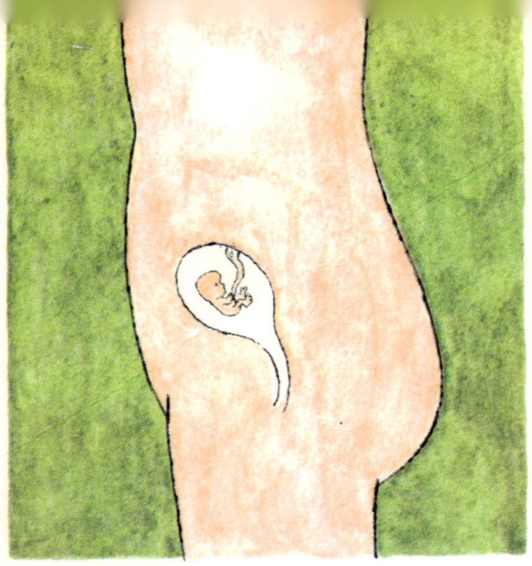

Second month—only one inch long, but now the baby looks like a baby.

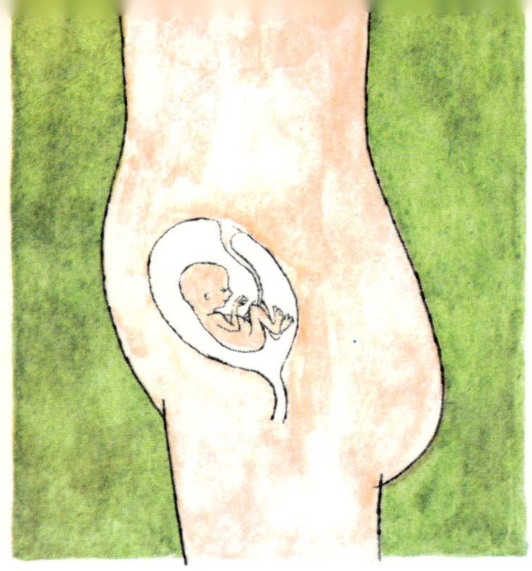

Third month—now the doctor can clearly hear the baby's heartbeat.

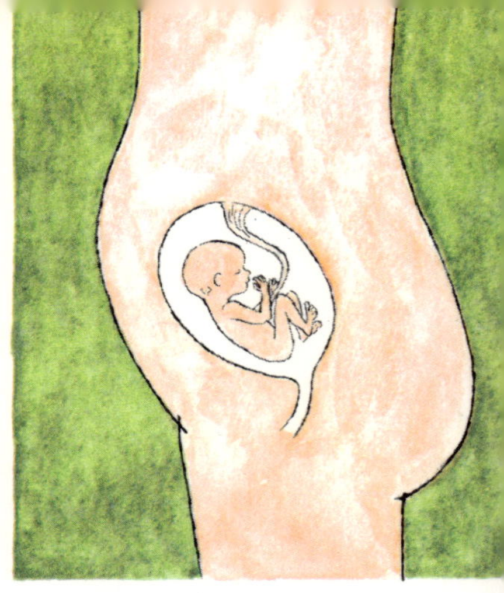

Fourth month—the mother may be able to feel the baby move.

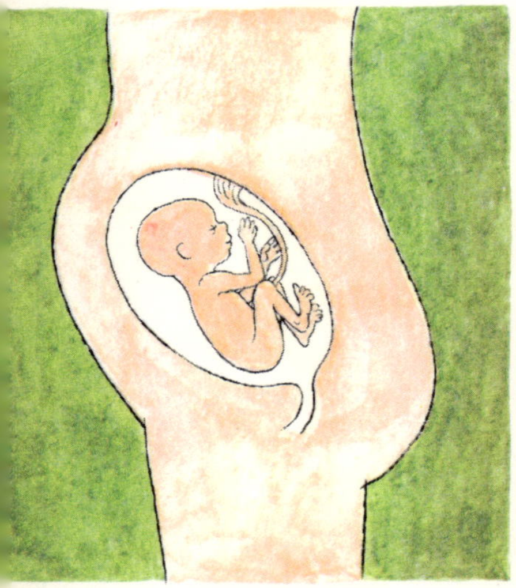

Fifth month—the baby weighs one pound—fingernails growing.

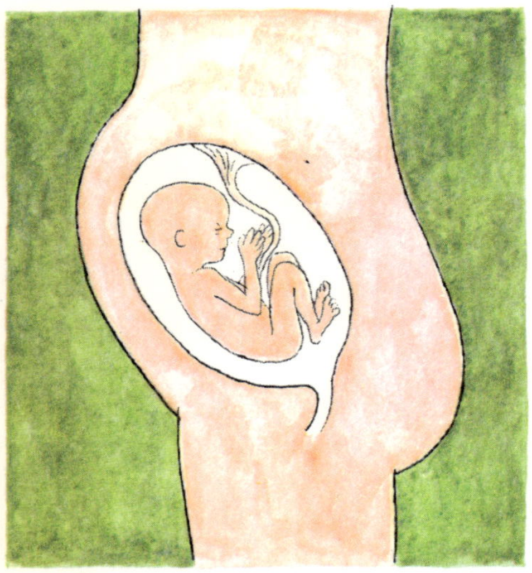

Sixth month—the baby is twelve inches long and weighs two pounds.

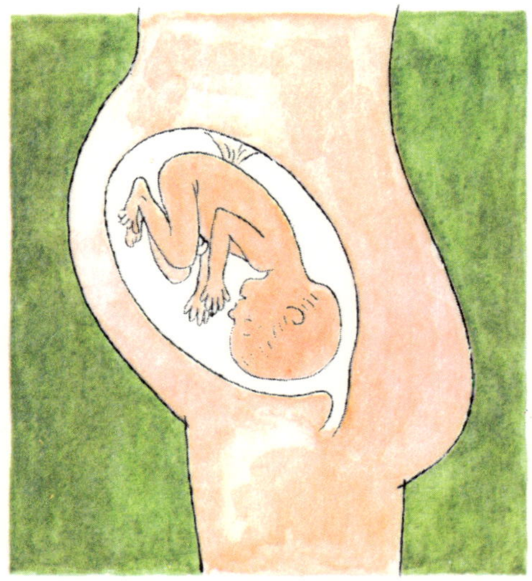

Seventh month—baby weighs three pounds—opens and closes its eyes.

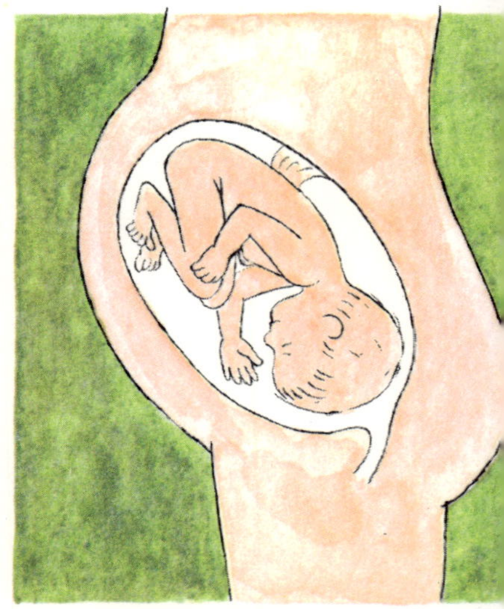

Eighth month—the baby has gained two pounds this month.

The BABY-TO-BE begins as just one cell, a fertilized egg cell so tiny that you can hardly see it. It splits and becomes two cells, the two become four, and they continue to multiply into a small cluster of cells called the embryo. Soon the embryo is settled into the lining of the mother's uterus. A strong sac filled with liquid forms around the embryo to protect it. Inside this warm sac it grows quickly, fed by the mother's body through a cord called the umbilical cord.

In the second month the embryo is beginning to look a little like a baby, with tiny arms, legs, eyes, and ears developing. From the third month on, when the embryo begins to move, it is called a fetus.

The fetus grows fast—at the end of four months it weighs eight ounces and is eight inches long. Teeth are forming inside its gums and there are a few hairs on its head. Another month passes—the fetus's bones are getting harder and its fingernails are growing.

At six months the baby is kicking, a very funny feeling for its mother. Now it is a foot long and weighs a pound and a half. It has learned a new trick—it can blink its eyes. At the end of the seventh month the baby weighs three pounds. Its trick of the month—it is learning to suck its thumb.

In the eighth and ninth months, the baby gains about a half pound a week. It is growing big and strong so it can live outside the mother.

Somewhere near the end of the ninth month the mother feels the muscles of her uterus beginning to squeeze around the baby. It's an exciting moment for her and the father—their baby is ready to be born. At the hospital, doctors and nurses are ready to help the mother give birth. The muscles of her uterus squeeze harder around the baby, pushing it slowly out of the uterus, through the vagina, into the world!

Ninth month—the baby is twenty inches long and weighs about seven pounds. It is completely formed and is able to live in the outside world. It is lying in the head-down position, and is ready to be born.

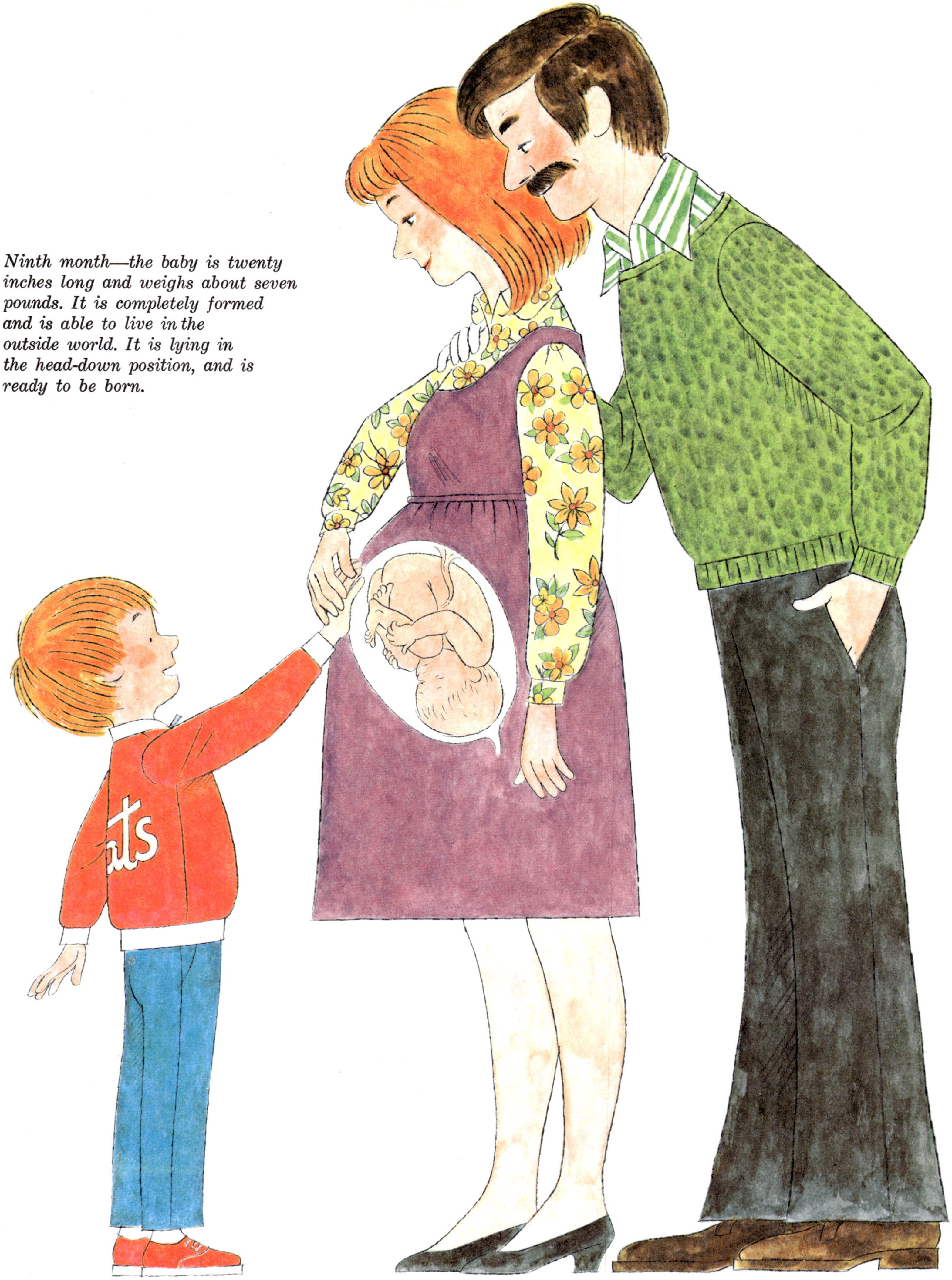

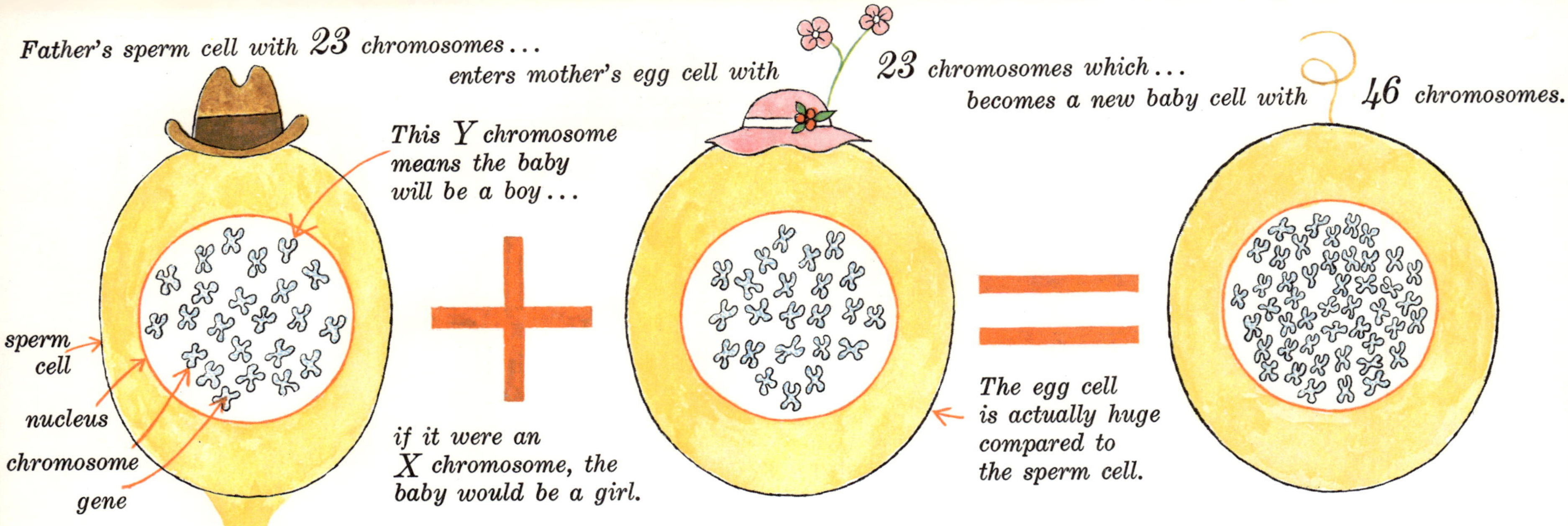

Your **HEREDITY** is what you inherit from your parents, your grandparents and maybe even your great-grandparents—the color of your hair and eyes and skin, the shape of your nose, how you smile. You inherit most of the things that make you look like you, and some of the things that make you think like you. Of course there are other influences on what you'll look like as an adult, and what kind of person you'll be. The food you eat, your exercise, what you learn and where you live are all important.

It takes millions of cells to make up a person's body, but everything you inherit is determined by just two cells—the sperm cell from your father and the egg cell from your mother.

Every cell in the body carries millions of genes. Genes are what determine your heredity. The genes are strung together like beads, forming 46 necklace-like fibers called chromosomes. The baby-producing cells—the father's sperm cells and the mother's egg cells—are the only body cells which do not carry 46 chromosomes—they each carry only 23. When a sperm cell enters the egg cell, the fertilized cell they form thus contains 23 pairs of chromosomes, or 46, the same number that all the other cells of the body have. The millions of genes in the 46 chromosomes determine the baby's inherited traits; there are genes for nose shape, genes for hair type and color, genes for eye color, etc. Because half are from the father and half are from the mother, the new baby will have some traits of each. And because the parents' genes came from the four grandparents, the baby inherits traits from the grandparents, too.

There are so many combinations of genes possible that no two babies are exactly alike—you know how different children in the same family can be. The only time this is not true is when identical twins are born. They come from a single fertilized egg cell which divides into two completely separate fertilized cells, each with the same genes. Each of these cells develops into a separate baby. The two babies are so much alike that even their parents may have trouble telling them apart.

This is an enlarged chromosome. It is made of a chemical called DNA. In it are arranged genes—millions of them—that determine just what traits you inherit.

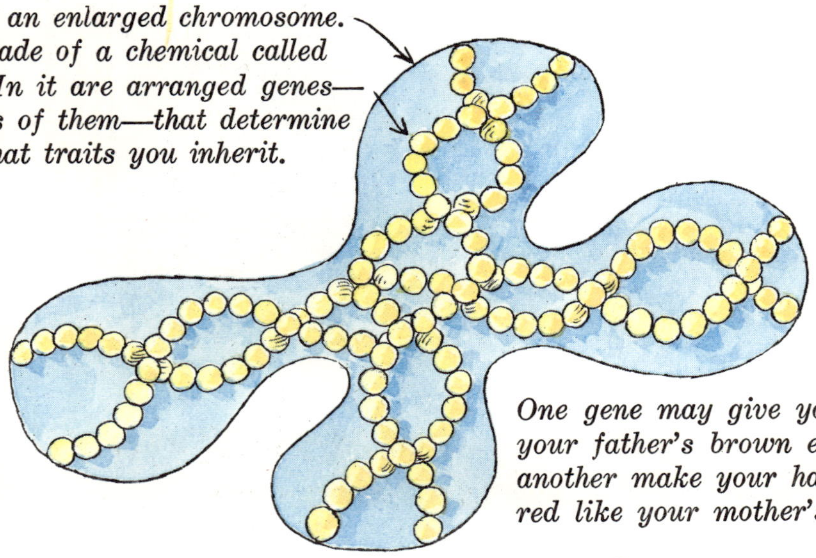

One gene may give you your father's brown eyes, another make your hair red like your mother's.

Most twins result from two sperms joining two egg cells. They are no more alike than any other brothers and sisters. But identical twins grow from one fertilized egg cell that splits in two, making two babies looking exactly alike.

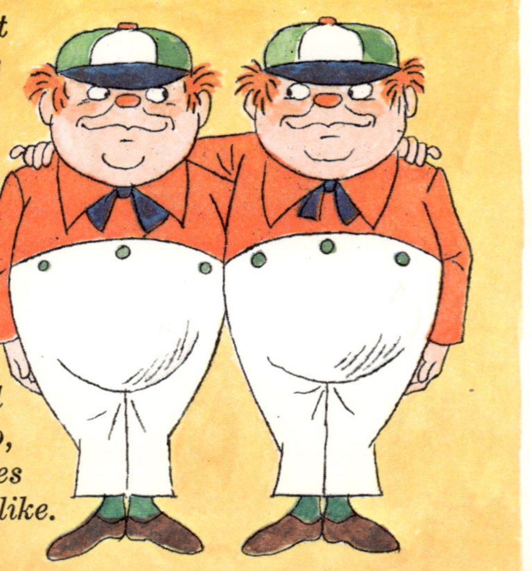

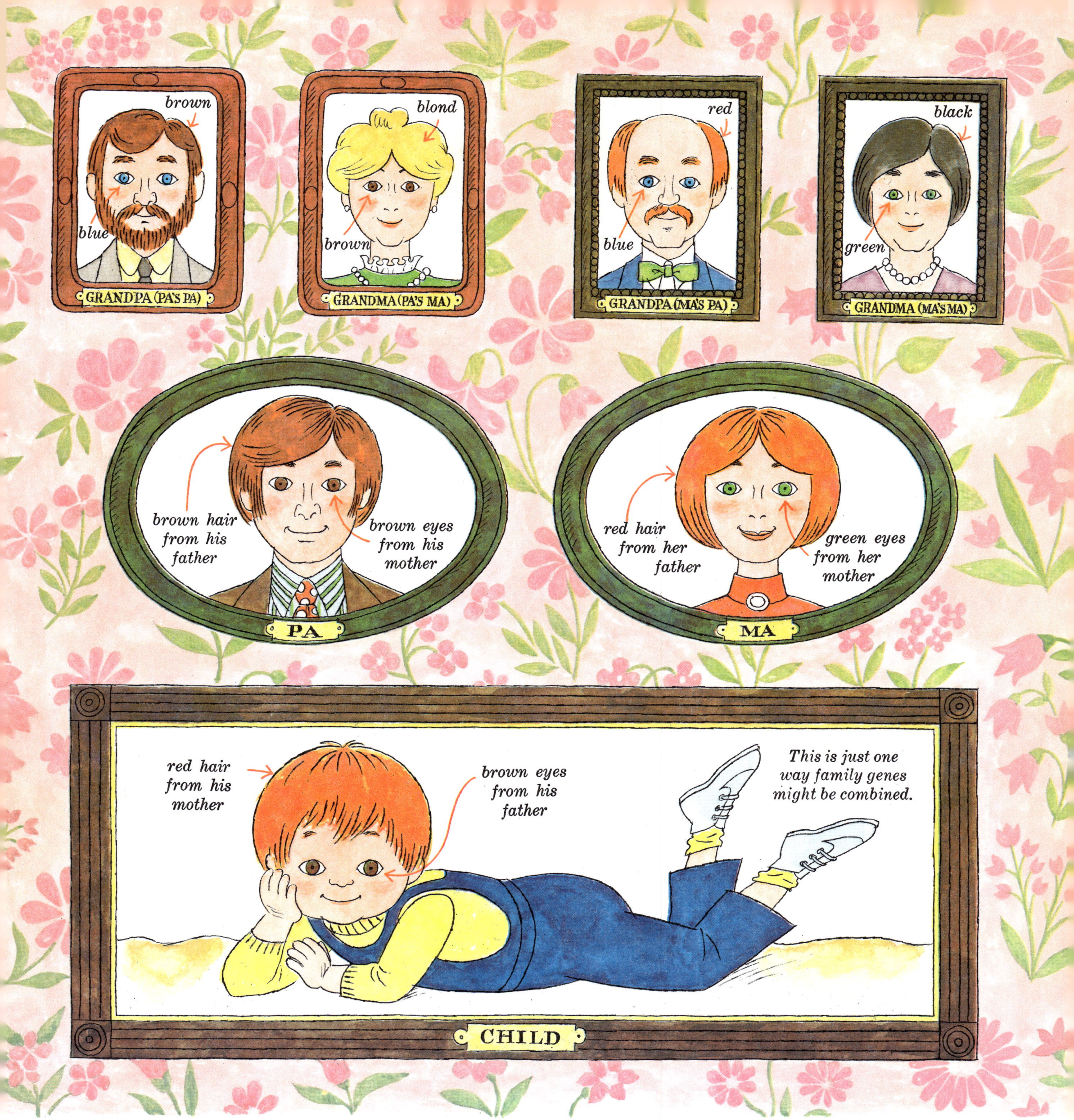
brown
blue
GRANDPA (PA'S PA)
blond
brown
GRANDMA (PA'S MA)
red
blue
GRANDPA (MA'S PA)
black
green
GRANDMA (MA'S MA)
brown hair from his father
brown eyes from his mother
PA
red hair from her father
green eyes from her mother
MA
red hair from his mother
brown eyes from his father
This is just one way family genes might be combined.
CHILD

From your parents and grandparents you inherit your eye color, your smile, the color of your hair, your nose shape, the size of your feet and hands, and many other traits.

When bone-ends join shaft of bone, growth is finished.

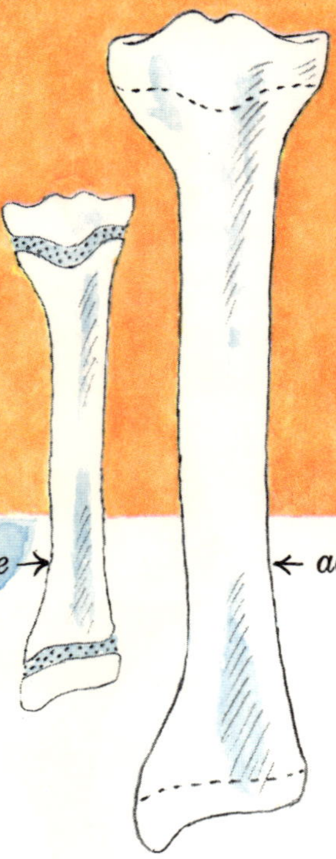

Bone length determines your height. Short bones mean you are short. Tall bones mean you are tall. While you are growing, your bones have spaces in them, between the shaft and the ends. Soft, clear cartilage fills the spaces. As new cartilage is added, the old hardens, becoming part of the bone shaft and making the bone longer. When the bone-ends join the bone shaft, growth stops—you have reached your full height.

At age 1, a baby weighs about three times as much as it did when it was born.

At age 3, a child is more than three feet tall. The body is still small compared to the head.

At age 6, children are about 45 inches tall and weigh about 45 pounds, one pound for each inch.

At age 9, both boys' and girls' arms and legs are longer compared to their bodies—boys and girls still look a lot alike.

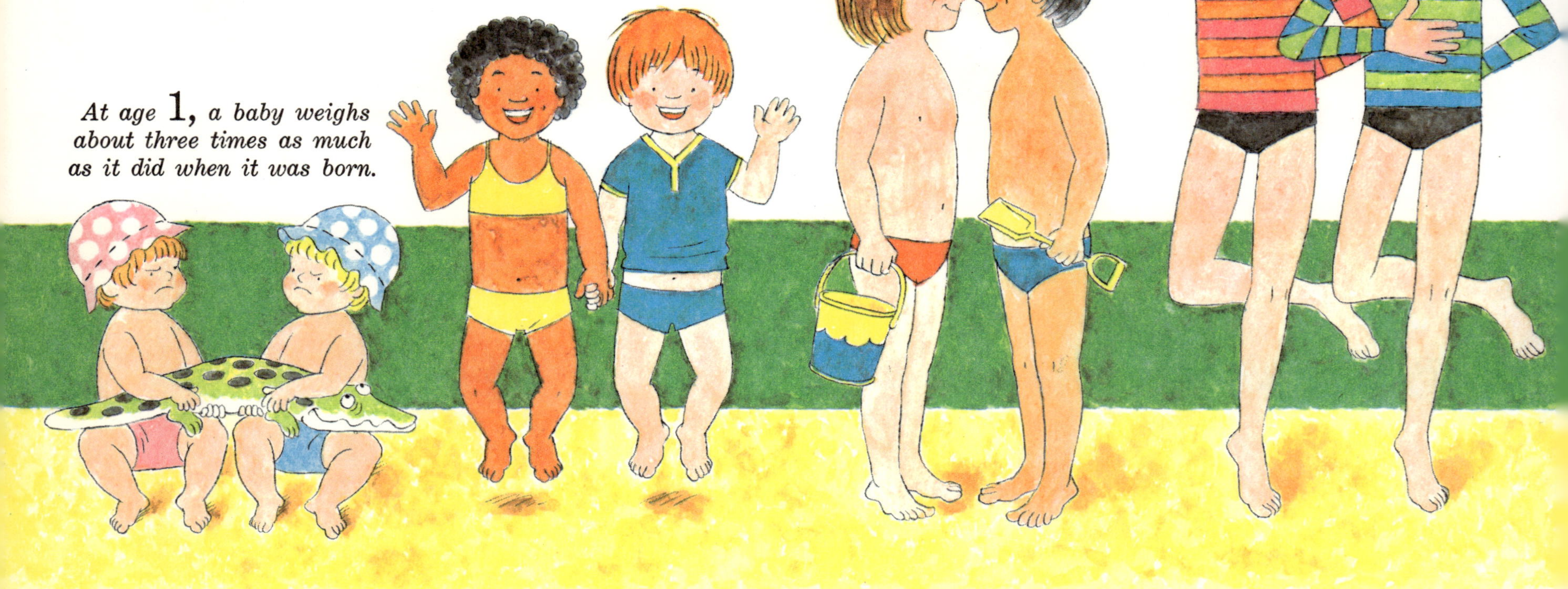

GROWING UP is something we all do, but we each grow in our own way. Some of us become tall and some of us stay short. Some grow quickly and some grow slowly. Some get heavy and some stay slim. Our growth pattern depends on the kind of body we inherit from our parents, what we eat, and how we take care of ourselves.

But although we all have our own individual growth pattern, there are averages of growth. A newborn baby weighs about seven pounds and is about twenty inches long. The baby grew very fast before birth and it continues to grow fast afterward. During the first two years it grows faster than it ever will again. A two-year-old weighs about twenty-eight pounds—four times as much as when it was born. If it continued to grow at that rate, multiplying its

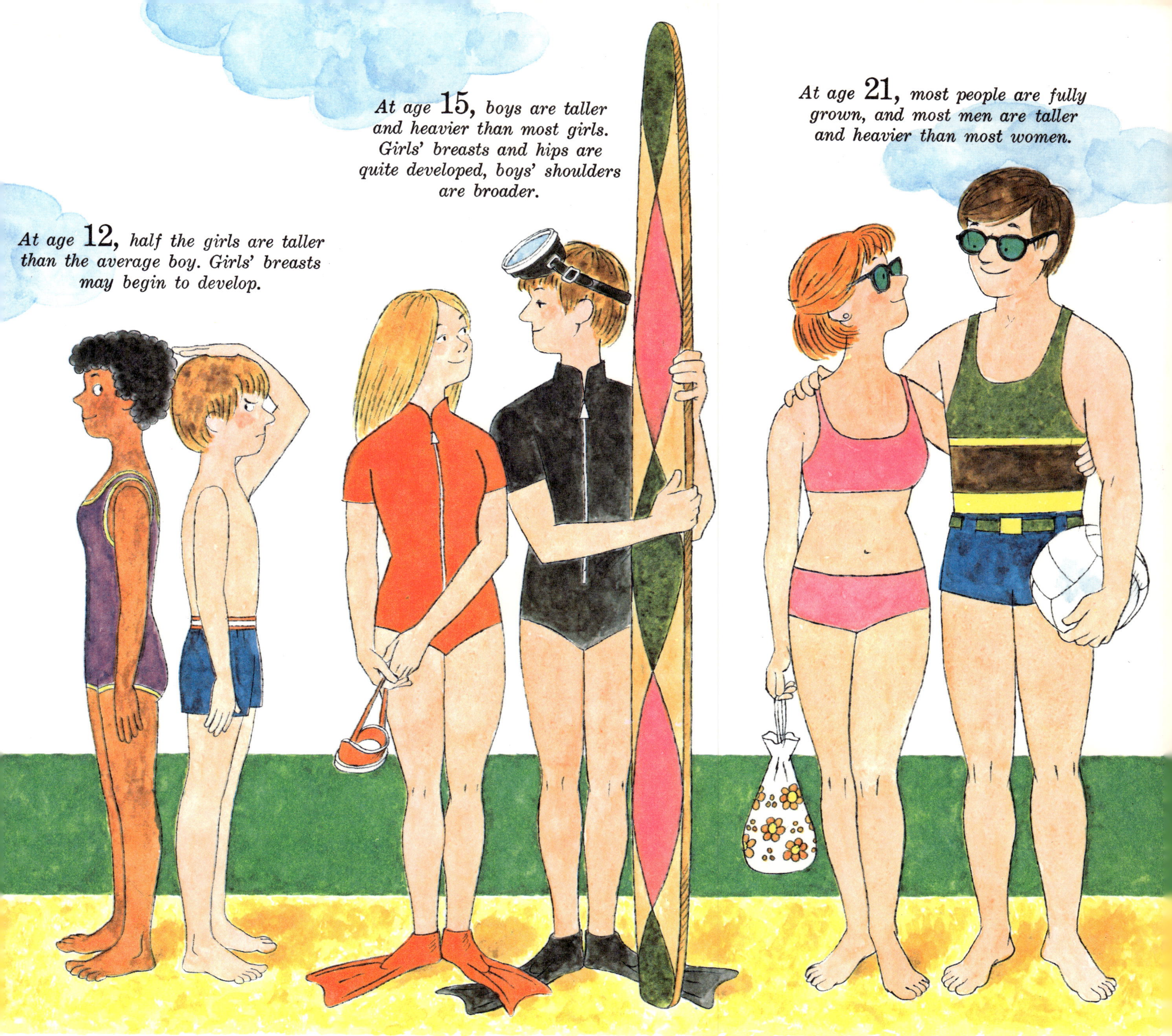
At age 12, *half the girls are taller than the average boy. Girls' breasts may begin to develop.*
At age 15, *boys are taller and heavier than most girls. Girls' breasts and hips are quite developed, boys' shoulders are broader.*
At age 21, *most people are fully grown, and most men are taller and heavier than most women.*

weight by four every two years, it would weigh more than 7,000 pounds at age ten! And if it grew taller at the same rate it did in its first two years, it would be more than twenty feet tall at age ten! So the growth rate slows after age two.

Boys and girls grow at about the same rate until age ten. They are then about the same height and their bodies have the same general shape. By age twelve many girls are taller than boys, and their breasts may have begun to develop and their hips to curve more. But by age fifteen most boys have caught up and passed the girls in height and weight. The girls' breasts and hips are quite developed by then, and the boys are getting muscular. By twenty-one most people are fully grown, and the men are usually somewhat heavier and taller than the women.

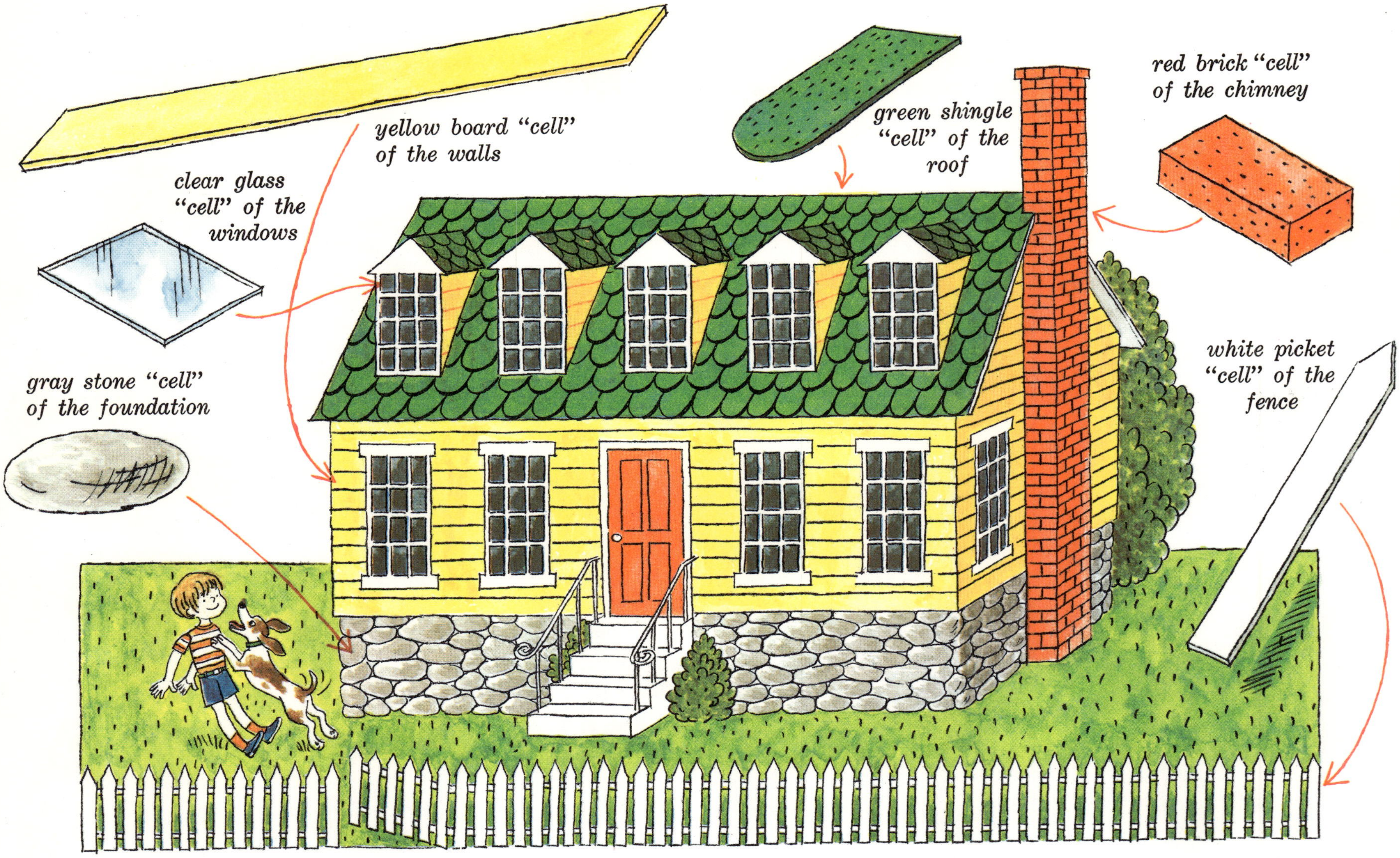

If you think of a house as a body you can see that the building materials are like cells. Many bricks make up a chimney and lots of shingles make up a roof, just as lots of bone cells add up to a bone and lots of brain cells make up a brain.

CELLS are the building materials of your body. Just as a big, complicated house is made up of small, simple building materials of different shapes and sizes, so your big, complicated body is made up of small, simple cells of different shapes and sizes with different jobs to do.

Billions of cells make up your body, and there are many different kinds of cells. But all the body's cells have some things in common. Every cell is made mostly of liquid—it is like a tiny droplet, protected by a thin, skin-like covering called a membrane. All the food the cell needs for living and growing comes in through the membrane, and the cell's waste products go out through the membrane. In the center of the cell is a part called the nucleus. This is the most important part of the cell, because it contains the cell's 46 chromosomes, the material the cell needs to reproduce itself.

Cells make your body grow not by getting bigger but by dividing in two, forming new cells that are exactly like the original ones in size and makeup. That is how a baby grows from a single fertilized egg cell to a full-grown person with billions of cells. Even when you are fully grown your cells will still keep dividing and making more cells, but only to replace cells that are worn-out or injured.

Just as similar building materials of a house are grouped together to make larger building units—boards with boards to make walls, tiles with tiles to make floors, pipes with pipes to make plumbing, and so forth—so similiar cells in the body are joined together to make larger body units called tissues. Muscle cells make up the muscles, bone cells make up the bones, nerve cells make up the nerves, skin cells make up the skin—even the blood is a tissue, a liquid tissue made up of blood cells.

We are all made of cells, ranging in size from tiny brain cells to three-foot-long nerve cells. Cells' shapes are different, too, because they have different things to do.

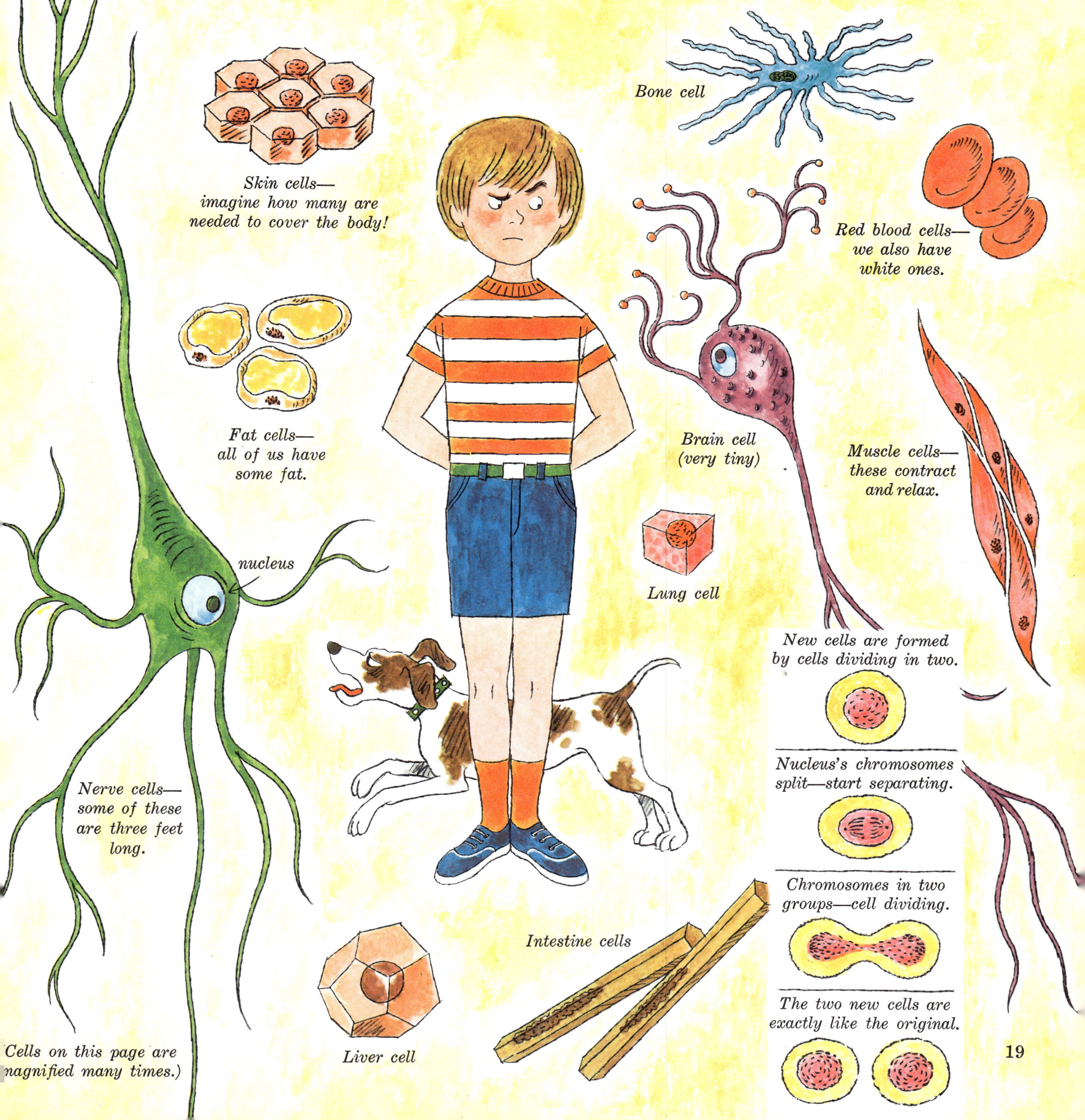

(Cells on this page are magnified many times.)

There are **206** bones in the body. The tiniest one (inside the ear) is this size and each of the thigh bones is about as big as this.

Put them all together and they spell S-K-E-L-E-T-O-N, the framework of bones that makes it possible for you to stand up straight.

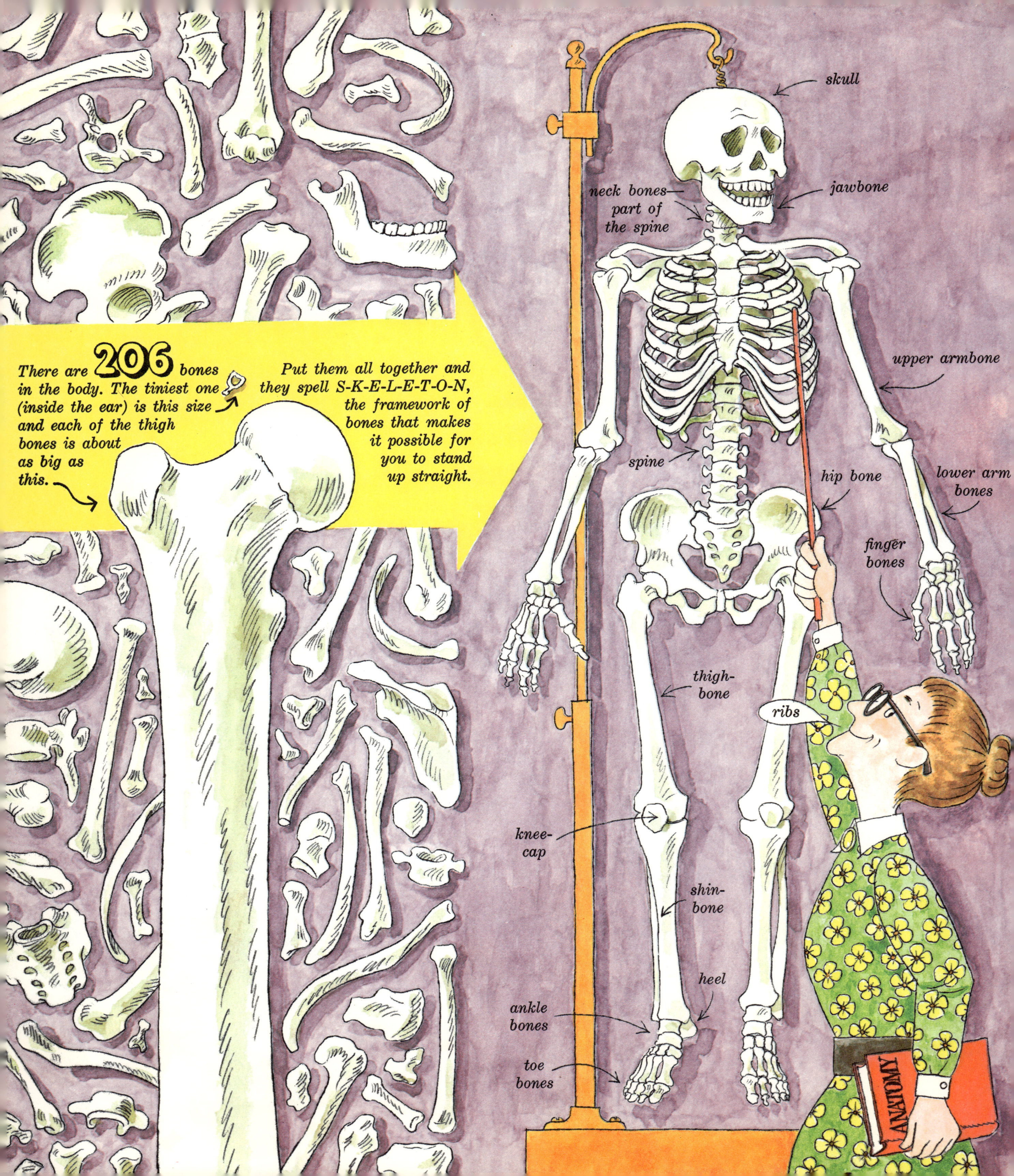

A framework is the skeletal structure of something—houses, bridges, skyscrapers, ships, and bodies, too.

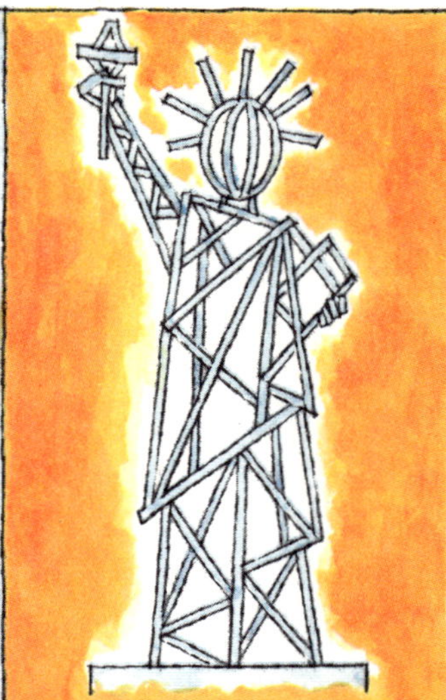

The steel framework of the Statue of Liberty.

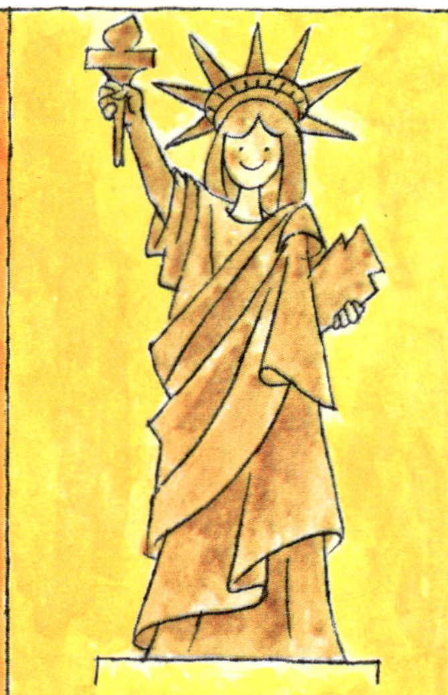

And here she is with her copper skin cover.

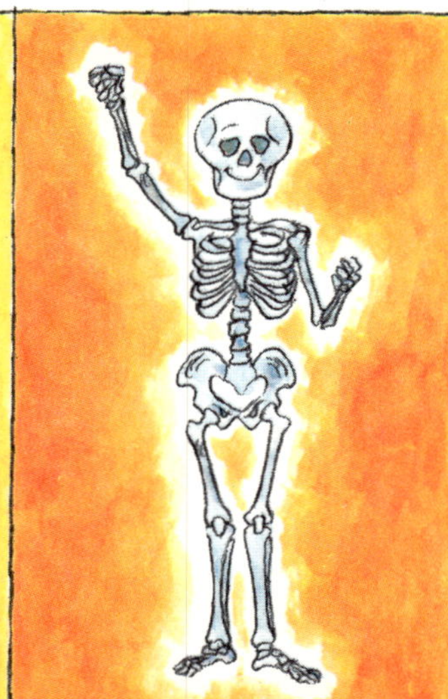

This is somebody's bone framework.

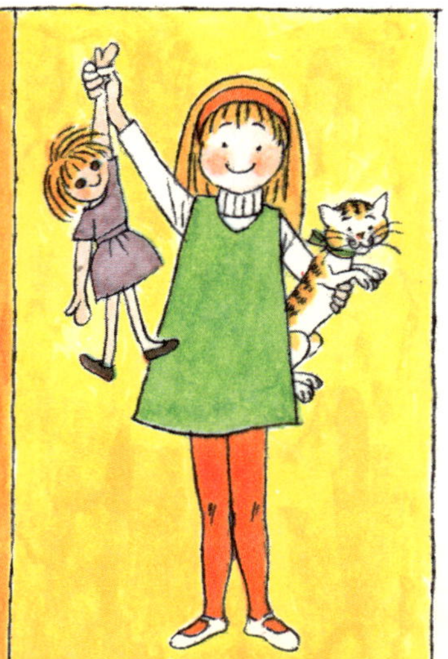

Now!—all covered with skin and clothes.

The BONES give the body its general shape; they are its framework. They support the body and protect the organs inside it.

There are several types of bones—long bones, such as those in the legs and arms; short bones, such as those in the wrists and ankles; flat bones, such as the ribs, breastbone, and skull; and irregular bones, such as those of the spine. All bones are hard on the outside and a little spongy on the inside.

Bones are made up mostly of the minerals calcium and phosphorus, which give them their hardness. If bones were made only of minerals they would be brittle and easily broken, so there is protein in bones too, to give them some flexibility.

Bones have spaces inside them filled with soft marrow. Yellow marrow, which is mostly fat, is found inside the middle part of long bones. There is red marrow in the ends of long bones and in ribs and some other flat bones. The red marrow is the place where the red and most white blood cells are made.

Even though the outside of a bone looks solid, it really has tiny openings in it, through which blood vessels enter and leave the bone. The blood carries away old used-up bone tissue and brings new supplies to help the bone cells replace it.

A baby's bones are not all fully formed when it is born. Some are still soft, clear cartilage. A newborn baby has no hard bones in its wrist. A two-year-old has two finished wrist bones, a five-year-old has five; only by the time a child is twelve have all eight wrist bones developed into hard, white, fully-formed bones.

Another interesting thing about the development of certain bones—at birth the skull and pelvis are made up of several small, separate bones. Later, these small bones grow together, and both the skull and pelvis become a solid bone.

And what's so scary about a skeleton?

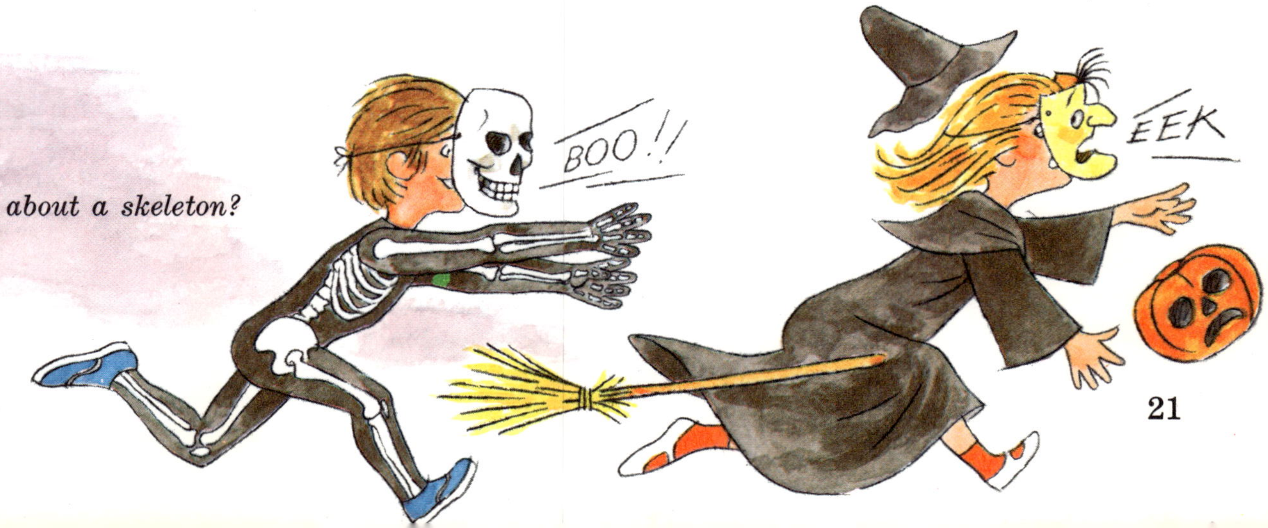

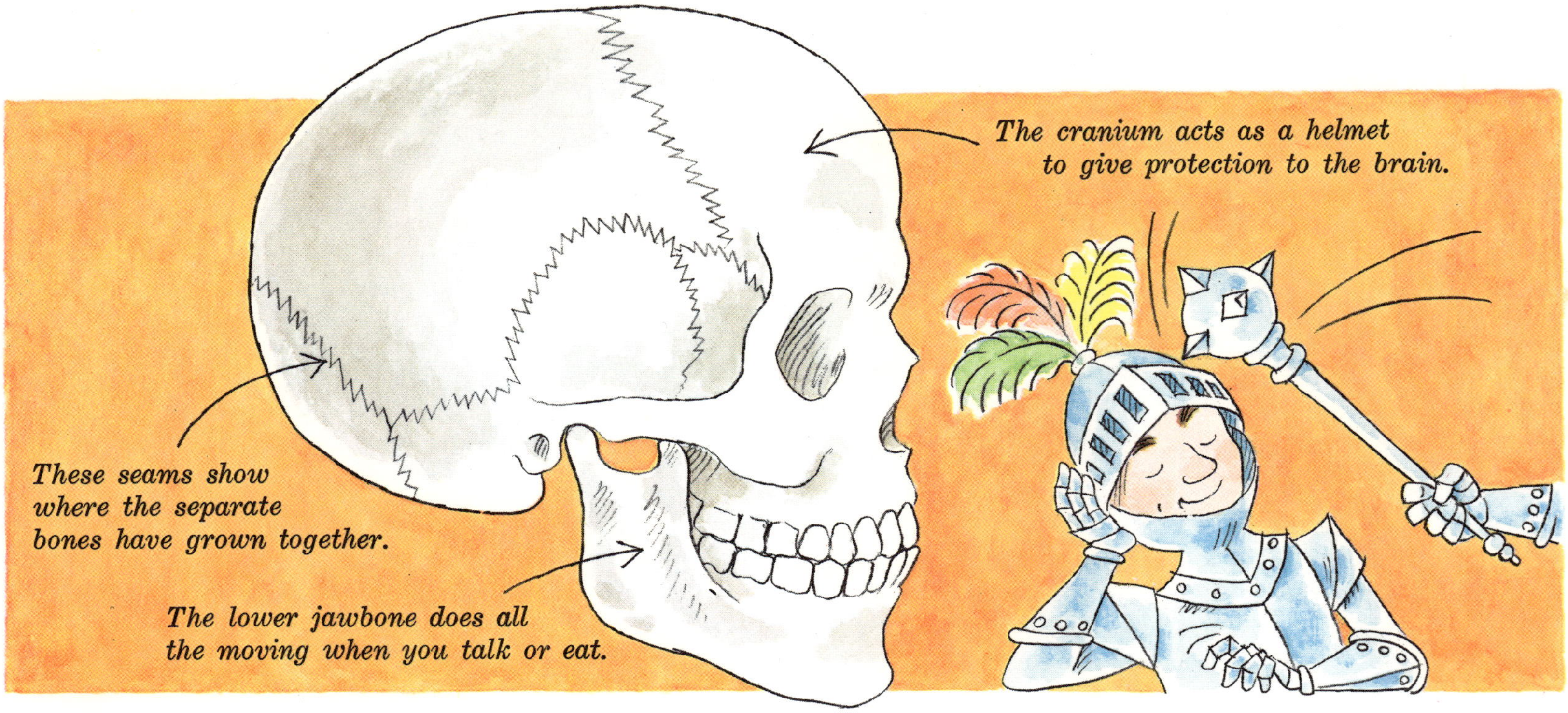
The cranium acts as a helmet
to give protection to the brain.
These seams show
where the separate
bones have grown together.
The lower jawbone does all
the moving when you talk or eat.

The SKULL sits on top of the spine. It is made up of twenty-two bones. The rounded top and back portions of the skull, which are called the cranium, form a strong bony roof to protect the brain. In a baby, the eight bones of the cranium are separate. They can shift, making it easier for the baby's head to squeeze through the birth canal. These bones grow together after a few years to form one solid bone.

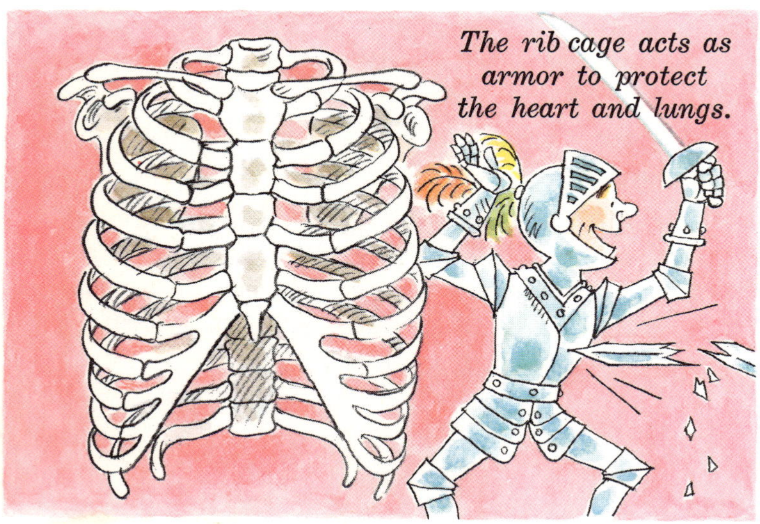

The RIB CAGE, a cage of bones, protects the heart and lungs. All twelve pairs of ribs are loosely fastened in back to the spine. The other ends of the ten upper pairs of ribs are also fastened in front to the breastbone, by flexible cartilage. The bottom two pairs are short, and do not connect in front. The flexible cartilage and the loose fastening at the spine let the rib cage expand and contract in breathing.

The rest of the skull bones, the face bones, form the shape of the face. Some are the cheekbones and the upper and lower jawbones, where the teeth are rooted. The only skull bone that moves is the lower jawbone. It is hinged to the skull so it can move up and down and from side to side for chewing. In the face bones there are places for the nose and eyes, and, of course, the mouth—between the two jawbones.

The PELVIS, made of the hipbones and the bottom of the spine, forms a basin which supports and protects the bladder, the lower intestine, and other organs in the bottom part of the abdomen. A woman's pelvis is somewhat wider than a man's so there will be room for a baby to pass through in childbirth. On each side of the pelvis, there is a socket for a thighbone to fit into.

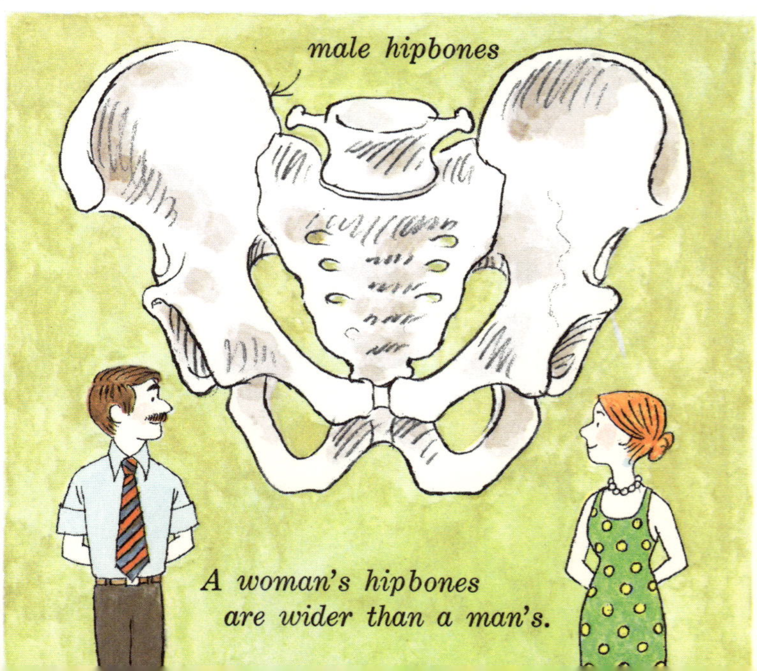

The SPINE, or backbone, can bend in all directions because it is a column of separate bones (called vertebrae) joined together by thick bands of tissue. The top seven vertebrae are the neck bones. The ribs are attached to the next twelve. Below these are the five vertebrae of the lower back, then two bones made of several vertebrae grown together.

Disks of cartilage act as cushions between the vertebrae, keeping them from rubbing against each other, and protecting the brain from the jolts of walking and running.

Each vertebrae has a vertical hole in it. These holes all line up with each other to form a vertical channel through the spine just behind the disks. Through this channel passes the spinal cord, well protected by the vertebrae.

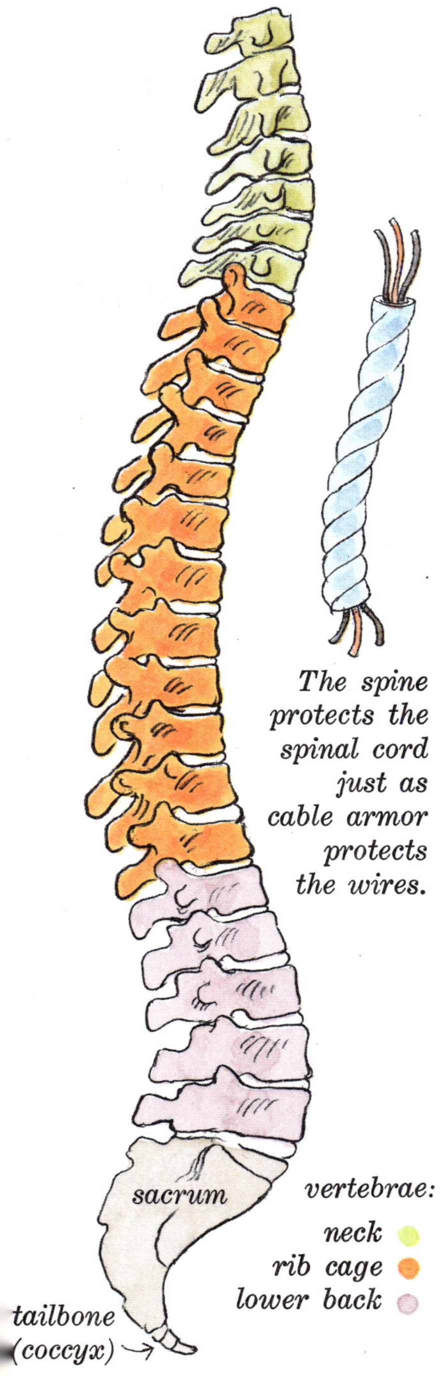

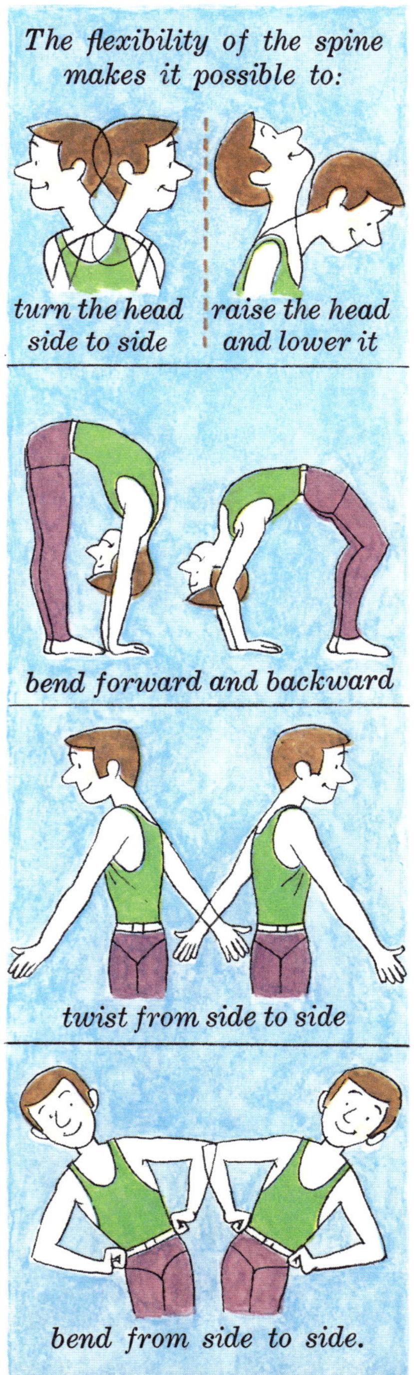

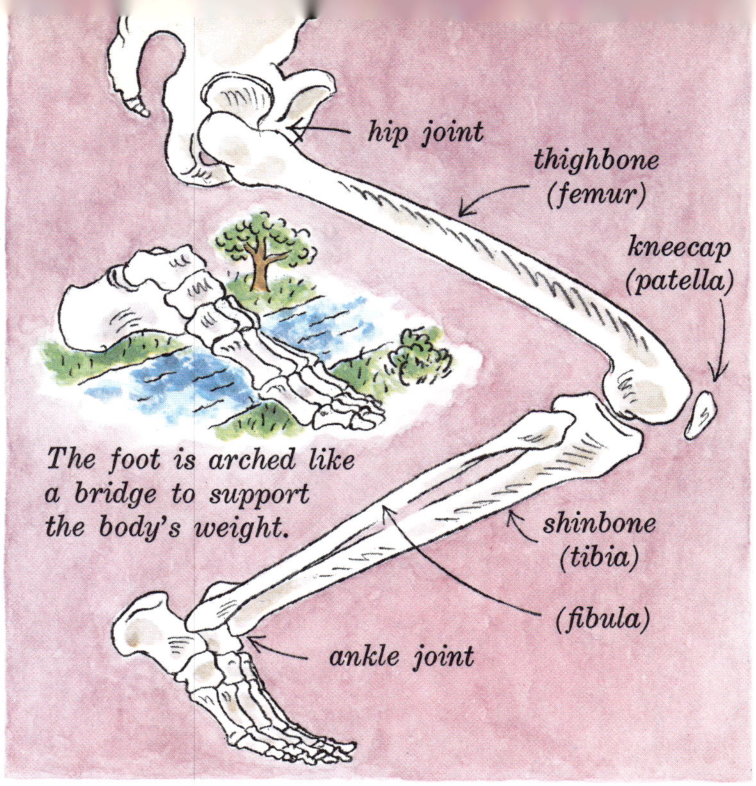

The LEG BONES are attached to the body at the hips. The ball-shaped top of the thighbone fits into a socket in the pelvis. This ball and socket joint allows the leg to move in all directions. The thighbone and lower leg bones are joined at the knee, forming a hinge joint that allows the lower leg to swing back and forth. The kneecap bone in front protects the knee joint. The lower leg bones are attached to the foot at the ankle, a joint that lets the foot see-saw up and down for walking.

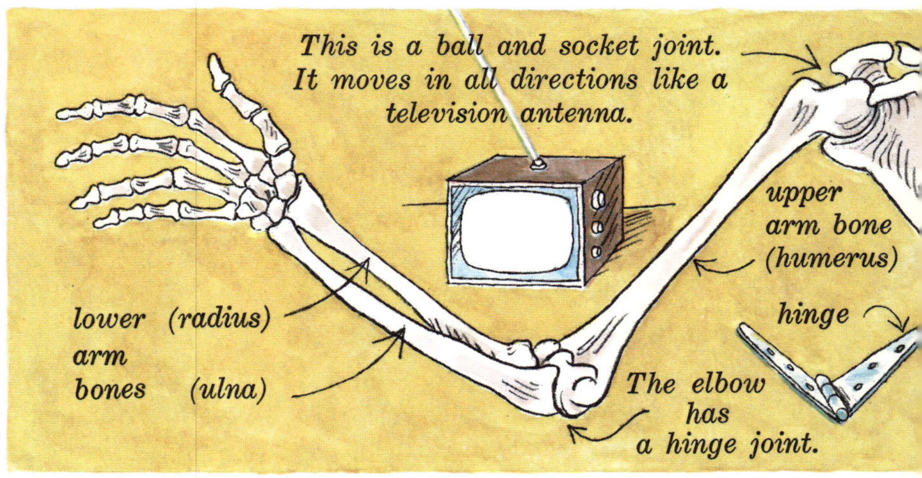

The ARM BONES are attached to the shoulder blade by a ball and socket joint. The upper arm bone and the lower arm bones join at the elbow in a hinge joint. The two lower arm bones allow a twisting wrist motion. When you hold your hand in front of you, palm up, the two bones are side by side. As you turn your palm down, one of these bones swivels around the other, until they are crossed.

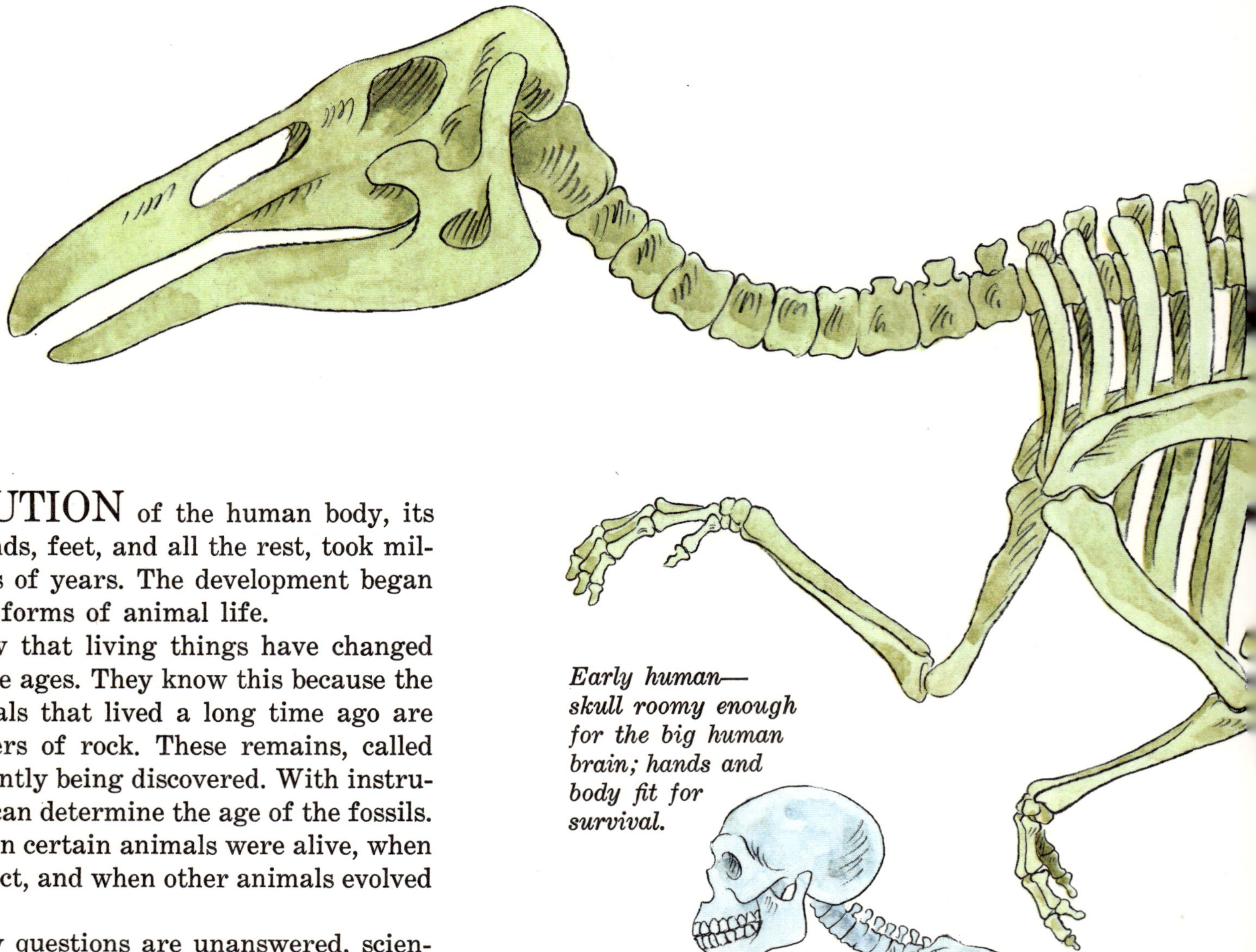

The EVOLUTION of the human body, its special brain, hands, feet, and all the rest, took millions and millions of years. The development began with the earliest forms of animal life.

Scientists know that living things have changed slowly through the ages. They know this because the remains of animals that lived a long time ago are preserved in layers of rock. These remains, called fossils, are constantly being discovered. With instruments, scientists can determine the age of the fossils. So they know when certain animals were alive, when they became extinct, and when other animals evolved to replace them.

Although many questions are unanswered, scientists now have a clear idea of how animal life developed on earth. They know that the earth was once covered with water, and that fish lived in the water. When land rose up, amphibian animals, those that could live both in water and on land, developed. Some amphibians came out of the water, returning only to lay their eggs. Later, reptiles, the first land animals, evolved. Among them were the great dinosaurs. Some reptiles survived and some died out. Then birds and mammals developed. They were warm-blooded—their bodies stayed at the same warm temperature in all weather.

At long last *we* arrived—humans, the most advanced animals so far. Our larger, more intelligent brain thinks up ideas. Our skillful hands carry out those ideas. Our body's bone structure, muscles, and upright posture help make it possible to accomplish the most difficult tasks. For better or worse, we predominate over all other living things on earth.

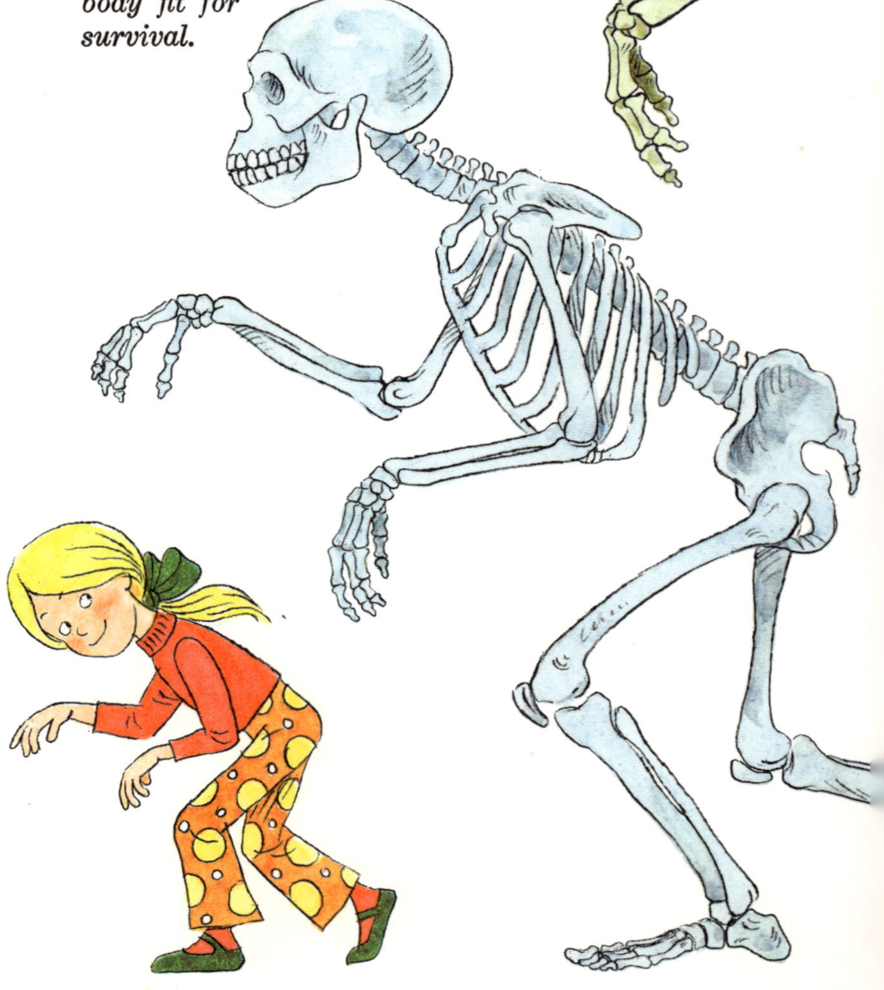

Early human—skull roomy enough for the big human brain; hands and body fit for survival.

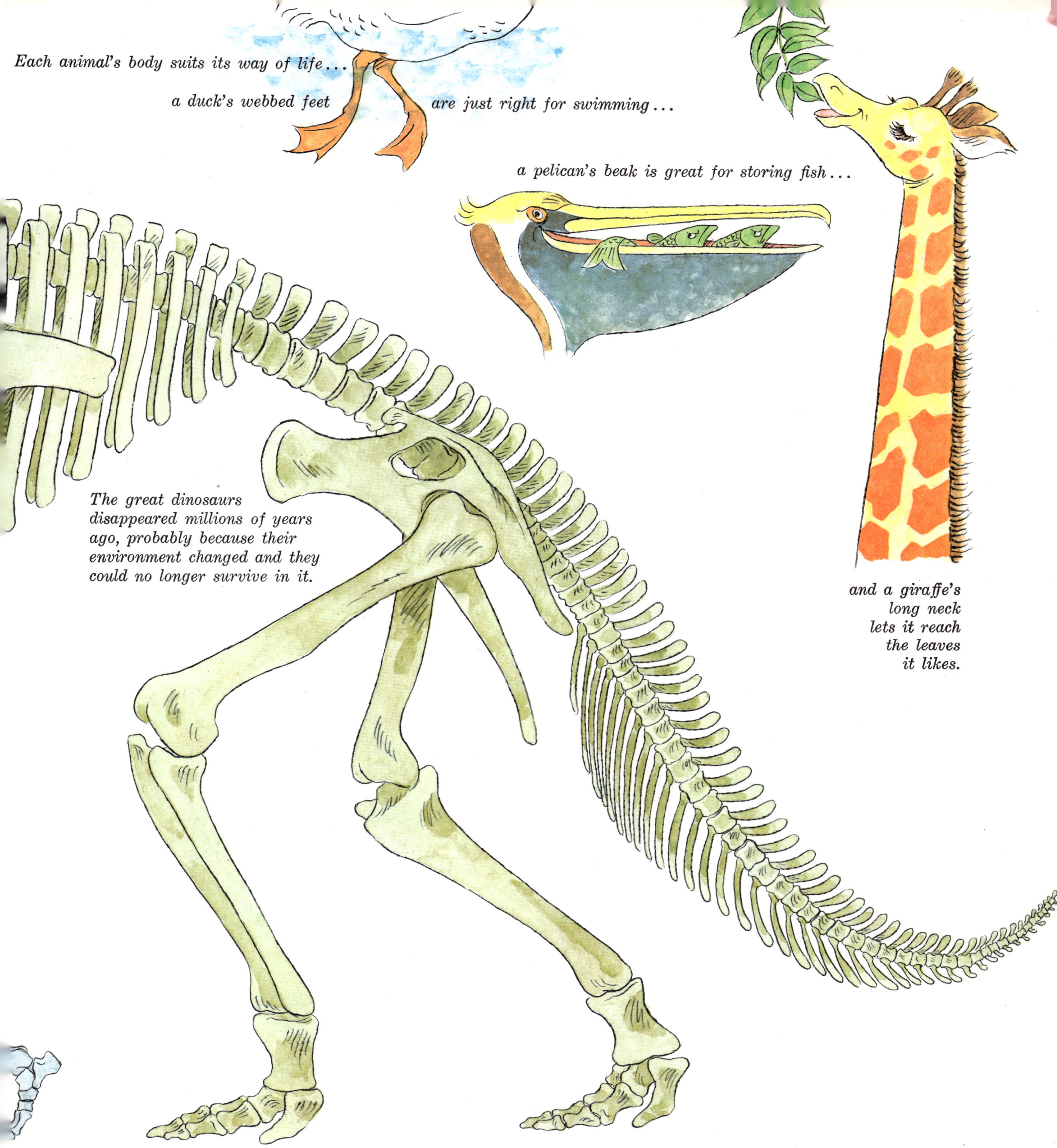

Each animal's body suits its way of life . . .

a duck's webbed feet *are just right for swimming . . .*

a pelican's beak is great for storing fish . . .

and a giraffe's long neck lets it reach the leaves it likes.

The great dinosaurs disappeared millions of years ago, probably because their environment changed and they could no longer survive in it.

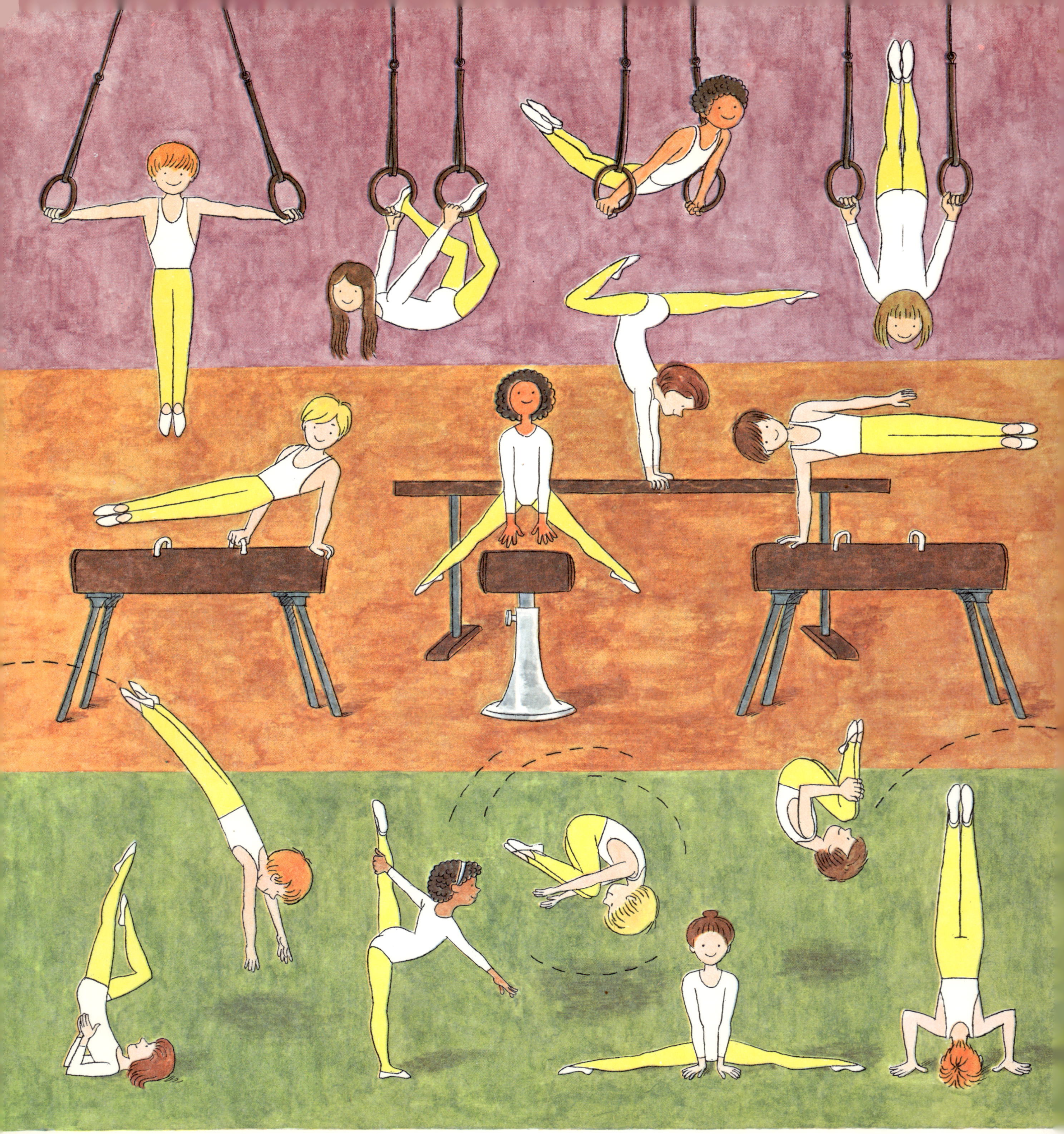

Your muscles, working together, make all the complicated movements of your body possible.

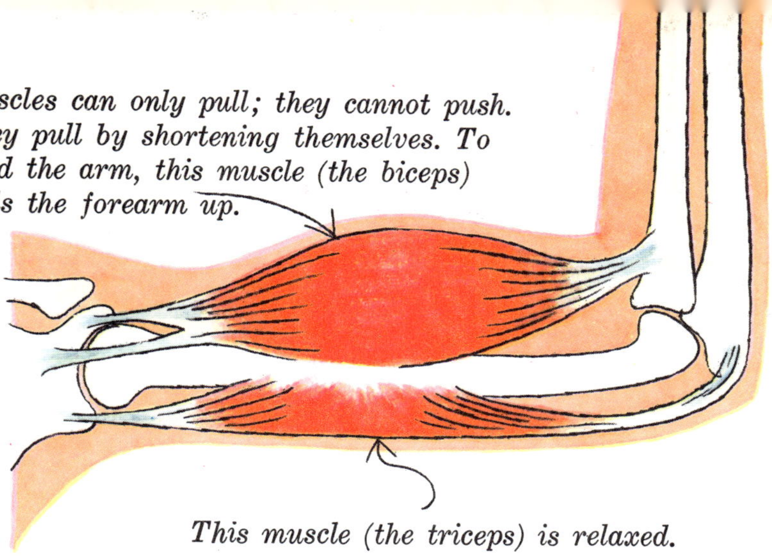

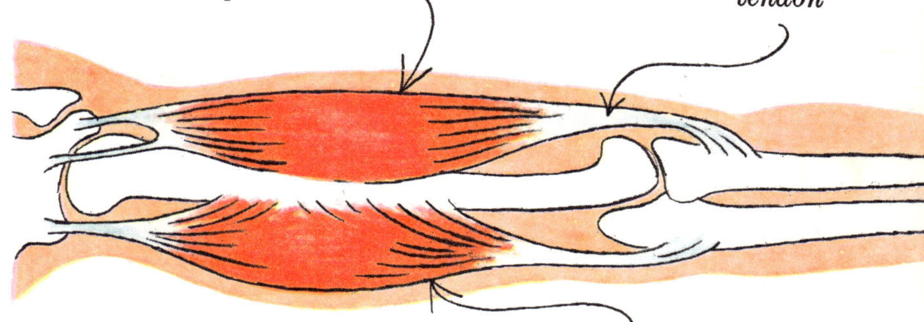

Your MUSCLES put all the parts of your body into motion. Your heart beats because of muscular action. Your lungs breathe mostly because of the action of your powerful diaphragm muscle. You can't say a word without using muscles, the muscles that make your lips and tongue move, and many other muscles of your mouth, throat, and jaw. Seeing needs muscles to move the eyes up or down or from side to side. Just think of eating. Jaw muscles help chew the food; tongue and throat muscles push the food down into the stomach; stomach muscles mix and mash the food to digest it; and intestinal muscles push the food along while the bloodstream absorbs nourishment from it. Walking, running, and playing use the powerful muscles of the arms, legs, and torso. Writing, painting, and tying a knot use the delicate muscles of the hand.

There are two kinds of muscles. One kind is the kind you can control, called voluntary muscles. They move only when you want them to. If you drop a pencil, your brain orders your voluntary muscles to bend your torso and move your fingers to pick it up.

The other kind of muscles is the kind you don't control. They are called involuntary muscles. Your stomach muscles don't wait for you to think about telling them to work—they mix and mash the food on their own. And your heart needs no reminder from you to keep pumping blood through your body. Involuntary muscles work automatically, keeping things going in the body, even when you're asleep.

The voluntary muscles are usually attached to the bones, one end to one bone and the other end to another. They move the bones by shortening themselves, or contracting. When a muscle contracts, it pulls on a bone and moves it. But that same muscle cannot *push* the bone back to its original position. (Muscles are a little like rubber bands—they can pull, but they can't push.) Another muscle is needed, in a place where it can move the bone back again by pulling. So voluntary muscles usually come in pairs, or in combinations that allow them to reverse every move they make.

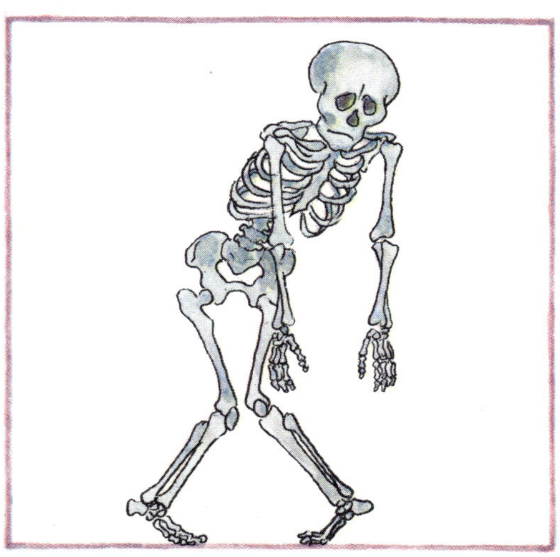
Bones aren't capable of moving . . .

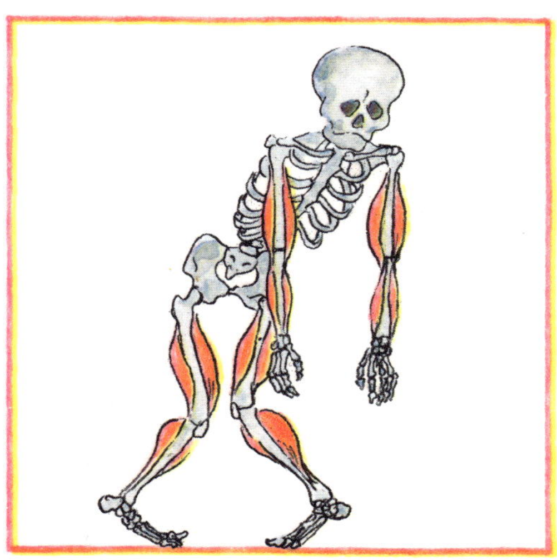
but when muscles are attached . . .

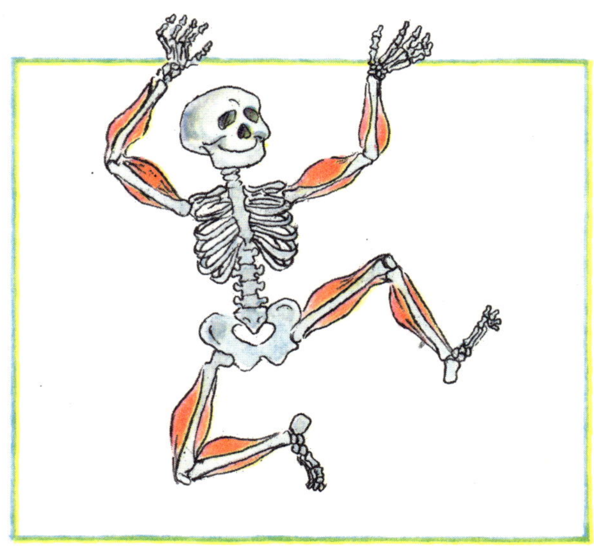
you can get all kinds of action!!!

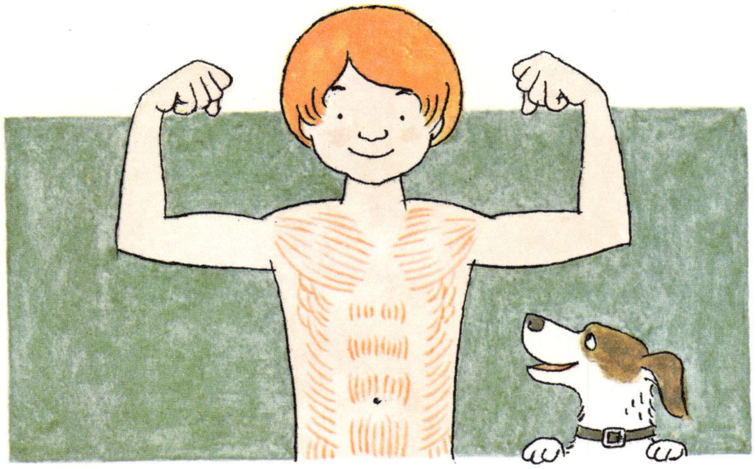

The **CHEST MUSCLES** and the abdominal muscles do many different things. Muscles on the upper part of the chest contract to pull the arms toward the body and to pull the shoulders forward. On either side of the chest, between the ribs, is a series of muscles that fasten one rib to the next. They are used in breathing. Some of them expand your chest when you inhale and others contract it when you exhale. Below the chest are several layers of flat abdominal muscles, running in different directions. They hold the inner organs firmly in place and protect them from injury where they are not shielded by bones. Some of these muscles act to bend the body and also help brace the body when you lift heavy things.

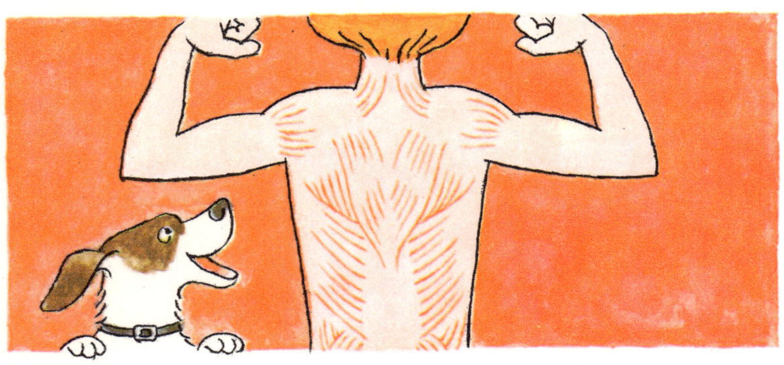

Two **BACK MUSCLES** cover almost the entire back, although there are other muscles beneath them. One is a large, flat, diamond-shaped muscle covering the upper half of the back. The top corner of the diamond is fastened to the base of the skull, the bottom corner is fastened to the middle of the spine, and the other two corners are fastened to the shoulder blades. This muscle can raise or lower the shoulders and can also pull them back. It can pull your head back and help it turn from side to side. It also helps in the motion of raising your arm above your head. The other large back muscle covers the lower half of the back. It reaches from the lower back to the upper arms. It pulls your arm back to throw a ball, use a tennis racket, or paddle a canoe.

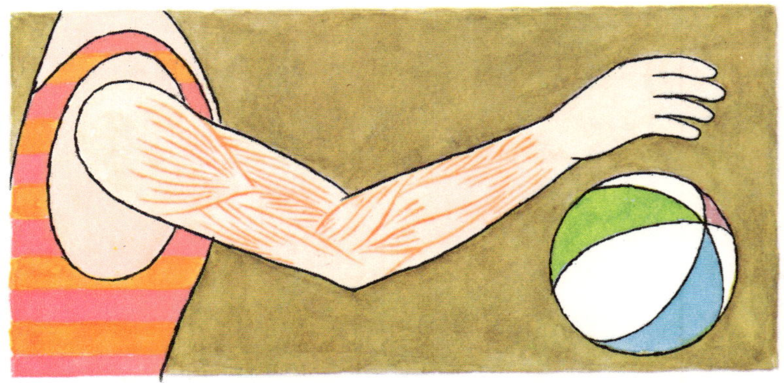

The **ARM MUSCLES** begin at the shoulder with a triangular muscle. It is wide at the top, where it is attached to the shoulder blade and collar bone, and it comes down to a point where it fastens to the upper arm bone. This muscle pulls the arm away from the body and helps turn it. You already know about the muscles of the upper arm (page 27) —the top one bends the arm and the bottom one straightens it. The forearm has many more muscles than the upper arm. Most of them end in tendons that run down into the hand. The muscles on the palm side of the forearm bend the fingers and wrist, and turn the hand palm-down. The muscles on the other side of the forearm straighten the fingers, pull the hand back at the wrist, and turn the hand palm-up.

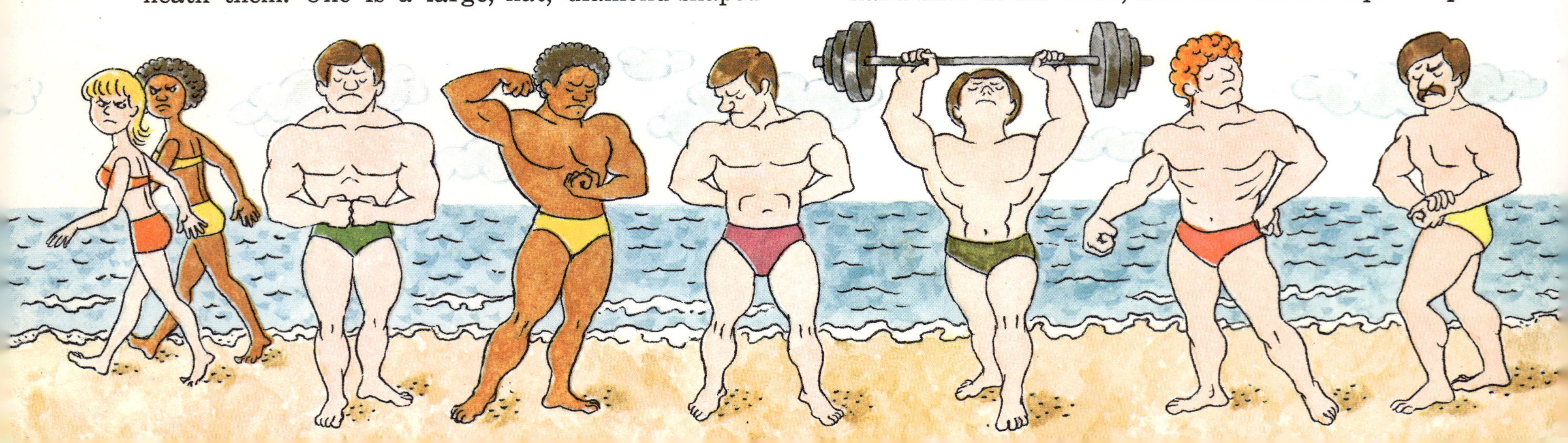

The LEG MUSCLES begin with a group of muscles at the pelvis. These muscles help pull you up straight after you bend over. They help straighten the leg, turn it outward, and pull it away from the body. The largest of the group is the one you sit on.

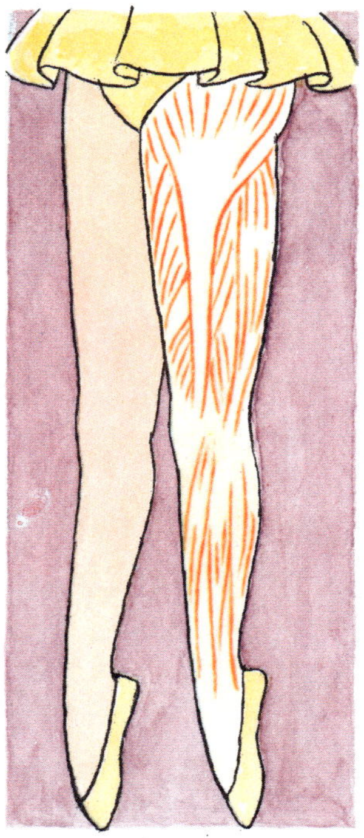

Muscles in the back of the thigh bend the knee. Muscles in the front of the thigh straighten the knee and pull it toward the chest. The body's longest muscle runs diagonally from the hip across the thigh to the inside of the leg below the knee. It bends the leg so you can sit cross-legged. Muscles that go from the lower leg to the foot control most of the foot's movements. Muscles in front pull the foot and toes up. The calf muscles in back pull the heel up.

There are many NECK MUSCLES. Two important ones come from behind the ears and slant to meet at the breastbone. Both contract to nod the head down. To make the head nod up and down, as though saying "yes," the large diamond-shaped muscle on the back is needed to pull the head up. Then the two neck muscles nod it forward again. These two important neck muscles also turn the head from side to side, as though saying "no." First one pulls the head one way, then the other pulls it the other way. These same muscles can tilt the head toward one shoulder or the other.

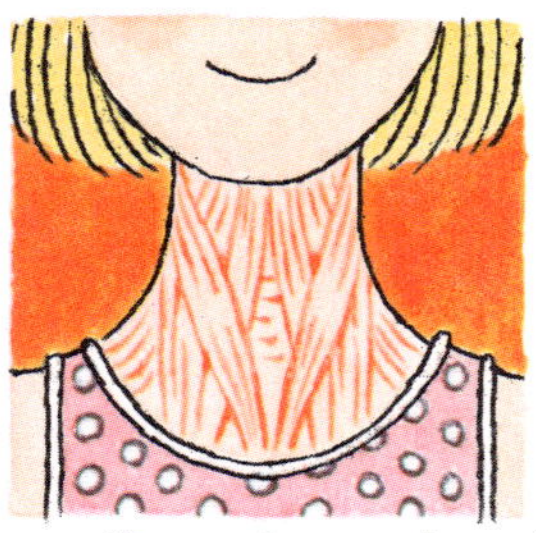

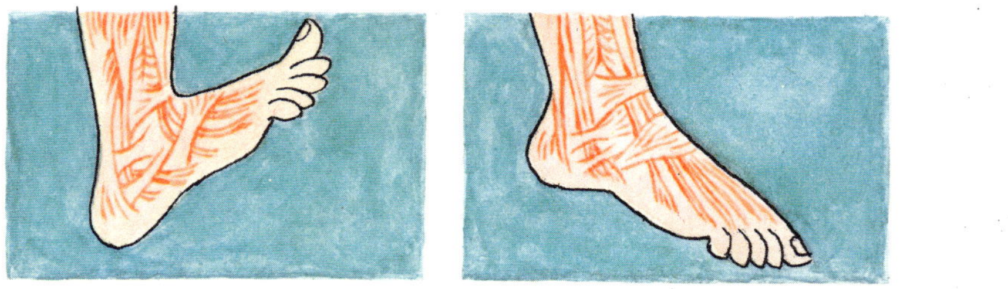

The FOOT MUSCLES play a very small part in moving the foot, as most of the muscles that move the foot begin in the leg. The foot has as many muscles as the hand, but far fewer delicate movements to make. A monkey's foot can grasp tree branches and do many other things. But humans use the foot mostly for walking, and the work of the foot muscles is confined mainly to supporting the bones that form the arch, and to wiggling the toes and spreading them.

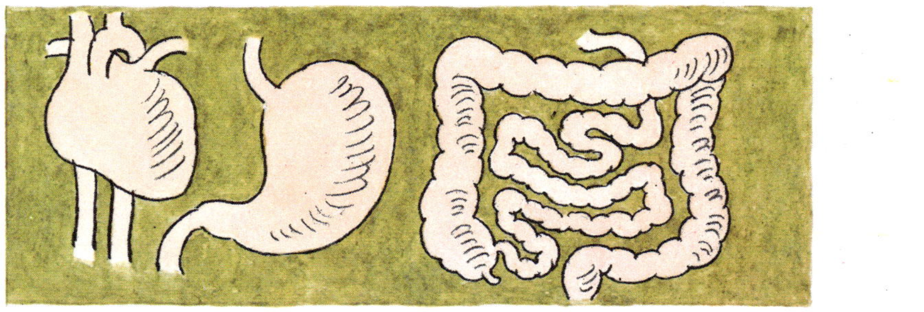

The ORGAN MUSCLES and those in the blood vessels are involuntary; they work without orders—keeping the bodily functions running automatically. Some of the involuntary muscles move slowly and smoothly; a single contraction may take minutes. The muscles in the digestive tract that mix and push the food along, and the muscles that widen or narrow the blood vessels to control the blood flow are some of these slow-moving involuntary muscles. The heart is also an involuntary muscle; it contracts and relaxes automatically, but its contractions are fast and sharp.

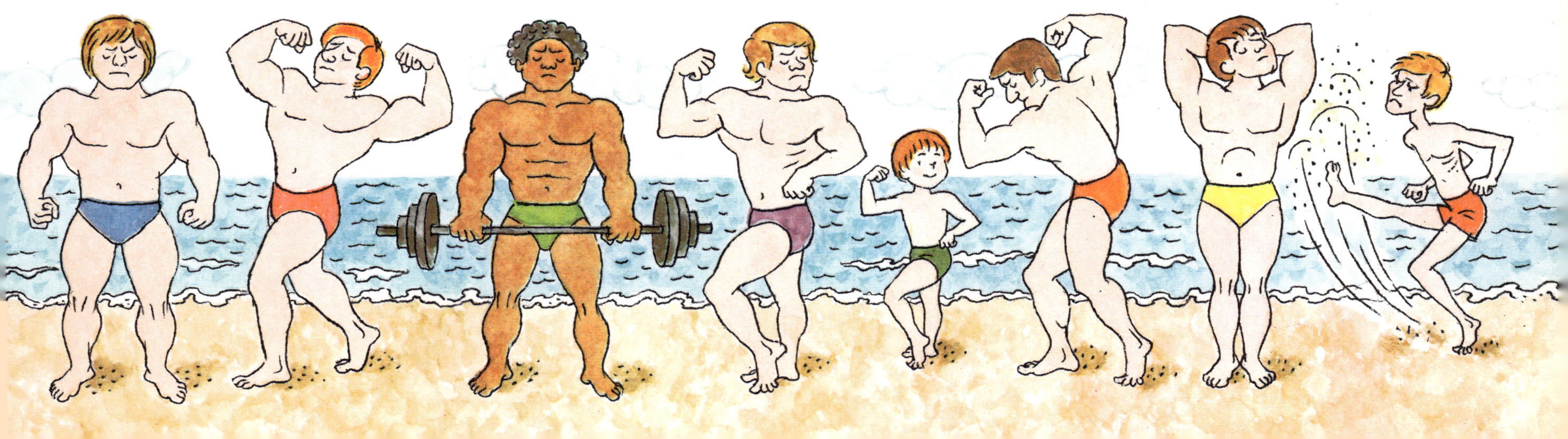

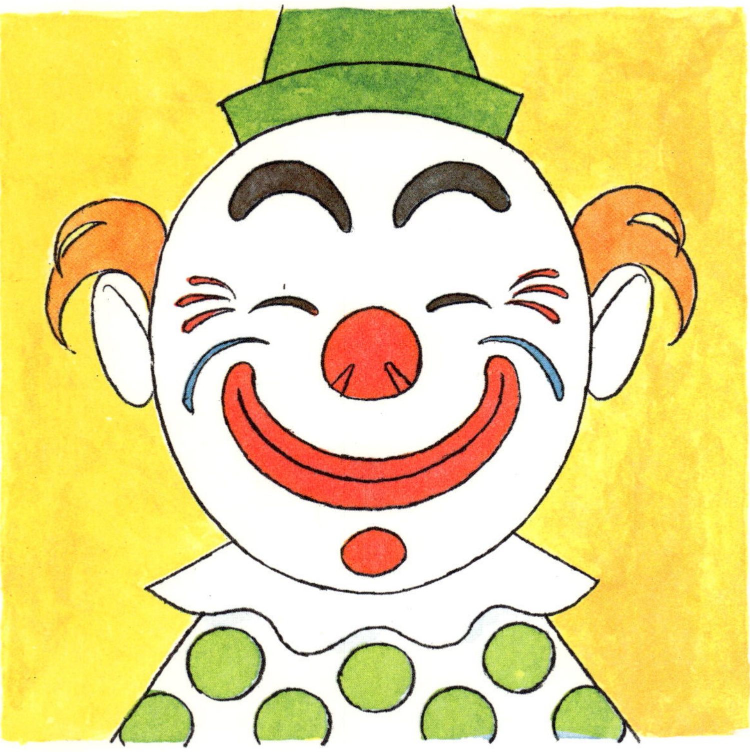

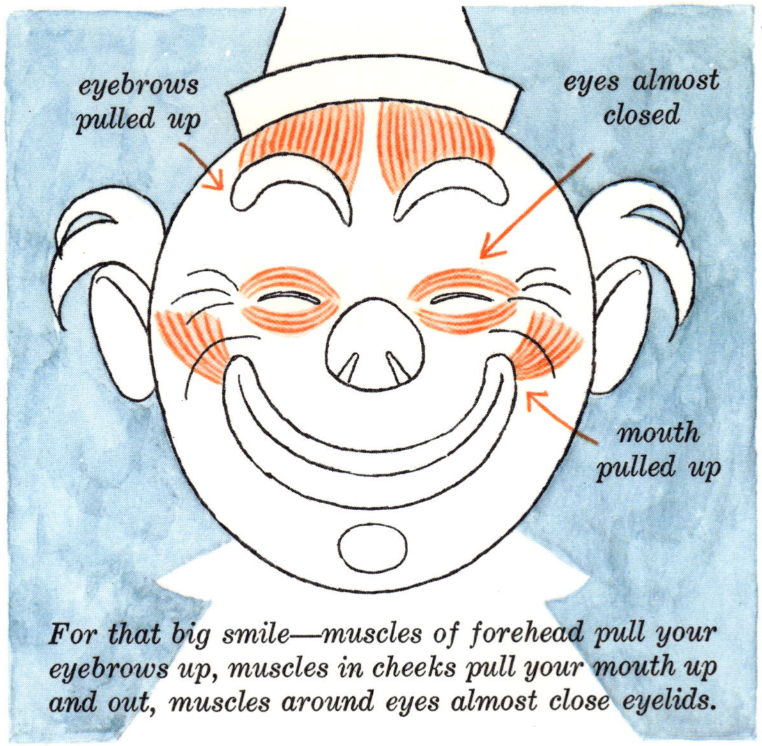

For that big smile—muscles of forehead pull your eyebrows up, muscles in cheeks pull your mouth up and out, muscles around eyes almost close eyelids.

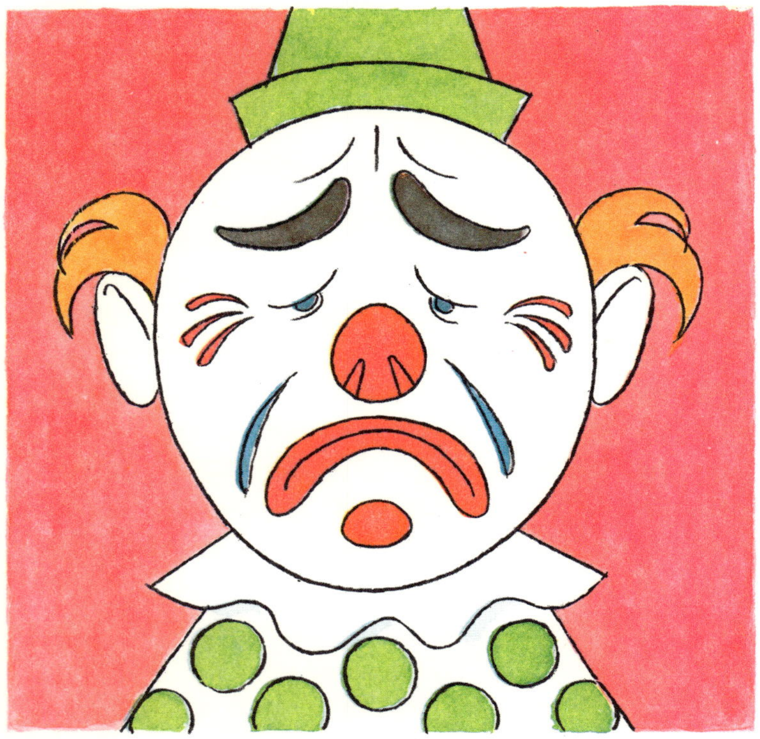

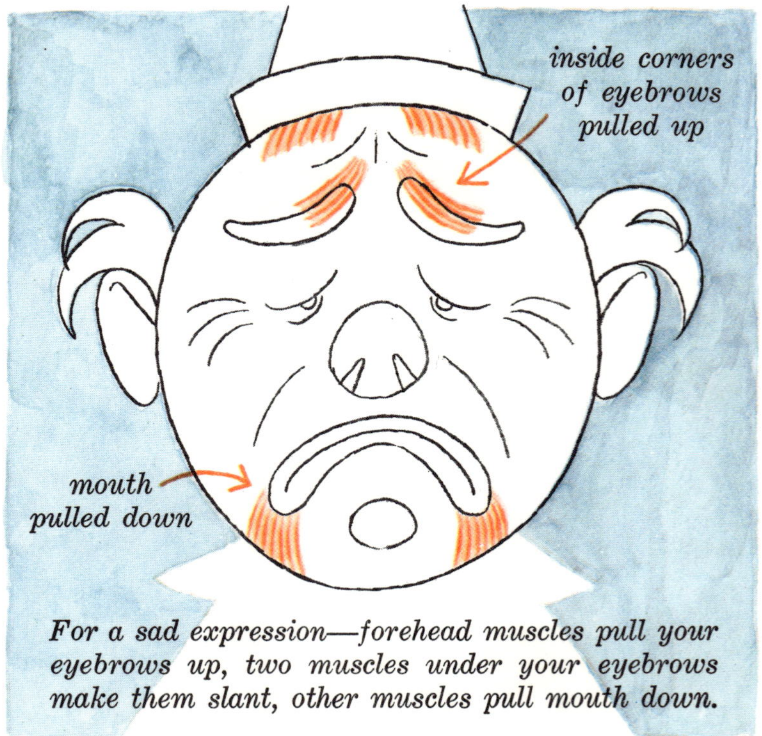

For a sad expression—forehead muscles pull your eyebrows up, two muscles under your eyebrows make them slant, other muscles pull mouth down.

The FACE MUSCLES have three main functions. The first is to move your lower jaw when you eat. The second is to move your lips when you talk or sing. The third is to move the features of your face to show emotions when you feel sad, happy, angry, surprised, or scared.

Most of the eating muscles are attached to the back part of your jaws, right in front of your ears. They open, shut, and move your lower jaw sideways, so your teeth can bite, chew, and grind your food.

Some eating muscles are used when you talk or sing, along with the ring of muscles around your lips. Say "oh" and "ee" into a mirror, and watch how the muscles change the shape of your mouth.

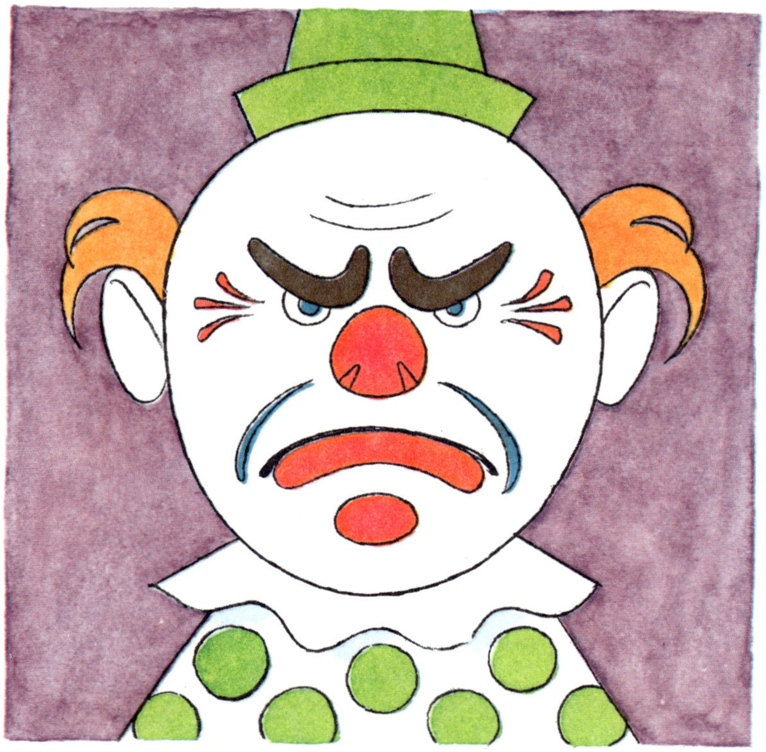

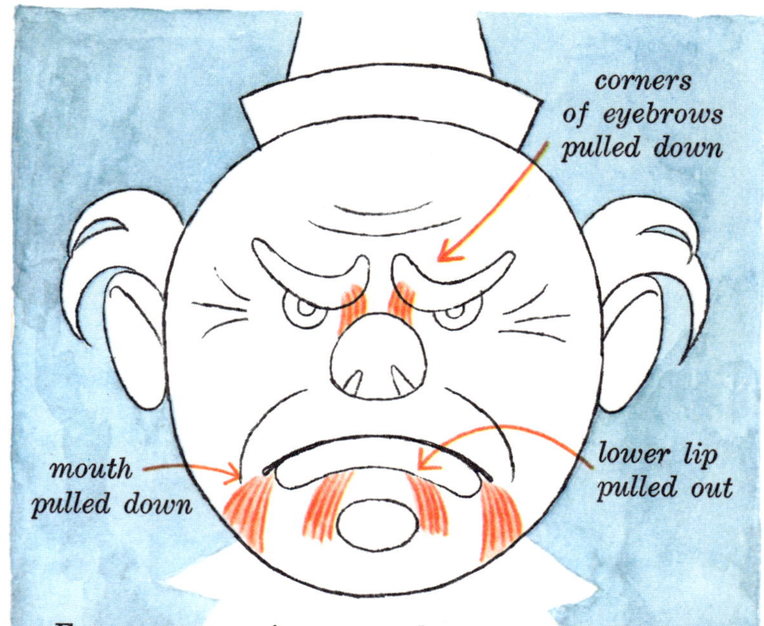

For an angry face—muscles on nose pull your eyebrows down, muscles from your neck pull your mouth down, muscles from chin pull lower lip out.

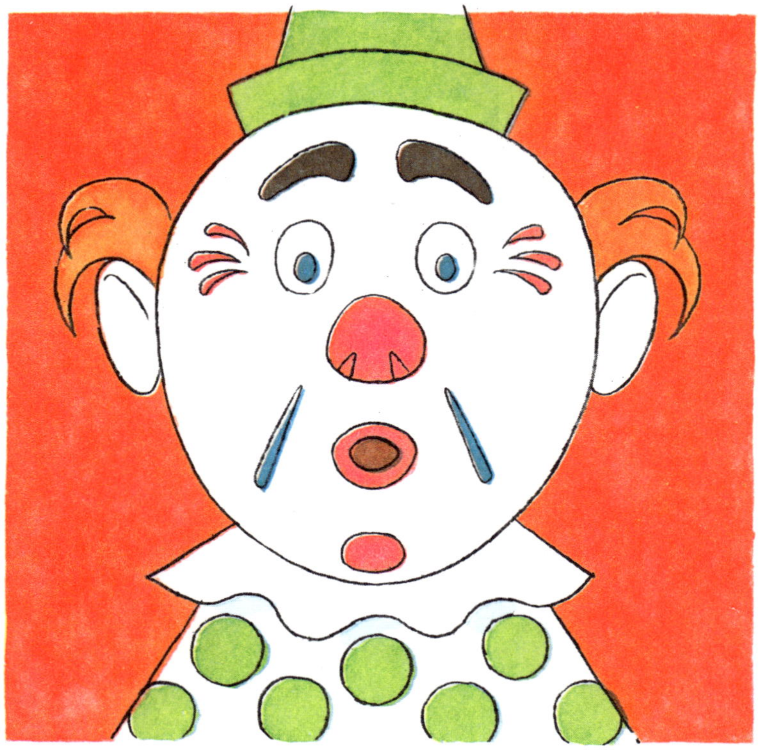

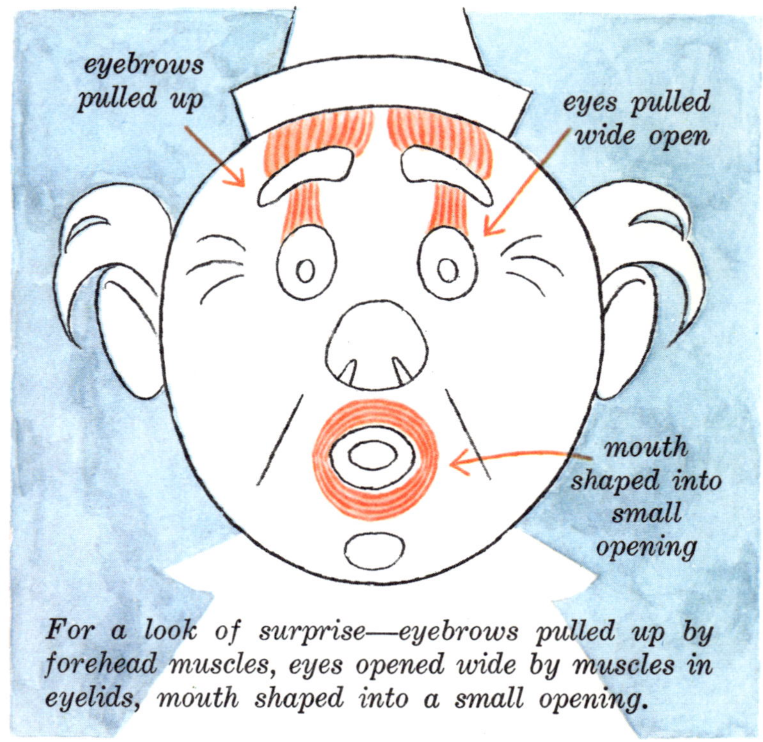

For a look of surprise—eyebrows pulled up by forehead muscles, eyes opened wide by muscles in eyelids, mouth shaped into a small opening.

To express emotion your face has sixteen muscles. They are mostly in pairs, with one muscle of a pair on each side of the face. The muscles that move your mouth to eat or talk also move it to show surprise. Muscles attached to the chest pull on the lower part of the face to express sadness. Other muscles pull the corners of your mouth up or down or sideways.

Muscles from your scalp pull your eyebrows up and wrinkle your forehead when you are surprised, and some make your eyebrows slant when you feel like crying. Rings of muscles around your eyes, like those around your mouth, change the shape of the eyes. With so many combinations of muscles your face can express just about anything you feel.

Daily EXERCISE keeps your muscles in trim. Muscles that aren't used very much get soft and loose and weak. They don't respond quickly and strongly when you want them to do something. If you exercise and use all your muscles regularly, they stay firm and strong, ready for anything. Firm muscles give your body a healthy look, and help you stand straight and move gracefully.

Exercise is important for your whole body. It makes your heart beat faster and keeps it strong. It gets your lungs breathing deeper, bringing more oxygen into your body. It makes you strong enough to do the things you enjoy without tiring. It helps you feel better, work better, and look better.

Here are some exercises to do every day that you might enjoy. Keep doing them regularly, along with running and playing some active outdoor games, and you'll stay in good shape.

Start slowly, doing each exercise just a few times. Gradually increase the number until you can do the full amount. Try to do the exercises smoothly and gracefully, to get the most out of them.

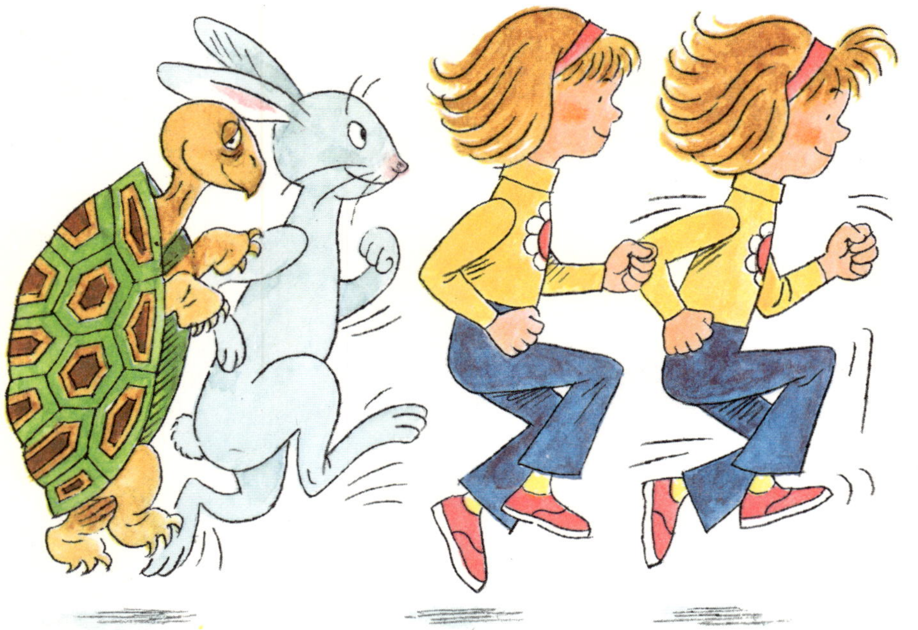

1. *TORTOISE and HARE*

This is a running exercise that you do by just running in place. First you run 50 steps in place slowly, as a tortoise would. Then run 50 steps as a hare would run, very fast. Repeat this 3 times.

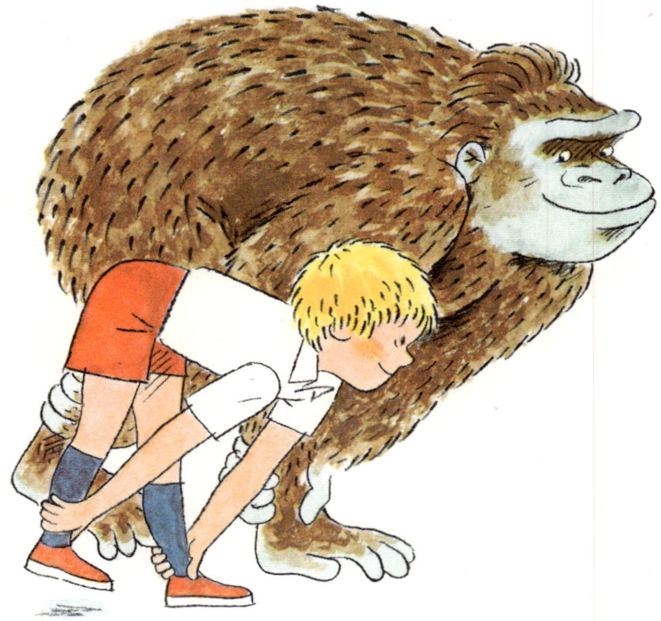

2. *GORILLA WALK*

Spread your feet apart about as wide as your shoulders. Bend at your waist and grab your ankles. Hold your ankles and walk stiff-legged.

3. *MEASURING WORM*

Get into push-up position, body and arms straight, hands on floor.

Keep hands still and walk feet up as close to hands as possible.

Keep feet still and walk hands forward to starting position.

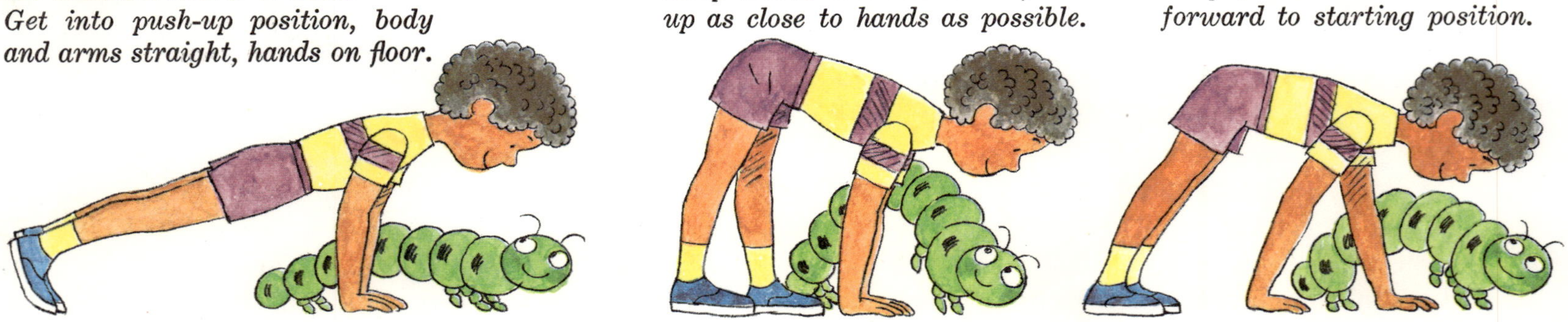

4. *RUSSIAN HOP*
Get into a squat position with your arms folded across your chest. Hop up and forward with both your feet. At the end of each hop you are back in the starting position. Hop around in a circle.

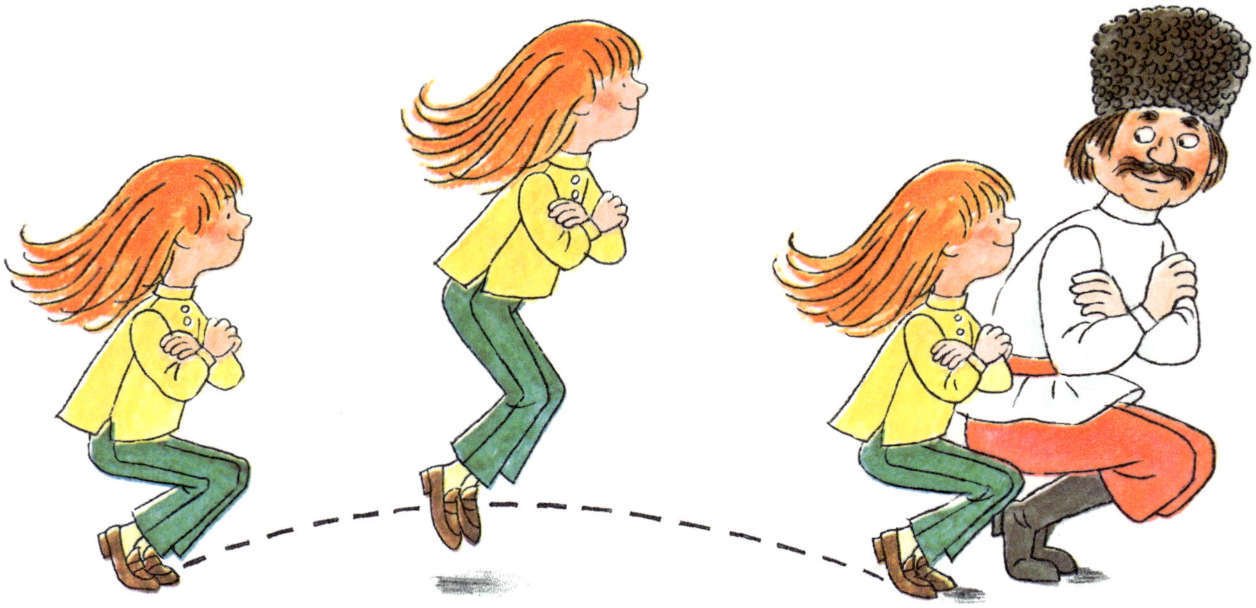

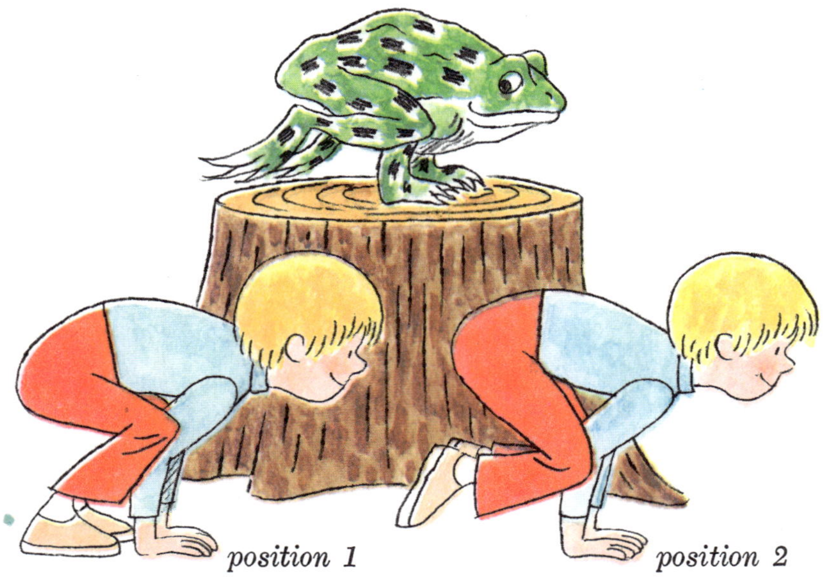

5. *FROG STAND Get into squat position, hands on floor. Lean forward, raise feet, balance on hands. Repeat 5 times.*

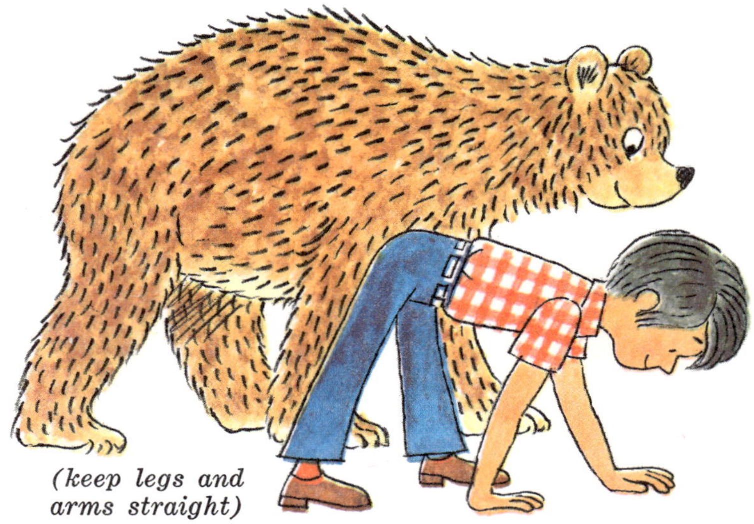

6. *BEAR WALK Bend, put hands on floor. Walk in circle, left arm and leg together, then right arm and leg.*

7. *WHEELBARROW*
This exercise is for two people. One gets on hands and knees. The other picks up the first person's legs by the ankles. They both walk forward, one on hands, the other on feet. Then they change places.

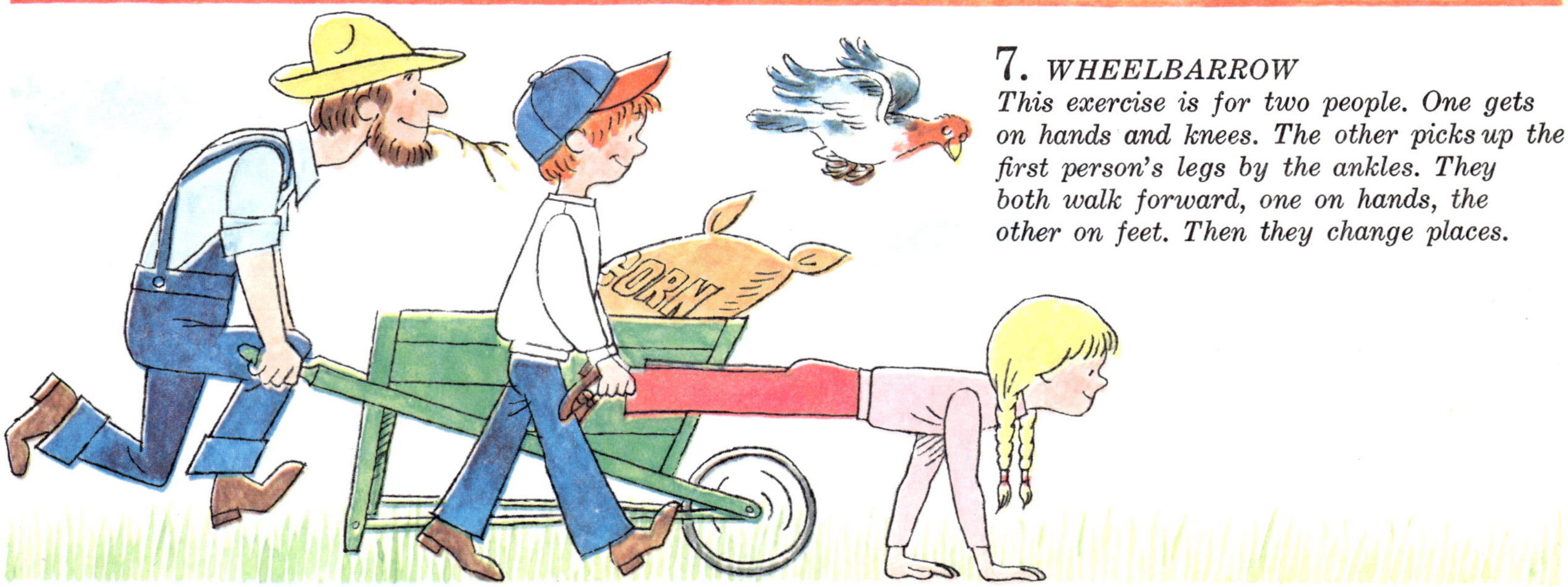

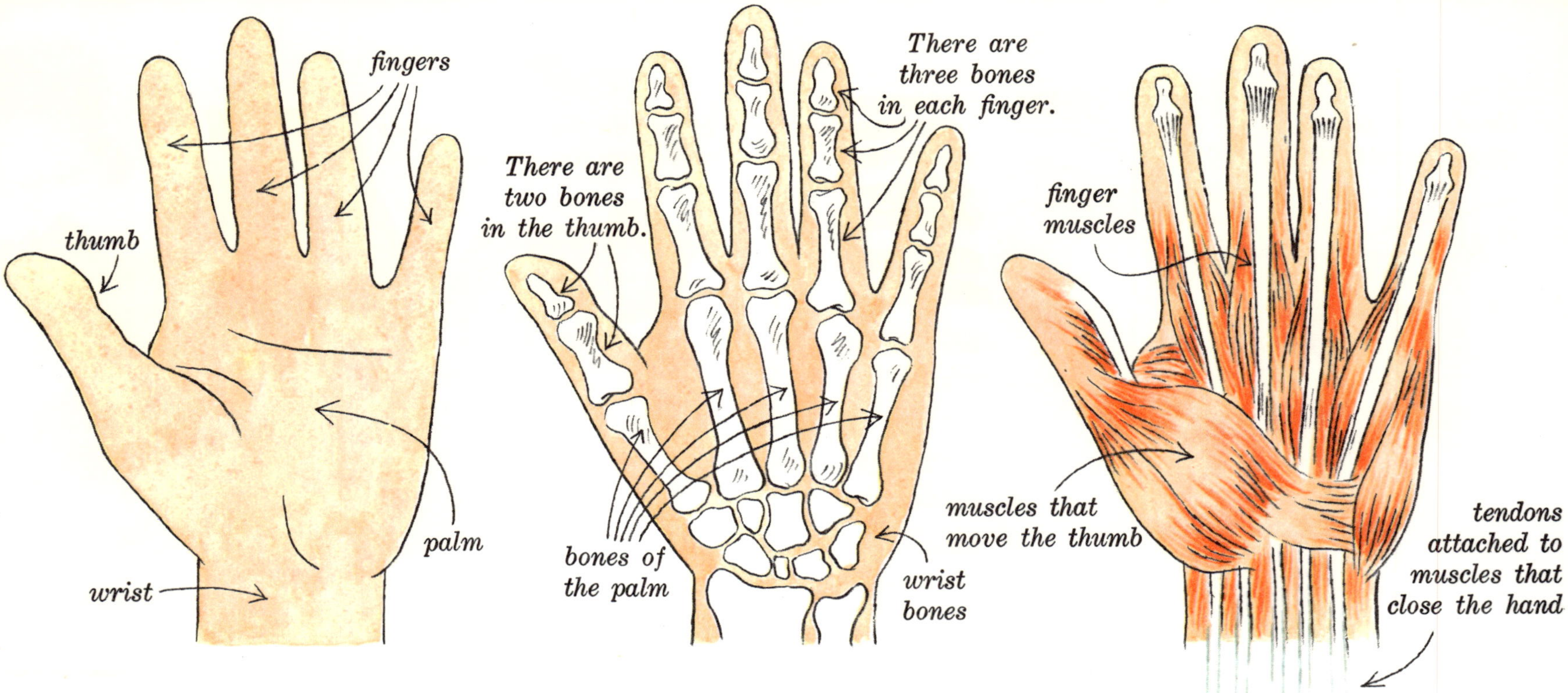

Your HANDS is one of the three main reasons why you, as a human, are more advanced than any of the other animals. Your brain, with its power to reason and develop ideas, and your ability to speak, so that you can talk to people about those ideas, are the other two reasons.

Your hands carry out the ideas and inventions your brain thinks of. It is not enough for someone to say, "I have just thought up a way to protect myself from bad weather—a house made of logs." It takes hands to make tools to cut down trees and trim them into logs. Hands are needed to pile the logs into position and cover them with a roof. And when the brain of a composer works out a beautiful piano piece, the trained hands of a pianist make it possible for all of us to hear what it sounds like.

Hands can pick up tiny pins, grasp heavy tools, pull doors open, push them shut, twist off bottletops, tickle people, write, paint, and play musical instruments. They can do so many different things, and make all the movements needed to do them, because of their very complicated structure.

Each hand has twenty-seven small bones—together the hands have fifty-four bones, over one quarter of the 206 bones in the whole body! There are eight bones in the wrist. They can slide over each other a bit, allowing the wrist to be very flexible and move the hand into many different positions.

The palm has five bones. The thumb bone is set at an angle to the four finger-bones, so the thumb can move toward the fingers, enabling the hand to pick up and hold things. (Try to pick up something with just your fingers. It's not nearly so easy as when you use your thumb, too!) The fingernails help to pick up small things the fingers can't get hold of.

Thirty muscles move the fingers of each hand. Because it has so many muscles, your hand can make all the small, careful motions you want it to.

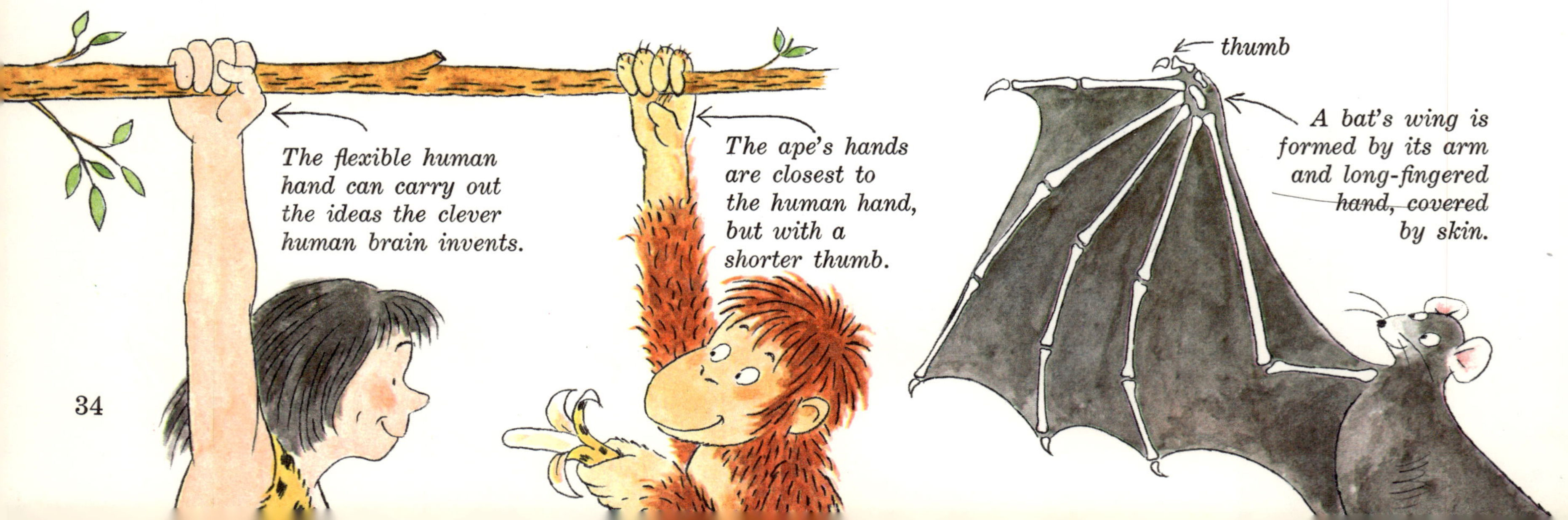

The flexible human hand can carry out the ideas the clever human brain invents.

The ape's hands are closest to the human hand, but with a shorter thumb.

A bat's wing is formed by its arm and long-fingered hand, covered by skin.

Hands can play musical instruments.

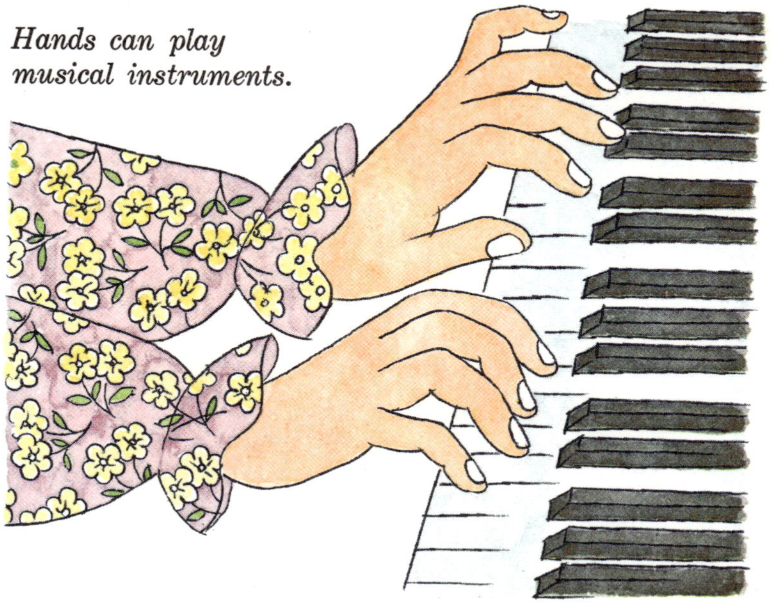

Hands do the difficult tasks when you are dressing.

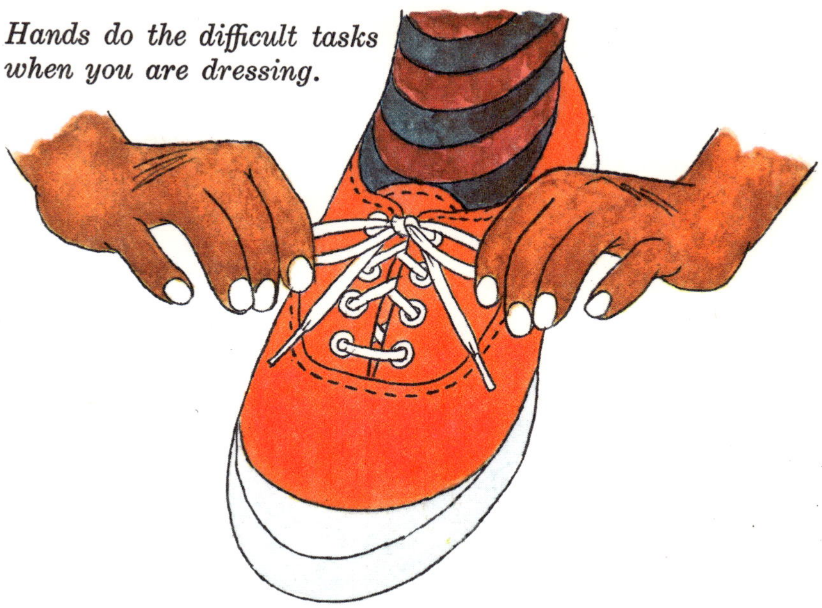

Hands can write, model, draw, and paint.

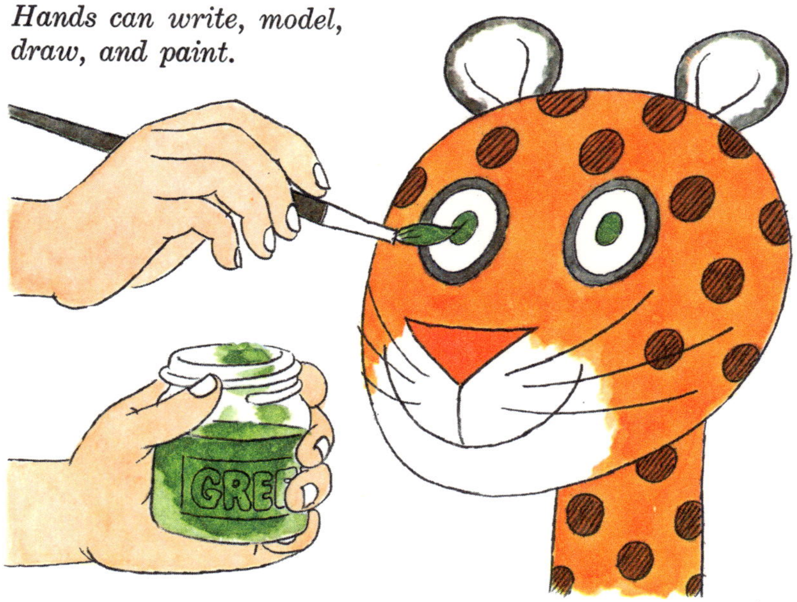

And hands can grip heavy weights and work with heavy tools.

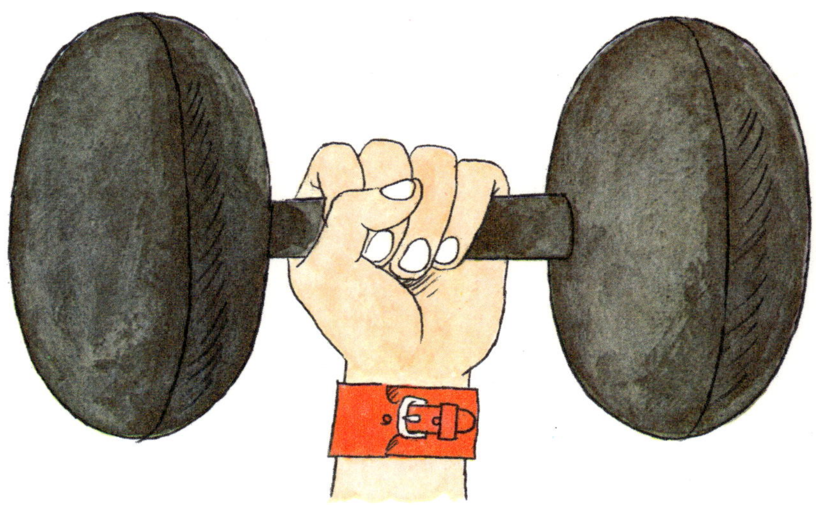

Deaf people can speak to each other with their hands. This is how they use their hands to spell out the alphabet.

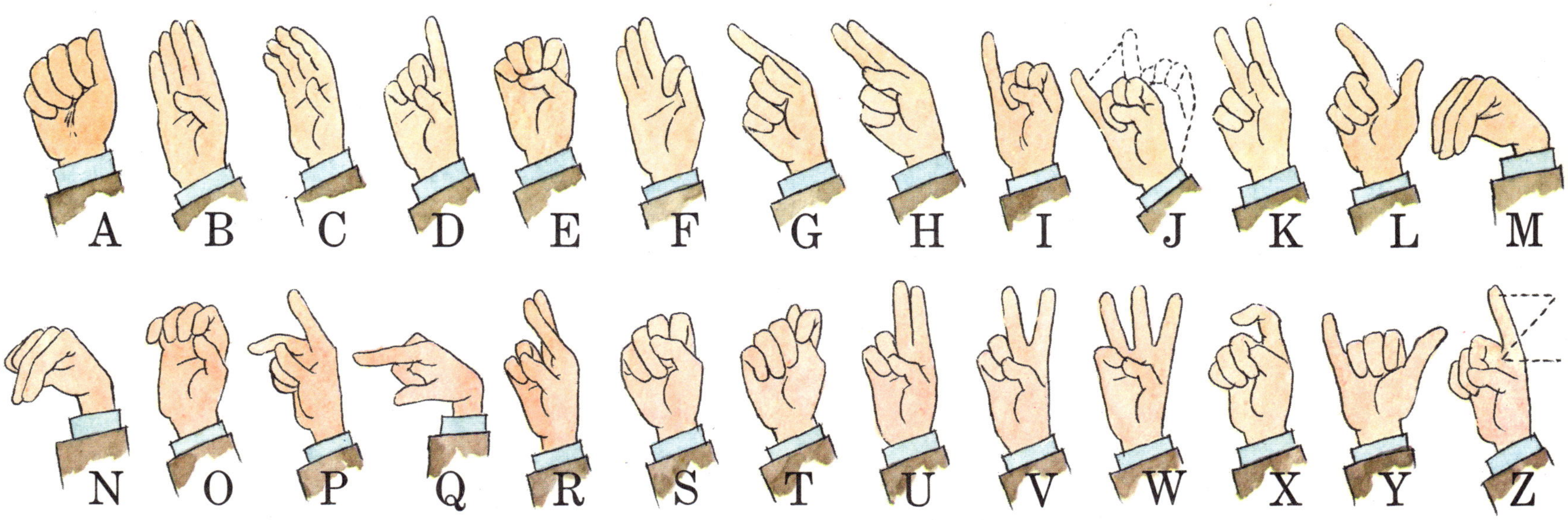

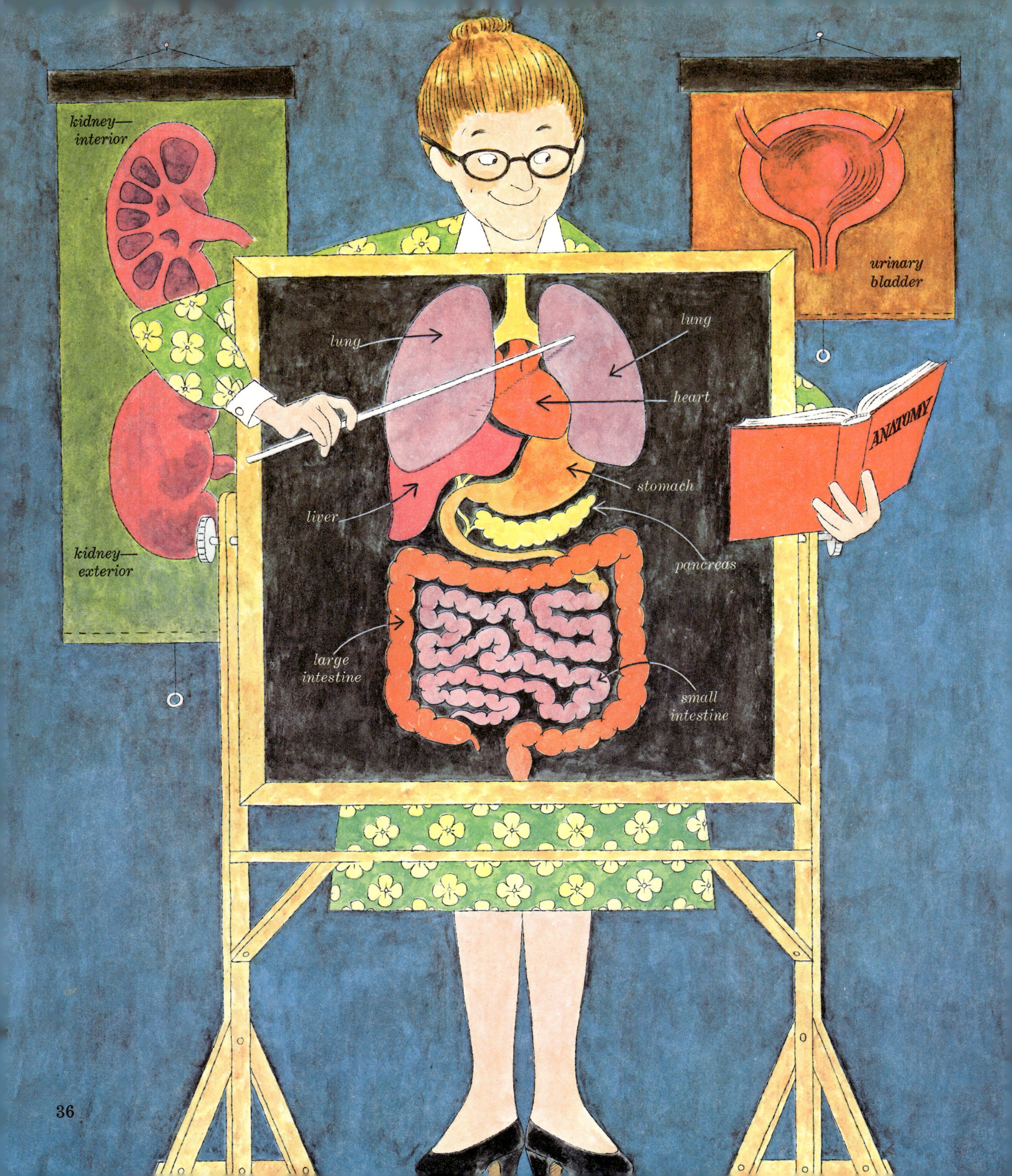
kidney—
interior
kidney—
exterior
urinary
bladder
lung
lung
heart
stomach
liver
pancreas
large
intestine
small
intestine
ANATOMY

An ORGAN is made up of a group of tissues joined together to do a special job. (Tissues are cells of the same kind grouped together—page 18.) The heart, eyes, lungs, stomach, intestine, and brain are some of the body's organs.

A group of organs working together to do a specific job is called a system. There are ten main systems in the human body. They work together in a wonderful way to keep the body going.

The *skeletal system*, the bones and the connective tissue holding them together, is the framework of the body. The *muscle system* moves the body's framework, pushes food through the body, and makes the blood circulate. The *nervous system*, the brain, spinal cord, and nerves, regulates all the other systems. It gives the muscles the signals they need to move. Through the senses of touch, sight, smell, sound, and taste, it makes us aware of our surroundings. It does the thinking.

The *digestive system*, the mouth, stomach, and intestines, takes in food to provide the energy the body needs to do all its work, separates out the usable food, and expels the waste from the body. The *respiratory system*, the windpipe and lungs, breathes in air and separates out the oxygen the body needs to burn the food it eats. It also breathes out carbon dioxide wastes collected from the cells. The *circulatory system*, the heart, the blood, and all the blood vessels, carries the food and oxygen to all parts of the body.

The *lymphatic system* uses a fluid called lymph to collect and carry away some of the waste materials from the tissues. The *urinary system*, the kidneys and bladder, removes liquid wastes from the blood and sends them out of the body. The *endocrine system* helps run the body by releasing chemical "messengers" into the bloodstream. They tell the different body systems how to operate to satisfy the body's needs at any moment. The *reproductive system* is the group of organs that allows humans to have babies—to make new human beings.

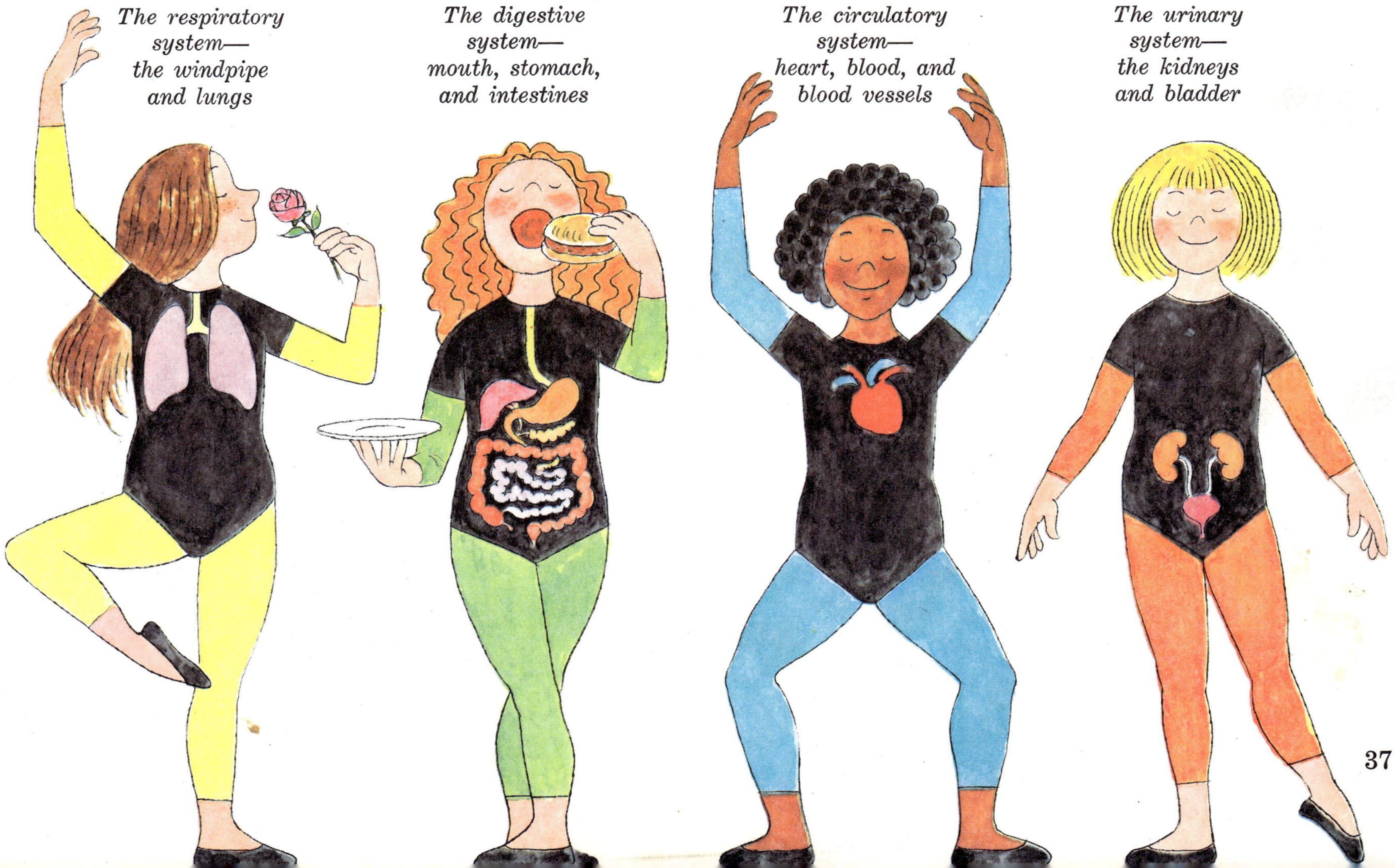

The respiratory system—the windpipe and lungs

The digestive system—mouth, stomach, and intestines

The circulatory system—heart, blood, and blood vessels

The urinary system—the kidneys and bladder

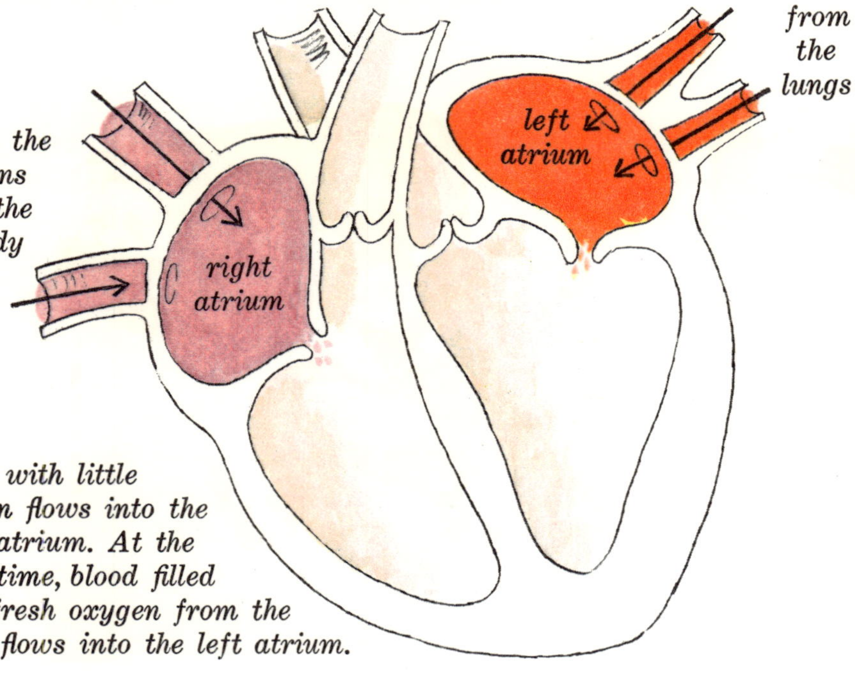

1.
Blood with little oxygen flows into the right atrium. At the same time, blood filled with fresh oxygen from the lungs flows into the left atrium.

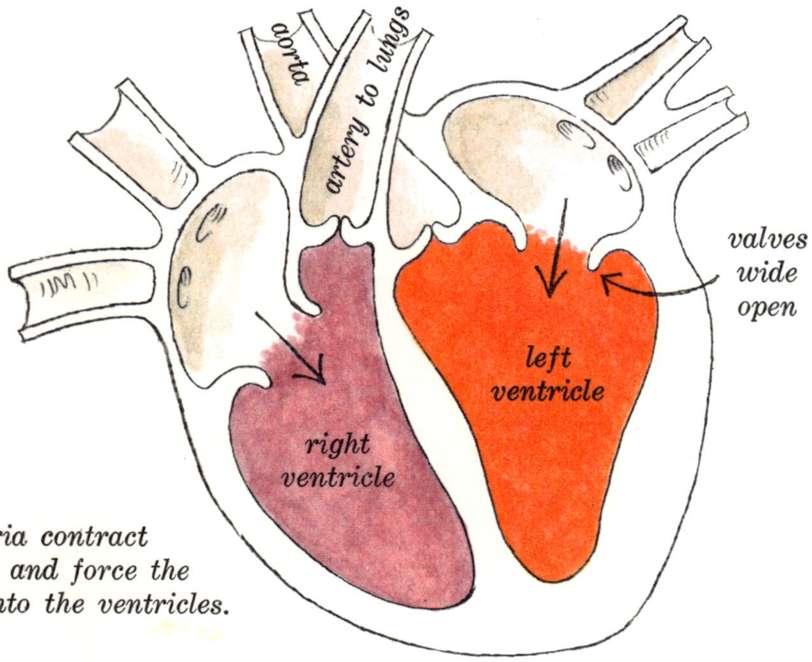

2.
The atria contract slightly and force the blood into the ventricles.

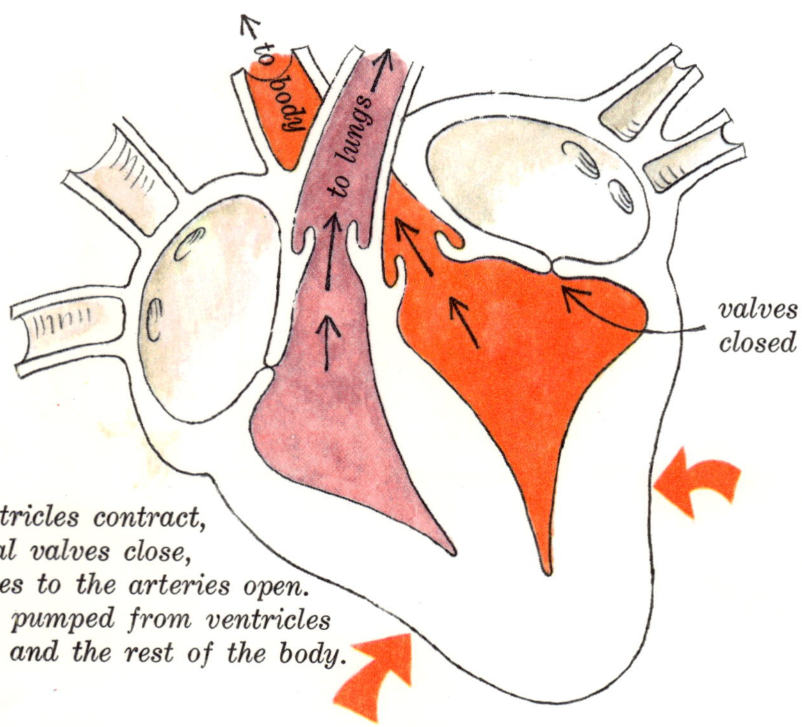

3.
The ventricles contract, the atrial valves close, the valves to the arteries open. Blood is pumped from ventricles to lungs and the rest of the body.

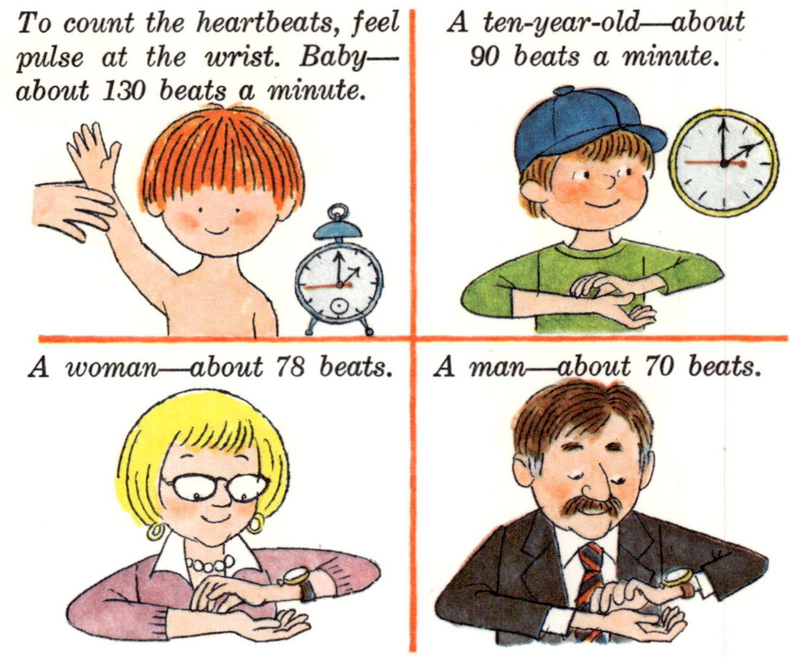
To count the heartbeats, feel pulse at the wrist. Baby—about 130 beats a minute.
A ten-year-old—about 90 beats a minute.
A woman—about 78 beats.
A man—about 70 beats.

Your HEART is a powerful pump, made of muscle, about the size of your fist. Inside, it is hollow and divided into four spaces, two above called atria and two below called ventricles. Blood entering the heart goes into the atria. Blood leaving the heart is pumped out of the ventricles. Blood vessels that carry blood to the heart are called veins; those that carry it away are called arteries.

The atrium and the ventricle on the left do one job, and the atrium and the ventricle on the right do another. On the left, blood from the lungs, full of fresh oxygen, enters the left atrium. It is pumped through a valve into the left ventricle. The valve, a sort of one-way door, opens to let the blood flow from the atrium to the ventricle, then closes, so the blood can't go back.

Then the heart contracts strongly, pumping the blood from the left ventricle through another one-

Here are some other pumps:

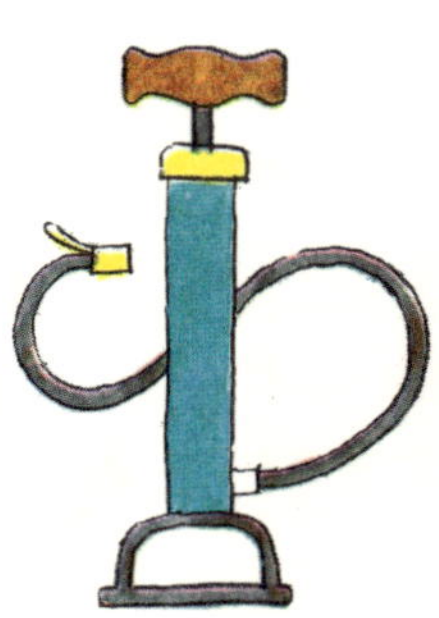

air pump

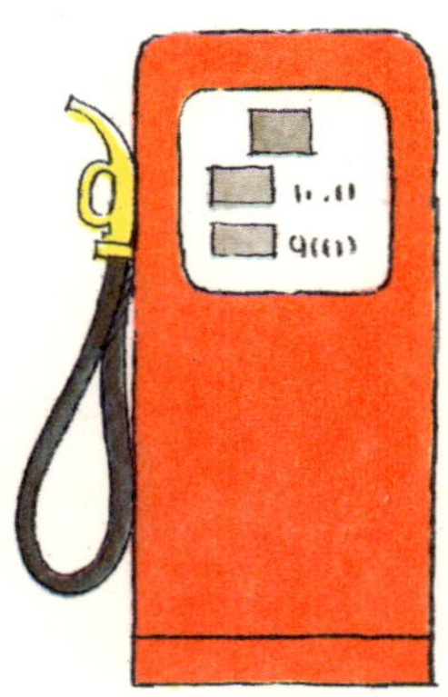

gasoline pump

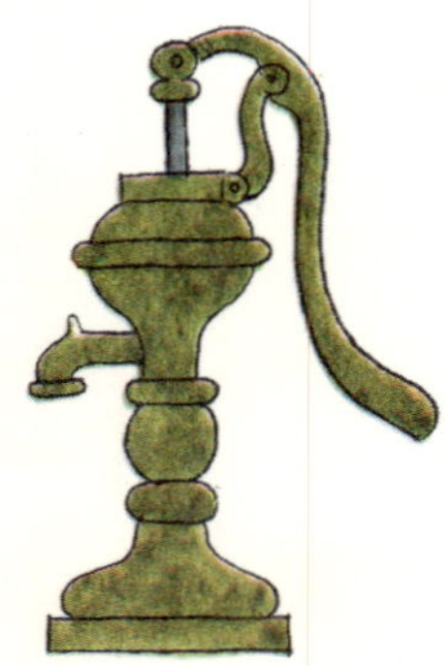

water pump

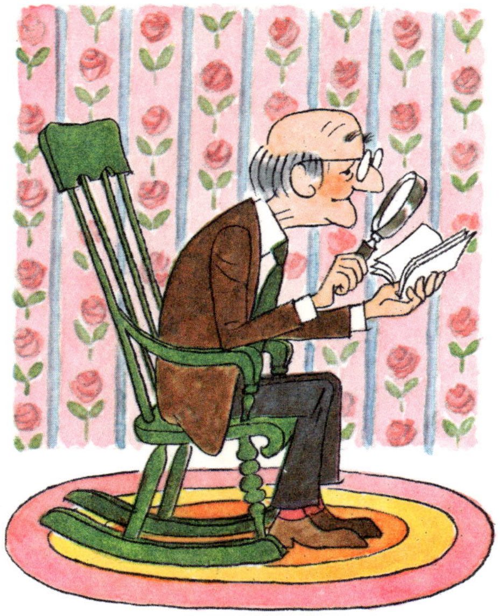

The heart beats at a relaxed rate when a person is sitting quietly.

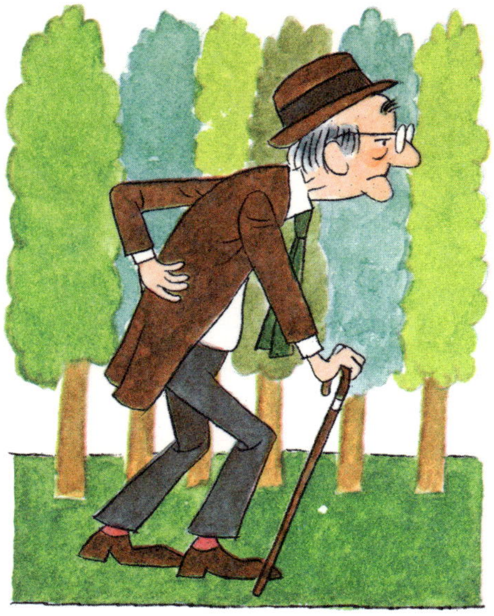

The rate of the heartbeat gets a little faster during mild exercise.

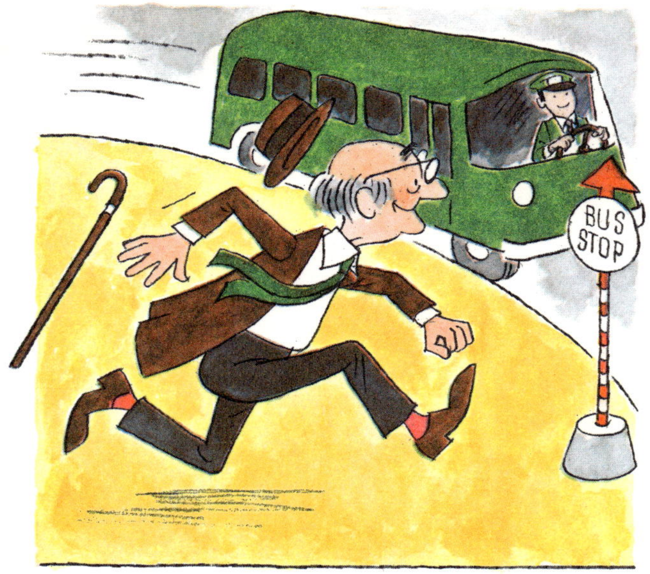

During violent exercise, when the body needs lots of energy, the heart beats very fast.

way valve into the aorta, the biggest artery, for a trip through the rest of the body.

After the blood has made the trip through the body, it returns to the heart, enters the right atrium, and is pumped through a valve to the right ventricle below. This blood was bright red and full of oxygen when it started its trip. Now it has given up most of the oxygen to the body's cells and has picked up carbon dioxide. Its color is bluish.

The same contraction of the heart that sends blood from the left ventricle into the arteries sends blood from the right ventricle to the lungs. There the blood gets rid of its carbon dioxide, picks up fresh oxygen, and returns to the left side of the heart for a new trip through the body.

The atrial muscles are smaller than those of the ventricles, because the atria have less work to do. They only pump blood into the ventricles below them. The muscle around the right ventricle is heavy and strong—it must contract with enough force to send the blood through both lungs. But the thickest and most powerful of all the heart muscles surrounds the left ventricle. It must contract with enough force to send the blood to every part of the body. The ventricles' powerful contractions are what we feel as the heartbeat.

A baby's heart beats about 130 times a minute, a ten-year-old's heart beats about 90 times a minute, a woman's heart beats about 78 times a minute and a man's about 70 times. That is when they are sitting or standing. If they play hard or exercise, it beats faster. An athlete's heart, during a race, beats as fast as 150 times a minute. There are several places along the course of the arteries where you can feel your heartbeat. A good one is at your wrist, where your doctor feels your pulse.

A doctor can use a machine to make a diagram of a patient's heartbeats. It helps show if the heart is working well.

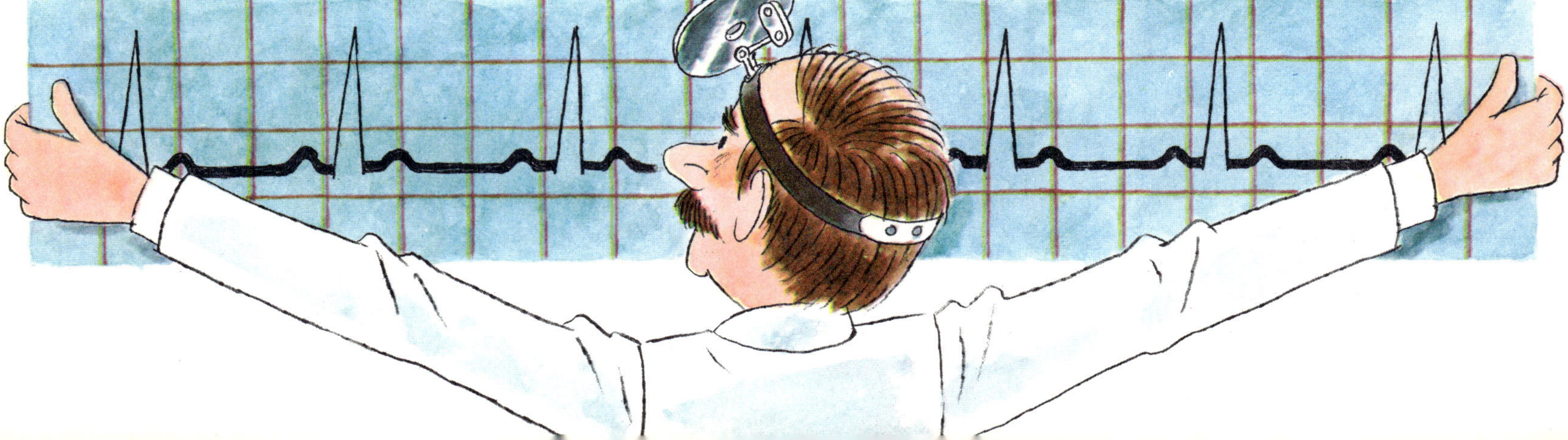

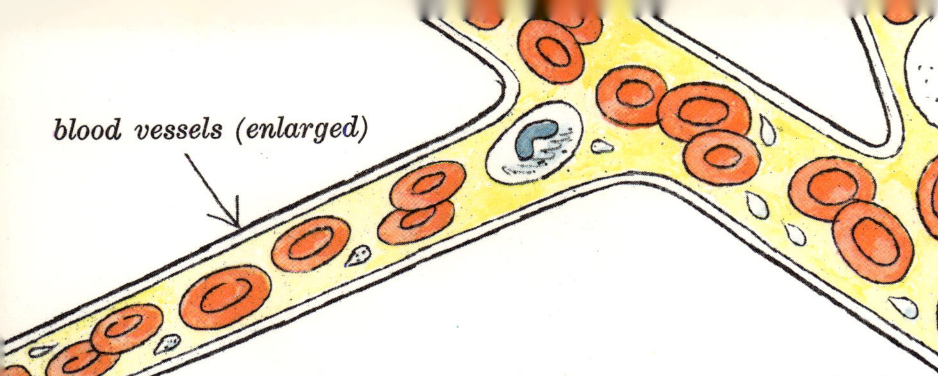

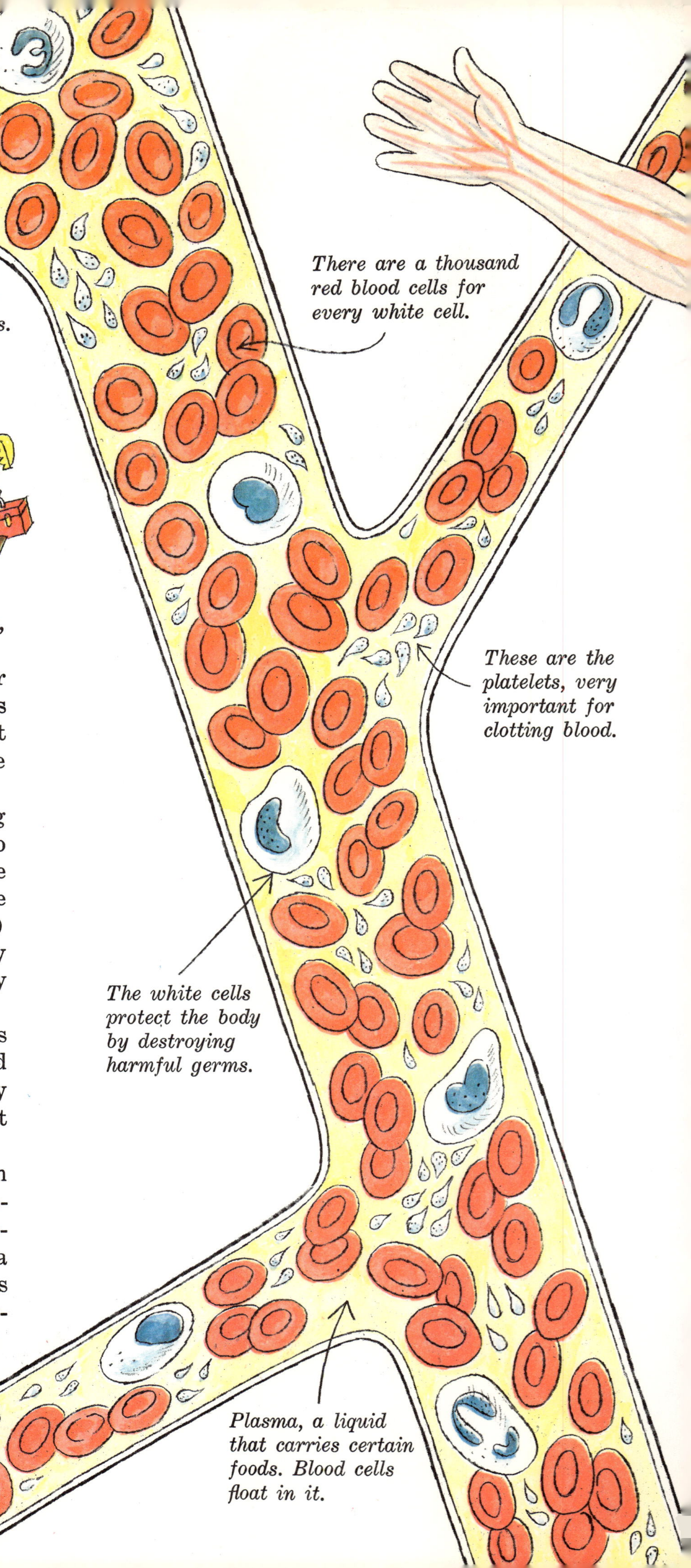

The red cells carry oxygen to body cells. *The white cells fight germs that infect the body.* *The platelets stop leaks by clotting at cuts.*

BLOOD is made up of plasma, red blood cells, white blood cells, and platelets.

Over half the blood is plasma. Plasma is a clear yellow liquid, mostly water, enriched with proteins and substances that can make the blood clot. It carries the foods the body needs and most of the wastes the body is getting rid of.

There are millions of tiny red blood cells floating in the plasma. They carry oxygen from the lungs to every part of the body and take waste carbon dioxide back to the lungs to be breathed out into the air. (The plasma also carries some of the carbon dioxide.) Red cells are made in the bone marrow. They only last a few months, so the bone marrow keeps busy making new ones.

The white cells fight disease. If infectious germs enter the body, white cells rush to the spot, surround the germs, and destroy them. New white cells, mostly made in the bone marrow, replace the white cells that die in the fight.

The platelets' job is to keep too much blood from leaking out—for instance, if you cut yourself. Platelets gather at the cut, combine with the clotting substance from the plasma, and form a clot, sealing off the leak. The clot dries and turns into a scab, the skin underneath heals, and the scab falls off.

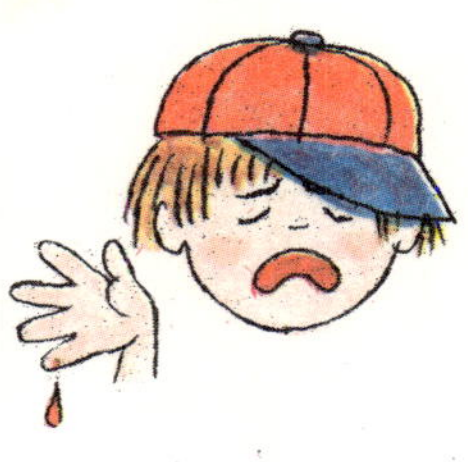

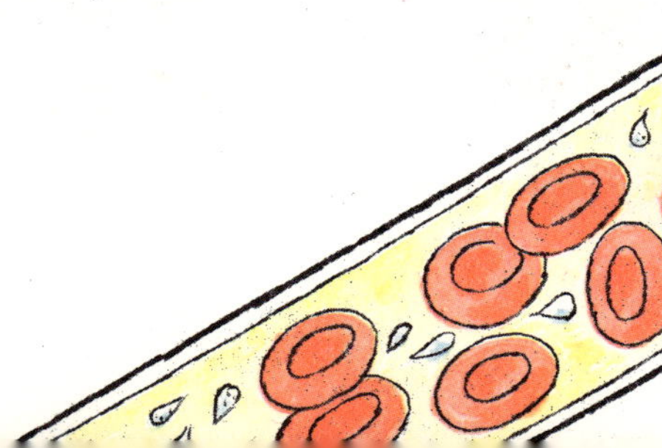

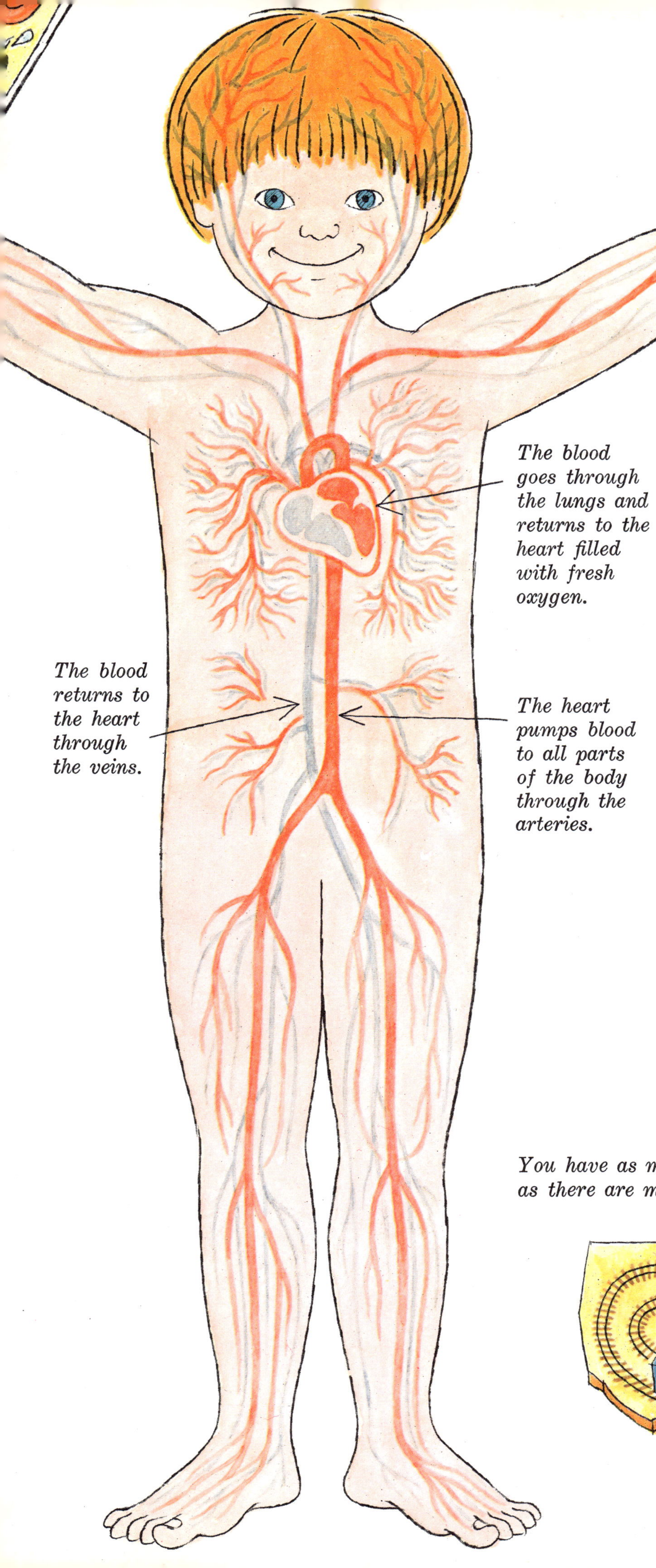

In its CIRCULATION, blood flows in a continuous stream through the body's system of blood vessels. The blood makes two separate round trips, a short one and a long one.

On the short trip, the right side of the heart pumps blood to the lungs. The blood gets rid of carbon dioxide, picks up oxygen, and returns to the left side of the heart.

On the long trip, the left side of the heart pumps blood through the rest of the body. Some of the blood goes through the coronary arteries, feeding the heart itself. Other arteries carry blood everywhere else—through the kidneys, where it is cleaned of the wastes it carries; to the small intestine, where it picks up tiny bits of food; to the rest of the arteries branching out smaller and smaller all through the body.

The smallest blood vessels, as fine as hairs, are called capillaries. Here the blood releases the oxygen and food it carries, giving it up to the individual cells. The cells give off carbon dioxide and other wastes to the blood as it continues through the capillaries, flowing to the tiniest veins, which join larger veins, which join even larger veins, as they get closer to the heart. The blood returns to the right side of the heart and will be pumped back to the lungs to begin the cycle again.

You have as many miles of blood vessels in your body as there are miles of railroad tracks in the U.S.!

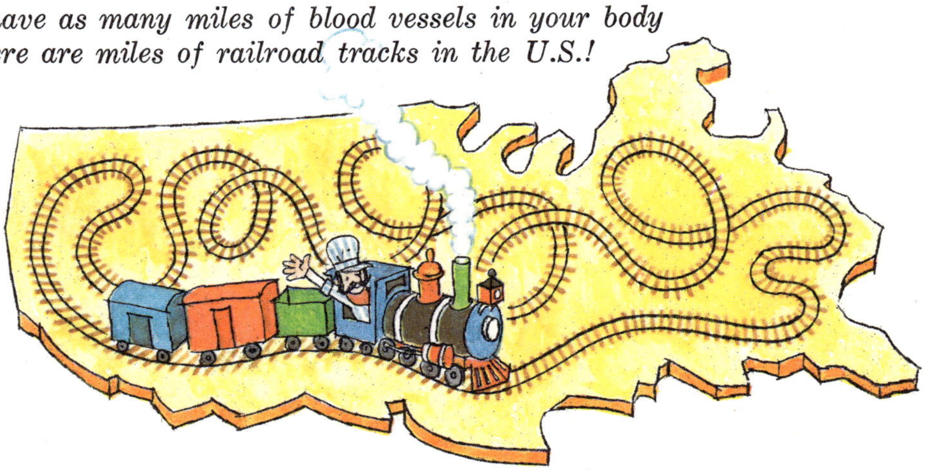

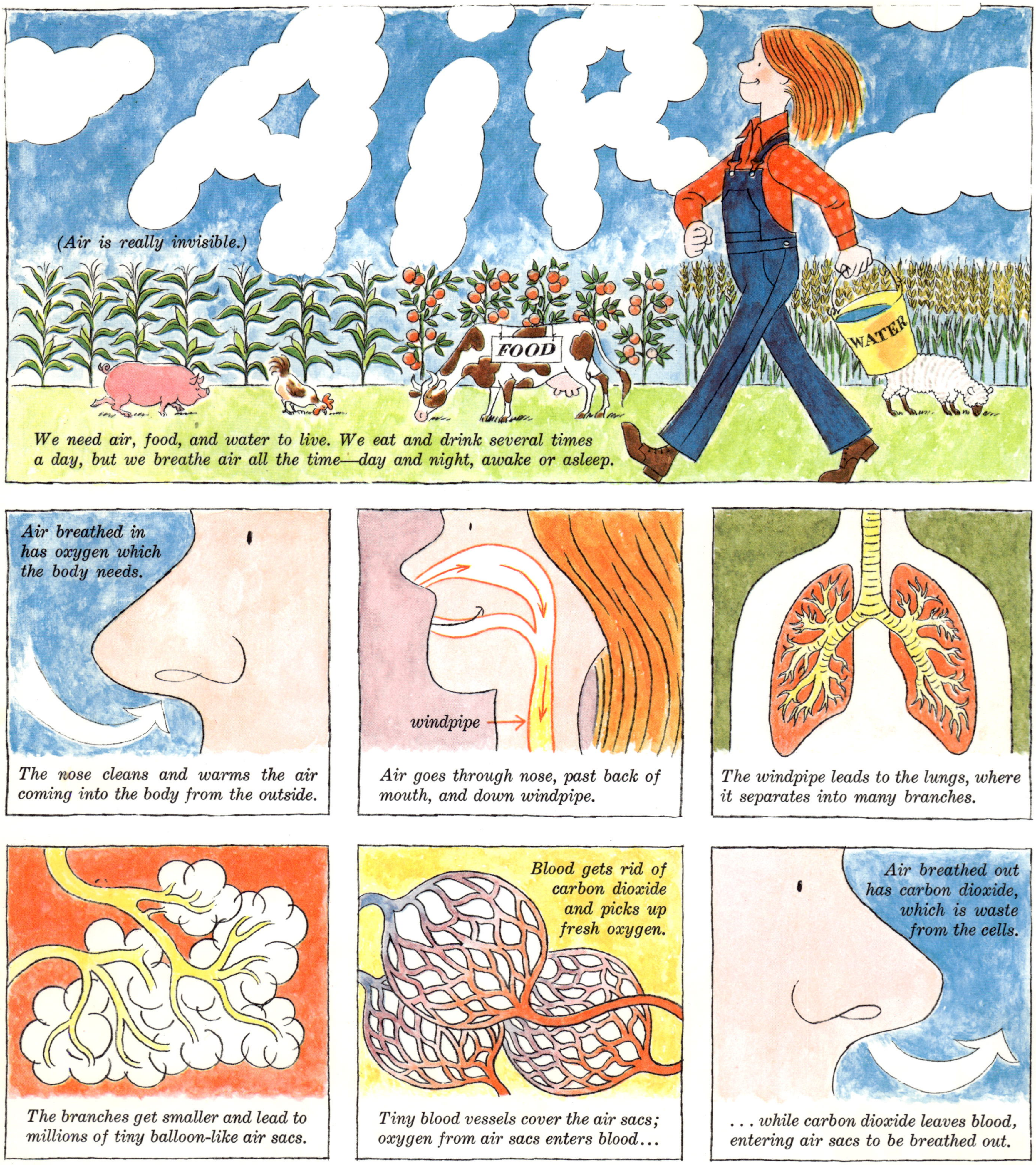
AIR
(Air is really invisible.)
FOOD
WATER
We need air, food, and water to live. We eat and drink several times a day, but we breathe air all the time—day and night, awake or asleep.
Air breathed in has oxygen which the body needs.
The nose cleans and warms the air coming into the body from the outside.
windpipe
Air goes through nose, past back of mouth, and down windpipe.
The windpipe leads to the lungs, where it separates into many branches.
The branches get smaller and lead to millions of tiny balloon-like air sacs.
Blood gets rid of carbon dioxide and picks up fresh oxygen.
Tiny blood vessels cover the air sacs; oxygen from air sacs enters blood...
Air breathed out has carbon dioxide, which is waste from the cells.
. . . while carbon dioxide leaves blood, entering air sacs to be breathed out.

The LUNGS receive the air you breathe in through your nose and mouth, air containing the oxygen your cells need to burn their food.

The nose has several jobs to do. Its hairs and sticky mucous lining help trap any dust or dirt in the air. If something irritating gets into the nose, the nose automatically sneezes, trying to push out the irritant with a blast of air. There are a lot of blood vessels close to the surface inside the nose. When cold air goes past them, the warm blood heats up the air. Even cold winter air will be close to body temperature after it has passed through the nose.

After the air goes past the nose and throat, it goes down the four-inch-long windpipe, where it is cleaned and warmed even more. The windpipe divides into two branches, one leading to each lung. Inside the lungs, each branch divides into smaller and smaller branches. They carry the air to the air sacs.

The lungs are made of millions of little balloon-like air sacs. A network of tiny blood vessels surrounds each of the sacs. Some of the oxygen in the air passes through the thin walls of the air sacs into the blood vessels, to be carried all over the body by the red blood cells. At the same time, carbon dioxide that has been collected from cells all over the body goes from the blood out into the air sacs. The carbon dioxide can then be breathed out of the body.

The lungs are surrounded and protected by the rib cage. Underneath the lungs is a big sheet of muscle called the diaphragm. When you breathe, the muscles attached to your ribs pull them out to make more space for your lungs. The diaphragm pulls down, making still more space. Air from outside the body goes into the lungs to fill the space. When you breathe out, the muscles relax, the rib cage space and the lungs get smaller, and the air is pushed out.

This is the rib cage, which protects the lungs. It expands and contracts when you breathe in and out.

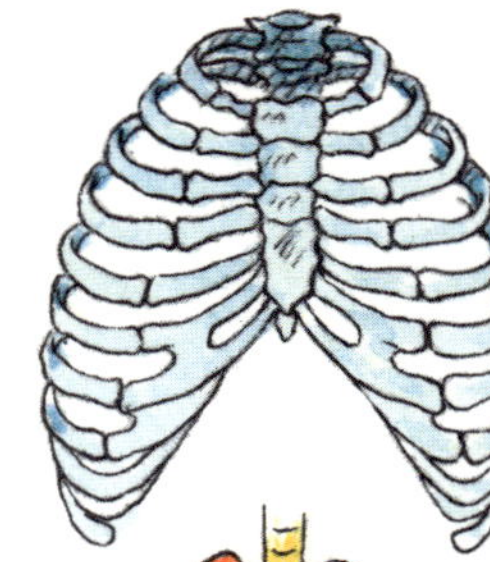

These are the lungs with the heart tucked in between them. All this fits into the rib cage.

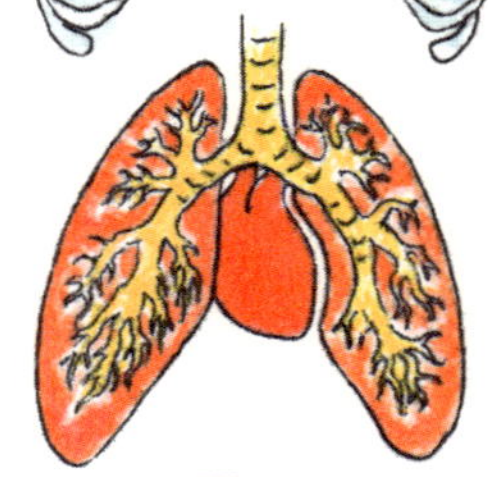

The diaphragm is a big muscle that goes up and down to help you breathe.

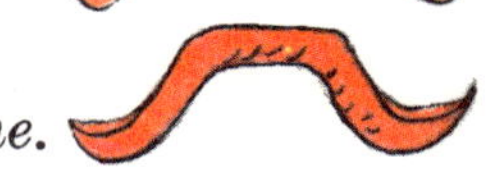

This is how they fit together—

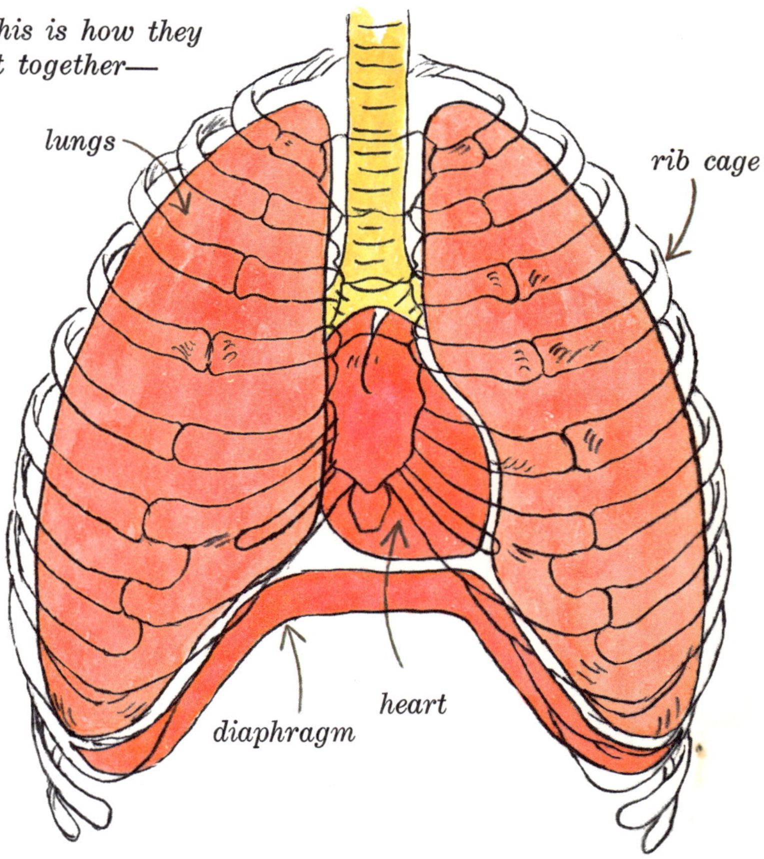

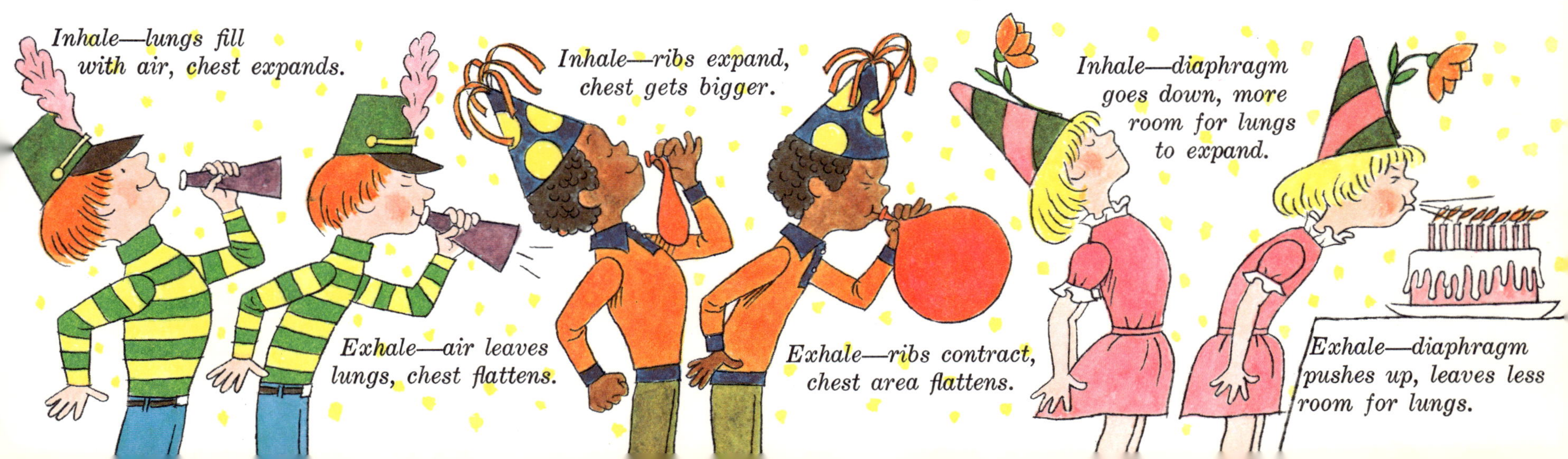

Looking down at the vocal cords when you sing . . .

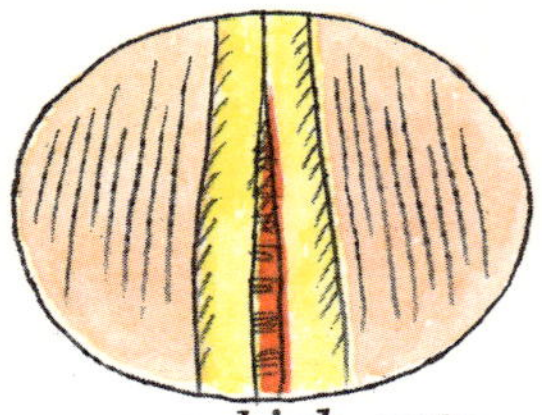

. . . a high note

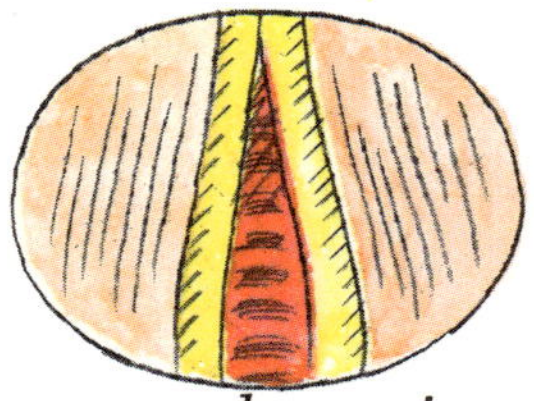

. . . a low note

The **VOICE** works like a woodwind instrument, such as a clarinet. When you blow into a clarinet the reed on top begins to vibrate, causing the air inside the clarinet to vibrate. The vibrating air comes out as sound. When you use your voice, air from your lungs blows past the vocal cords in your throat. They begin to vibrate and cause the air in your throat, mouth, and nose to vibrate. The vibrating air comes out of your mouth as your voice.

Your vocal cords are inside your voice box, at the top of the windpipe and right below the base of the tongue. When you are silent and just breathing, the vocal cords are relaxed in an open V-shape. When you speak or sing, muscles pull the vocal cords tight or let them relax to make a variety of sounds. To sing a high note, the muscles pull the cords tight, bringing them together at the open part of the V. Air from the lungs sets the tight cords vibrating at a high pitch. To sing a low note, the cords are looser and the V-shape is more open. Air from the lungs sets the loose cords vibrating at a lower pitch.

Some people have high voices and some have low voices. Grown-ups' voices are usually lower in pitch than children's. The difference is in the length and thickness of the vocal cords. When a boy gets to be about fourteen years old, his voice box gets bigger, his vocal cords grow longer and thicker, and suddenly he has a low voice like a man. When a girl gets to be about fourteen, her voice gets a little deeper and fuller, too, but it doesn't change as much as a boy's.

The lips, tongue, roof of the mouth, and teeth shape the sounds coming from the vocal cords into words. For instance, to pronounce "L" you put your tongue up to the roof of your mouth. To pronounce the sound "TH" you put your tongue between your teeth. And to say "O" you hold your lips in an O-shape.

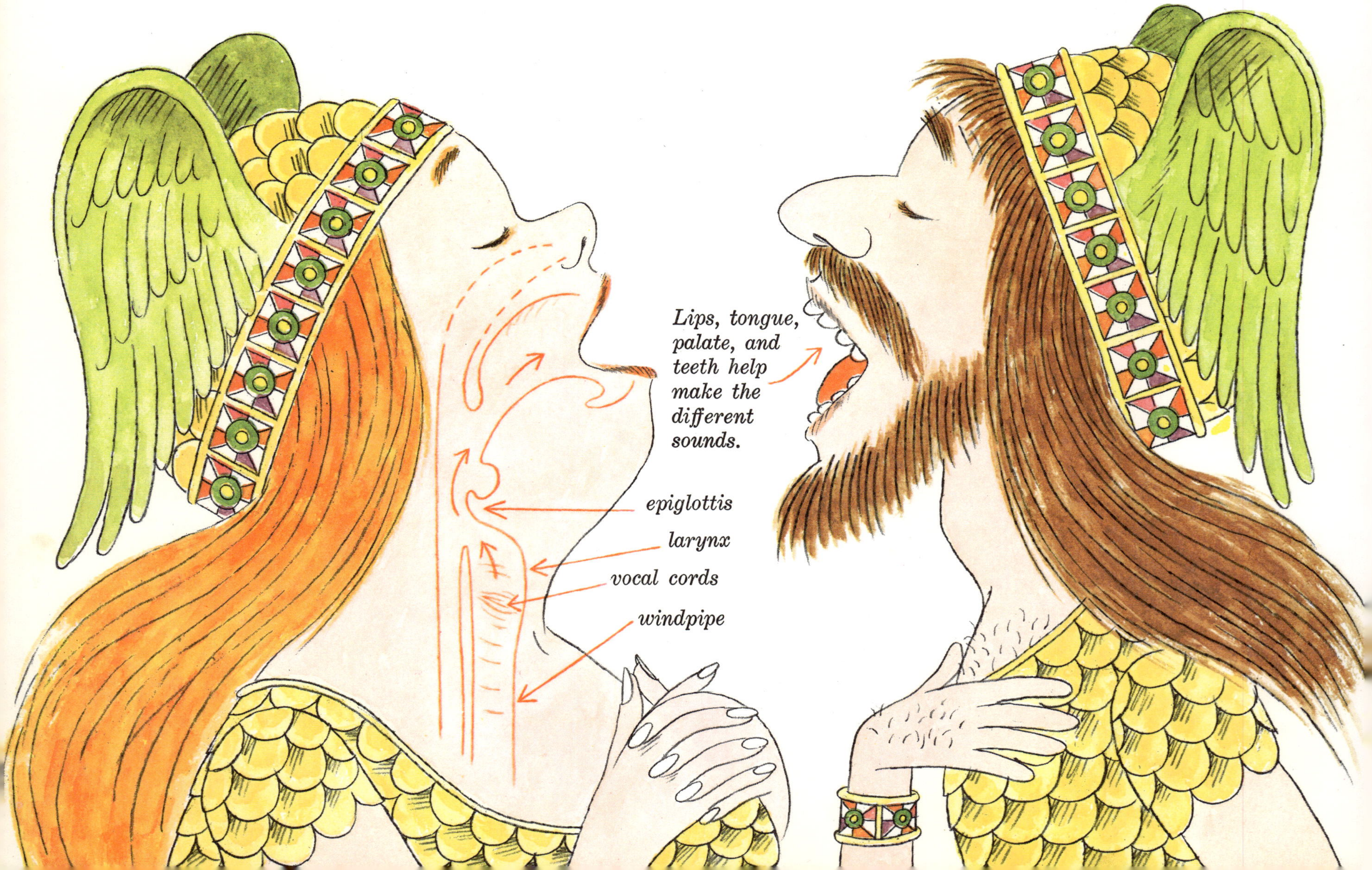
Lips, tongue, palate, and teeth help make the different sounds.
epiglottis
larynx
vocal cords
windpipe

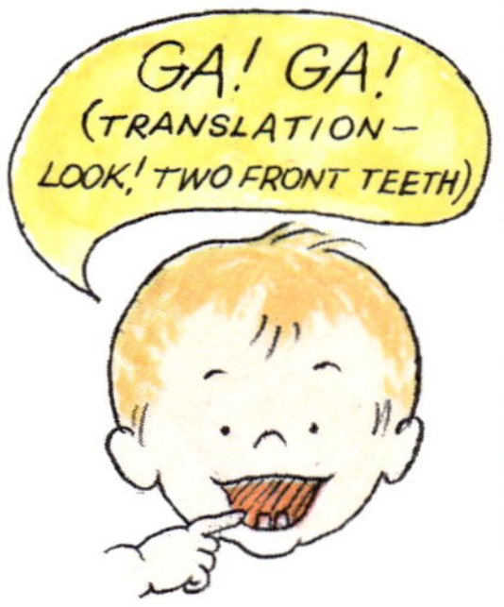

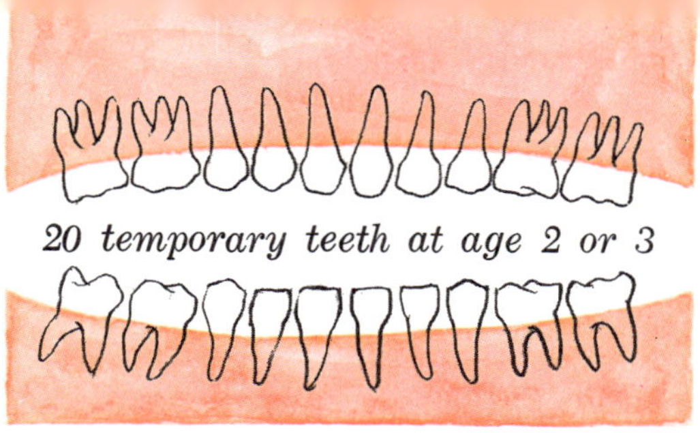

20 temporary teeth at age 2 or 3

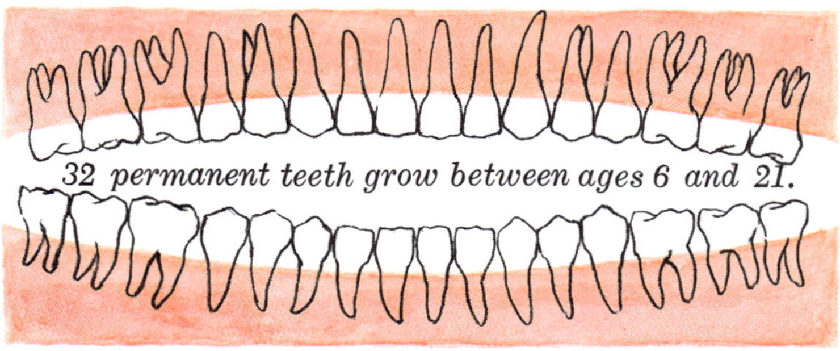

32 permanent teeth grow between ages 6 and 21.

Around age 6, the permanent teeth begin to grow in, one by one. As a new tooth pushes up under a baby tooth, the baby tooth gets loose and finally falls out, making room for the new tooth to grow.

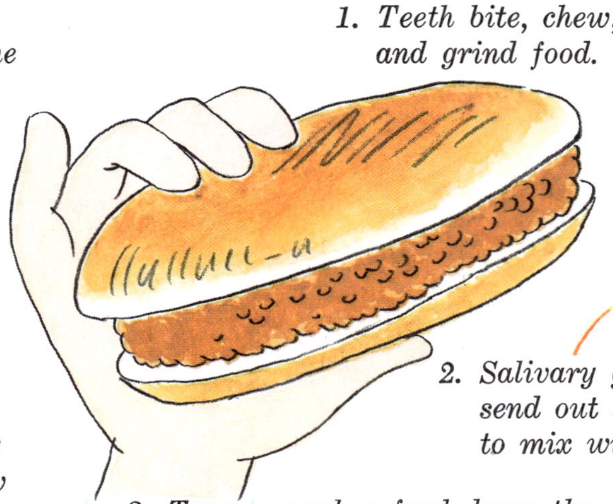

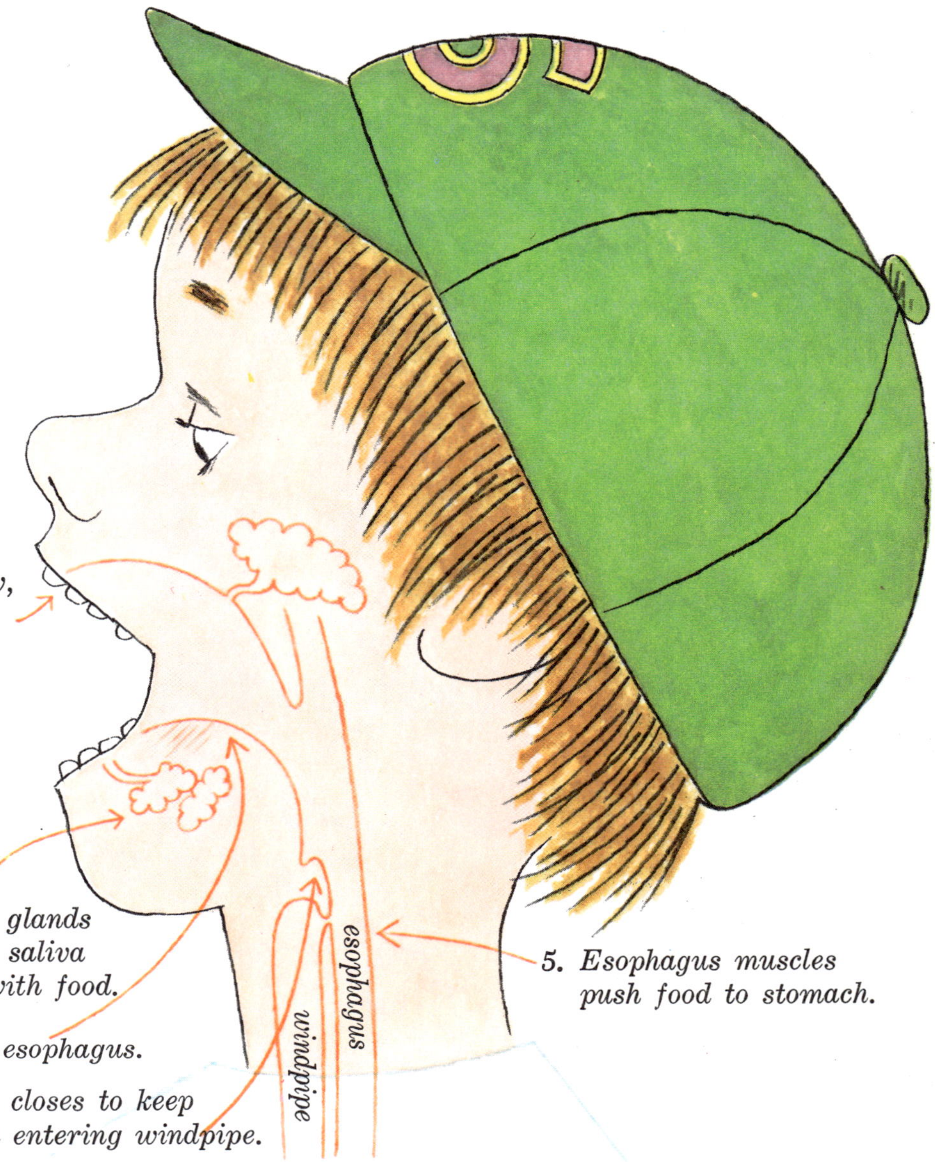

Your MOUTH is used for speaking, singing, and sometimes for breathing. It is also where the digestion of food begins.

Digestion means breaking food up into the tiniest particles, moistening and mixing it with chemical juices your body produces, and finally reducing it to a liquid that can nourish the cells.

You know how small a cell is and how big a sandwich is. The job of the digestive system is to get part of the sandwich into the cell to feed it.

That process starts with your mouth. Your sharp teeth bite off pieces of food. Then your flat-topped teeth chew the food into smaller pieces. Your lower teeth, set in the lower jawbone, move up and down and from side to side, grinding the food against your stationary upper teeth. The more you chew, the smaller the pieces become. Of course, soft foods like applesauce and pudding, and liquid foods like milk and juice don't have to be chewed.

While all the chewing is going on, a liquid called saliva is flowing into your mouth and mixing with the food. It comes from three sets of glands inside your mouth called salivary glands. Not only does the saliva moisten the food and make it easier to swallow, but it also helps you taste it. You can't taste dry food until liquid mixes with it and carries the "taste" chemicals of the food to the bottoms of the taste buds on your tongue.

Your tongue moves the food around to be chewed and ground, mixes it with the saliva, then pushes it to the back of your mouth ready to be swallowed.

Swallowing has some complications. There are two tubes in your throat. One, the esophagus (eh-SOF-uh-gus), leads down to your stomach and the other, the windpipe, leads down to your lungs. Food must not go down into the lungs. To prevent this, there is a little flap called the epiglottis (ep-ih-GLOT-is) that closes off the windpipe when you swallow.

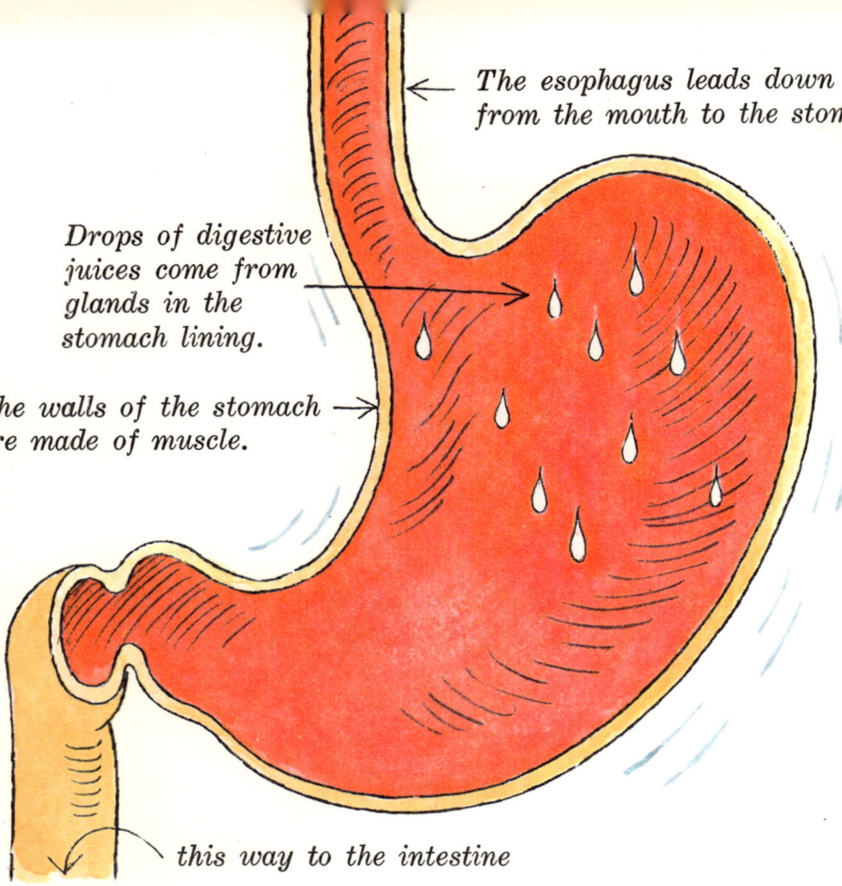

The STOMACH is a pouch with walls of tough muscle. It is about ten inches long and lies on the left side of the abdomen, under the ribs.

The stomach can stretch like a balloon. When you are hungry, with no food in your stomach, it is as skinny as a hot dog. But when it is full, after a big meal, your stomach looks like a blown-up, rounded, J-shaped balloon.

The food that comes into the stomach is already chewed up and wet, but before it leaves it must be turned into a smooth, fine paste. That is the job of the stomach. When all of the food has been swallowed into the stomach, a muscle at the top of the stomach and a muscle at the bottom close off the stomach. These muscles are called sphincter muscles. (A sphincter muscle is like a small thick rubber band, wrapped around an opening. When a sphincter relaxes, things can pass through; when it tightens, nothing gets in or out.) So when the sphincters close off the stomach, the food is locked in. It cannot get back out at the top or escape at the bottom.

Then the stomach goes to work on it. Digestive juices, from glands in the stomach lining, drip on the food to break it down and dissolve it, and the powerful stomach-wall muscles mix and mash and crush and squeeze the food.

After about three hours of this action the sphincter leading to the intestine opens, and the stomach muscles push the pasty food out into the small intestine.

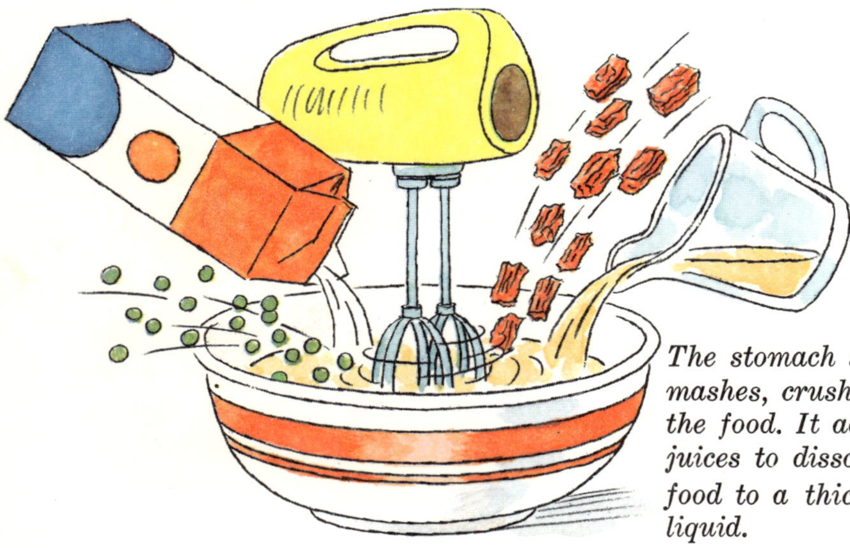

The stomach stirs, mashes, crushes the food. It adds juices to dissolve food to a thick liquid.

Your stomach likes food that has been well chewed.

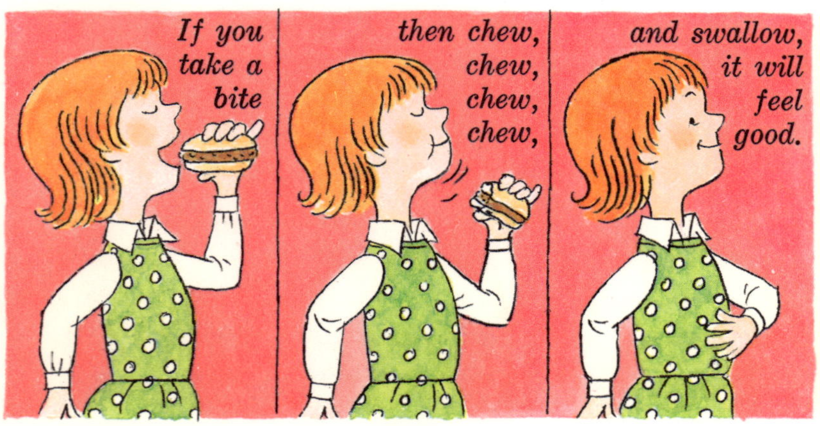
If you take a bite
then chew, chew, chew, chew,
and swallow, it will feel good.

Unchewed food makes the stomach work too hard.

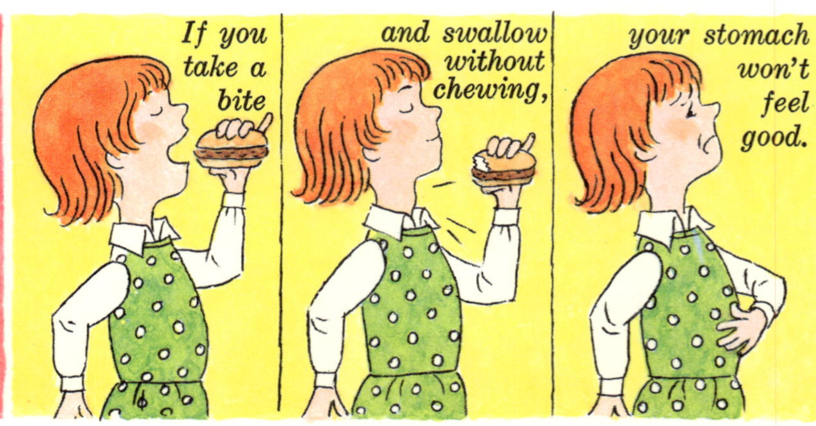
If you take a bite
and swallow without chewing,
your stomach won't feel good.

The INTESTINES are divided into two main sections, the small intestine, narrow and more than twenty feet long, and the large intestine, much wider but only about five or six feet long. The intestines are all coiled up in a small space so they can fit into the abdomen with all the other organs.

The pasty food moves from the stomach into the small intestine. While the food is in the first ten inches of the intestine, bile from the liver and gall bladder, and pancreatic juice from the pancreas come through a tube and are mixed with the food. These juices continue the digestion of the food until it is broken down into even finer particles. Muscles in the intestines keep mixing and pushing the food ahead.

Along its entire length the small intestine is lined with millions of tiny, hairlike projections called villi. Each of the villi has many little blood vessels. As the food moves around and between the villi, almost all the useful tiny food particles are absorbed into the bloodstream. The little blood vessels carrying the food join larger ones and the food is eventually delivered throughout the body by the bloodstream.

The large intestine then receives what is left of the food, a watery mixture. After the large intestine has absorbed the useful liquid from the mixture, unwanted semisolid waste is left. The waste leaves the body through the rectum at the end of the large intestine.

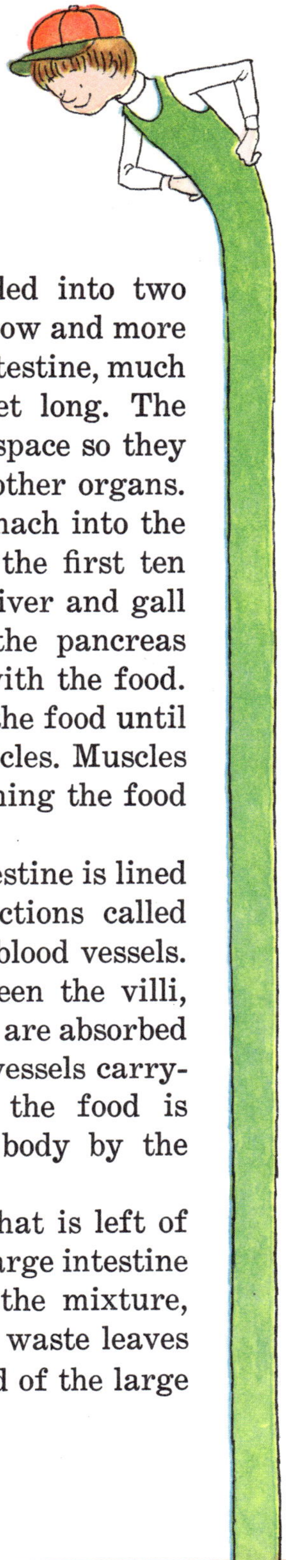

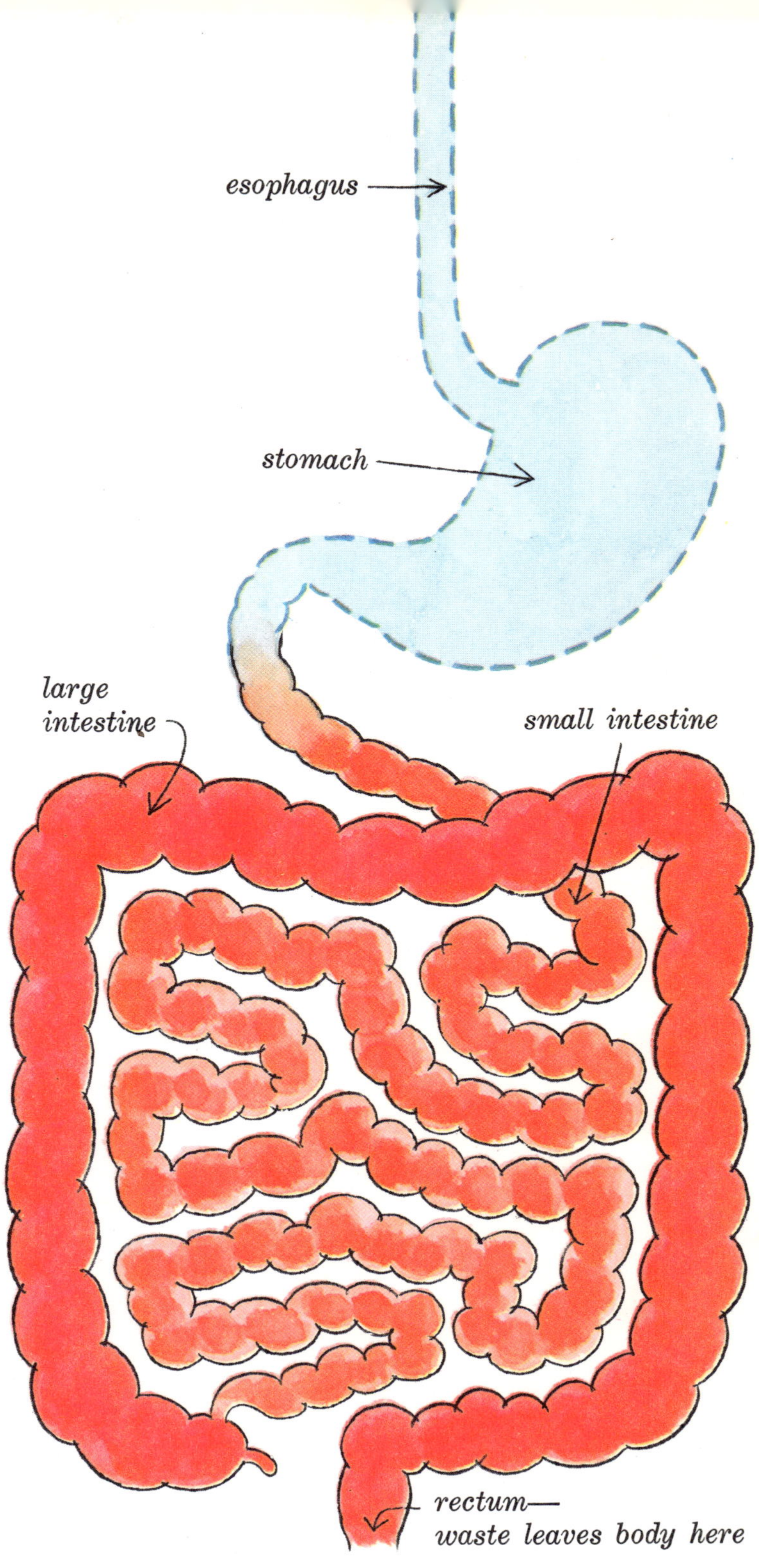

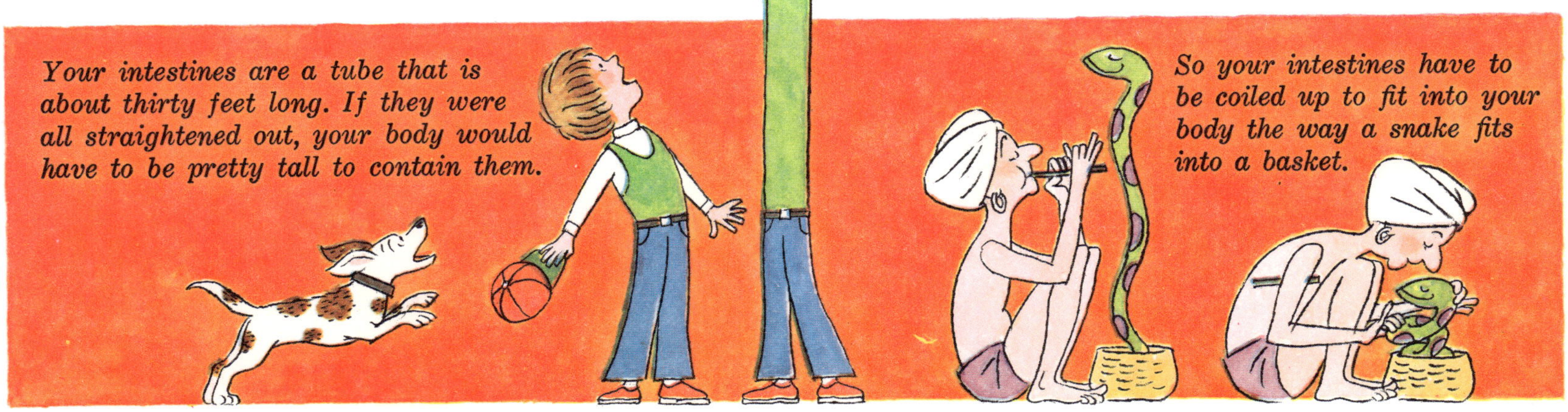

Your intestines are a tube that is about thirty feet long. If they were all straightened out, your body would have to be pretty tall to contain them.

So your intestines have to be coiled up to fit into your body the way a snake fits into a basket.

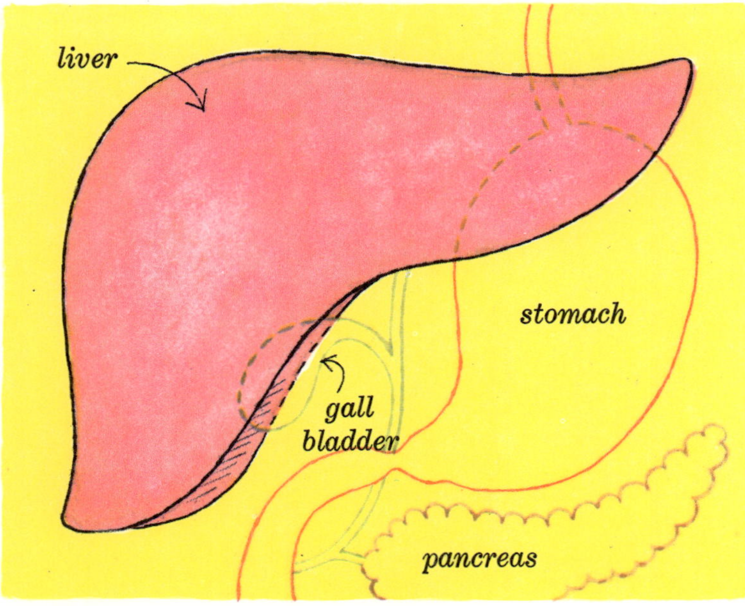

The LIVER, the largest organ inside the body, is four times heavier than the heart. It is a very unusual organ—almost all of its cells are exactly alike and if part of the liver is destroyed more liver cells will grow until the missing part is replaced. The liver has two blood supplies. One is a large vein bringing many kinds of food material directly from the intestine. The other is an artery from the heart bringing oxygen—fuel the liver needs for its work.

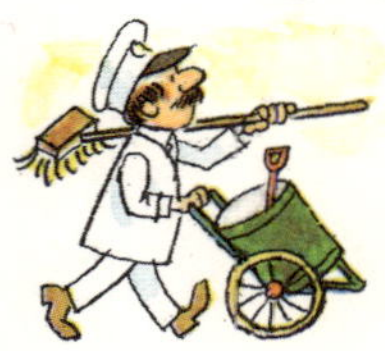

The liver cleans the blood.

The liver is a food processor, store house, and distributor. When the liver receives the food-filled blood it does many things with it. First it removes waste and gets rid of it through the kidneys. Then it destroys anything harmful or poisonous in the food.

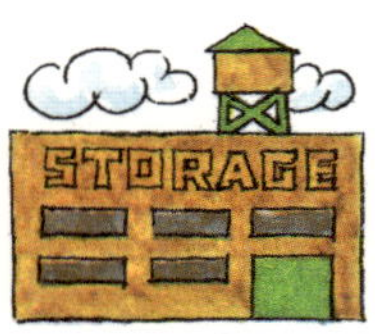

The liver is a warehouse.

The liver then takes sugar out of the blood and stores it for future use. When the body needs the sugar, the liver will take it out of storage.

The liver also stores certain vitamins and minerals; vitamin A for good vision, vitamin D for growing bones and teeth, and the B vitamins and iron needed to make red blood cells. So if you happen to eat more of these vitamins and minerals than your body needs right away, your liver will store them for later use.

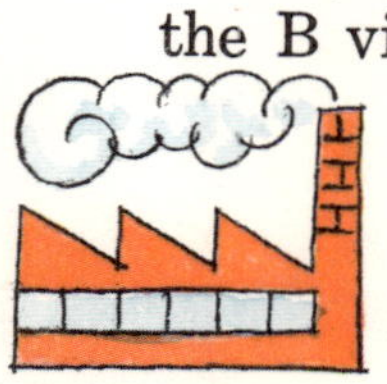

The liver is a factory.

The liver manufactures bile, which digests fats.

The GALL BLADDER is a small pear-shaped storage pouch about four inches long attached to the underside of the liver. It is connected to the middle of a tube called the bile duct which runs from the liver to the first part of the small intestine. When digestion is not going on in the small intestine, bile made by the liver flows through the bile duct and into the gall bladder for storage. When

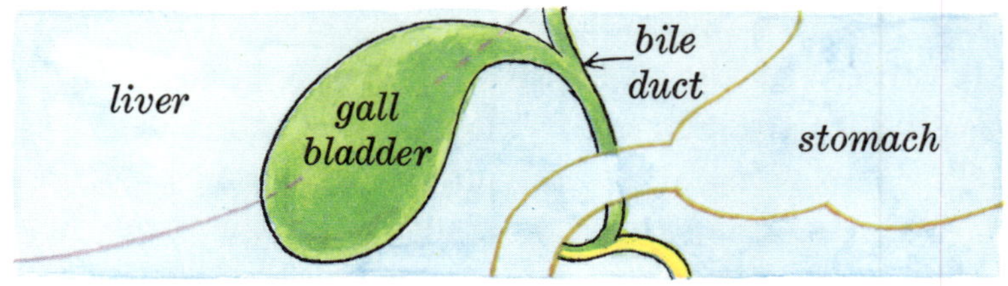

digestion *is* going on in the small intestine, the gall bladder squeezes the bile it has in storage into the intestine. Any bile the liver is making flows right past the gall bladder and on through the bile duct into the small intestine.

The PANCREAS lies below the liver and behind the stomach. It is a gland six or seven inches long, wide at one end and narrow at the other. It has two kinds of cells and does two entirely different jobs. One kind of cell makes pancreatic juices, which flow from the pancreas into the bile duct, joining the bile from the liver on its way to the small intestine. These pancreatic juices are made up of substances called enzymes which are needed in the digestion of most foods.

The other kind of cell is located in small rounded groups, lying like islands among the other cells of the pancreas. This other kind of cell makes a substance called insulin and sends it out into the bloodstream. Insulin is necessary to help the body convert sugars into energy. It also helps keep the proper level of sugar in the bloodstream by helping the liver store extra sugar until it is needed by the body.

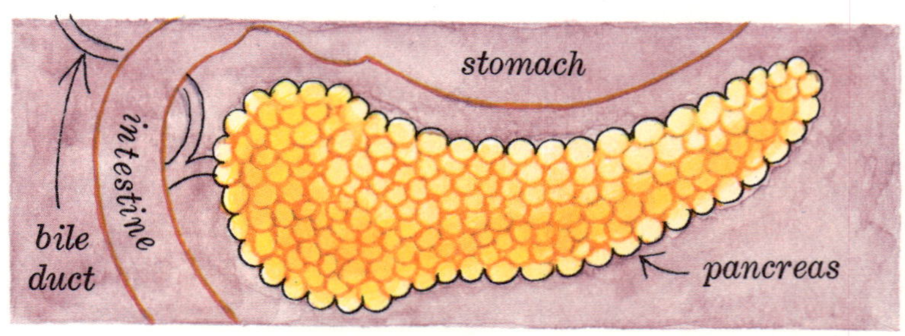

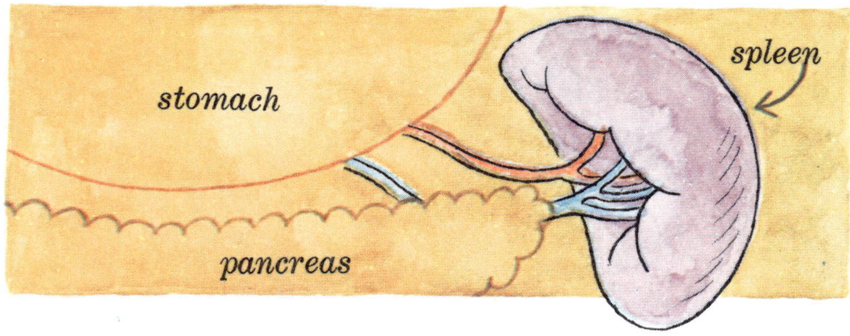

The SPLEEN is a sponge-like organ about as big as a fist. It lies behind the left part of the stomach and is protected by the lower left ribs. The spleen stores a large amount of reserve blood, rich in red blood cells. The spleen contracts about twice a minute and squeezes out a little of this blood at a time. On a hot day or during heavy exercise, when the blood gets low in oxygen, the spleen contracts harder and sends out more blood. It also removes worn-out red cells from the blood, and filters out harmful bacteria and other substances.

The LYMPHATIC SYSTEM is a system of vessels that runs through all parts of the body as the blood vessels do. They carry lymph, a watery fluid that is mostly plasma containing white blood cells. Lymph drains from the blood vessels and the tissues, carrying away the waste materials.

There is no pump, like the heart, to move lymph through the vessels—body motion keeps it going. Harmful material, passing through the lymphatic

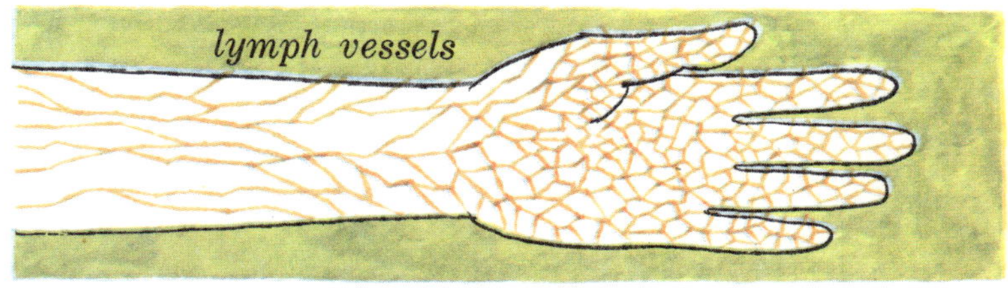

system, is filtered out by little glands called lymph nodes. The cleaned lymph returns to the bloodstream through veins near the neck.

The KIDNEYS are in the back of the abdomen, one on each side of the spine. They are bean-shaped, and about four inches long. All the blood in the body goes through the kidneys to have the wastes filtered out. The filtering system is millions of tiny blood vessels, tangled into little balls, each covered by a thin membrane sac. More than a million of these little balls make up the outer part of the kidneys.

Blood from a large artery is pumped through all those tiny balls of blood vessels. Any impurities filter out through the walls of the blood vessels and into the membrane sacs. The clean blood continues through the blood vessels, returning to the heart. The waste material is combined with water to form urine, which passes through tiny tubes to the hollow center of the kidney. One tube from the center of each kidney carries the urine to the bladder.

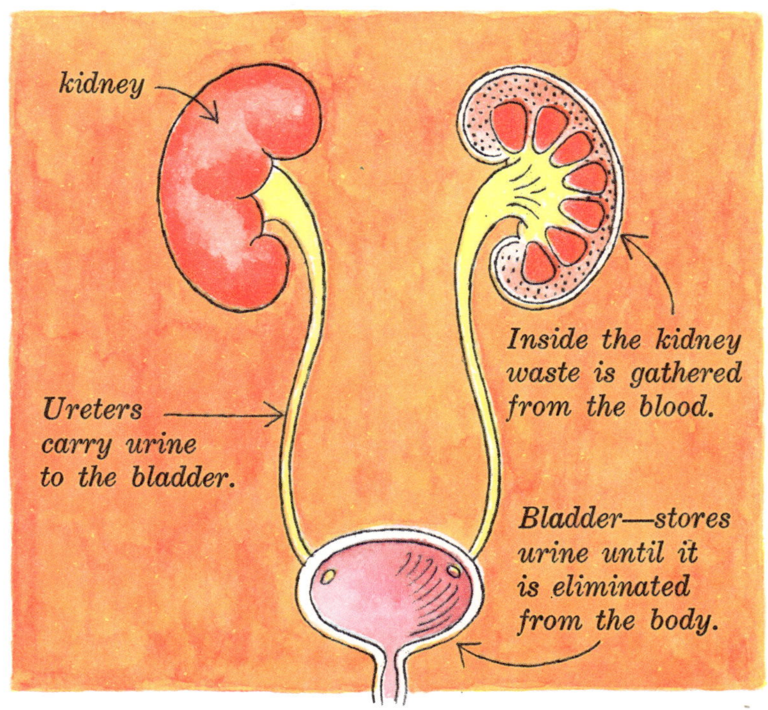

The BLADDER, centered in the lower part of the abdomen, is a hollow muscular sac. It can expand to hold about a pint of urine. A tube leads from the bladder to the outside of the body. A sphincter muscle around the outlet of the bladder keeps the urine from escaping. Usually, when the bladder fills half way, there is an urge to empty it. Then the sphincter muscle relaxes, the bladder contracts, and the urine is pushed out of the body. All this happens to us automatically as babies, but later we learn to control these actions ourselves. Only about fifteen drops of urine come from the kidneys every minute, but it adds up to over a quart a day to be eliminated by the bladder.

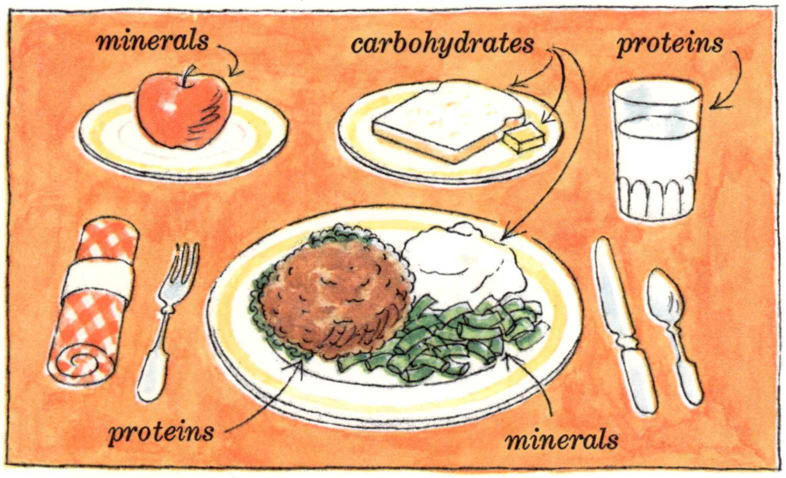

The FOOD you eat must be of a wide variety to keep you well nourished and healthy. You need foods that help you grow, foods that keep you healthy, and foods that give you energy. You should eat a variety of foods because each kind of food can only give you some of the things you need—no one food contains all the proteins, vitamins, minerals, carbohydrates, and fats your body must have. A good meal not only looks and tastes good, it is also balanced—it includes some of the body-building foods, some of the energy foods, and some of those that help protect your health.

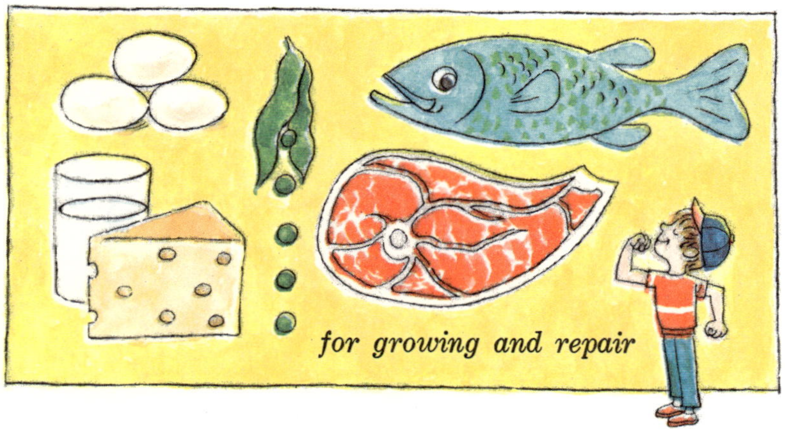

PROTEIN is the main body builder—you must have a lot of it while you are growing. Every cell in your body needs protein to build *more* cells. The faster you grow the more protein you need. Even when you stop growing you still need protein for building new cells to replace those that become worn-out and discarded. Foods from animals—meat, fish, poultry, eggs, milk, and cheese—are the best sources of protein. Beans, peas, and nuts of all kinds also have a lot of protein.

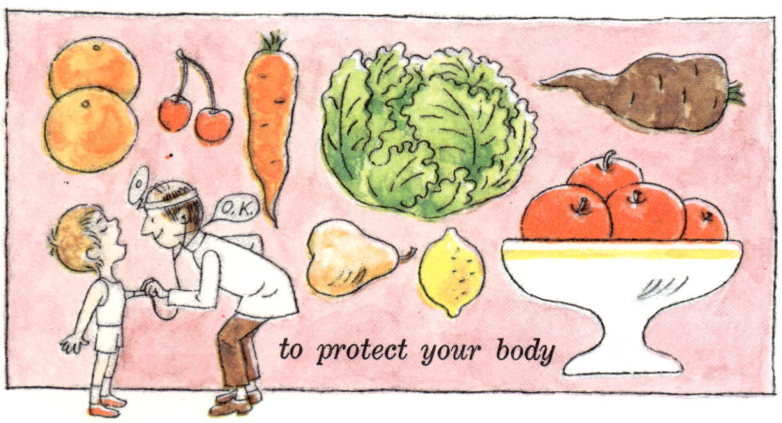

VITAMINS and MINERALS help you keep healthy and resist infections, colds, and other sicknesses. You need them for building strong bones and teeth and for having a good appetite and digestion. You need them for building a normal blood supply and for helping cuts and bruises heal quickly when you hurt yourself. Some foods that have the best supply of vitamins and minerals are all kinds of leafy salad greens, vegetables, fruits, fruit juices, and dried fruit; and liver and kidneys.

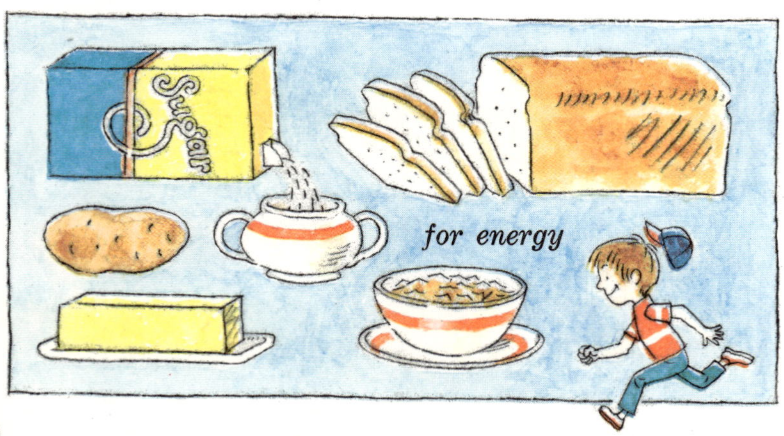

CARBOHYDRATES and FATS supply your body with the energy you need for work and play. Protein also gives you energy, but if you eat enough carbohydrates and fats the protein will be saved for more useful, body-building work. Some good sources of carbohydrates are bread, cereal, potatoes, spaghetti, noodles, rice, and sugar and other sweets (most sweets, however, are not good for the teeth). Some sources of fats are margarine, butter, cooking oils, and some salad dressings.

Part of the food we eat is used to give our cells what they need to divide and create new cells. So, what we eat becomes us.

The grass and stuff the cow eats becomes the cow . . .

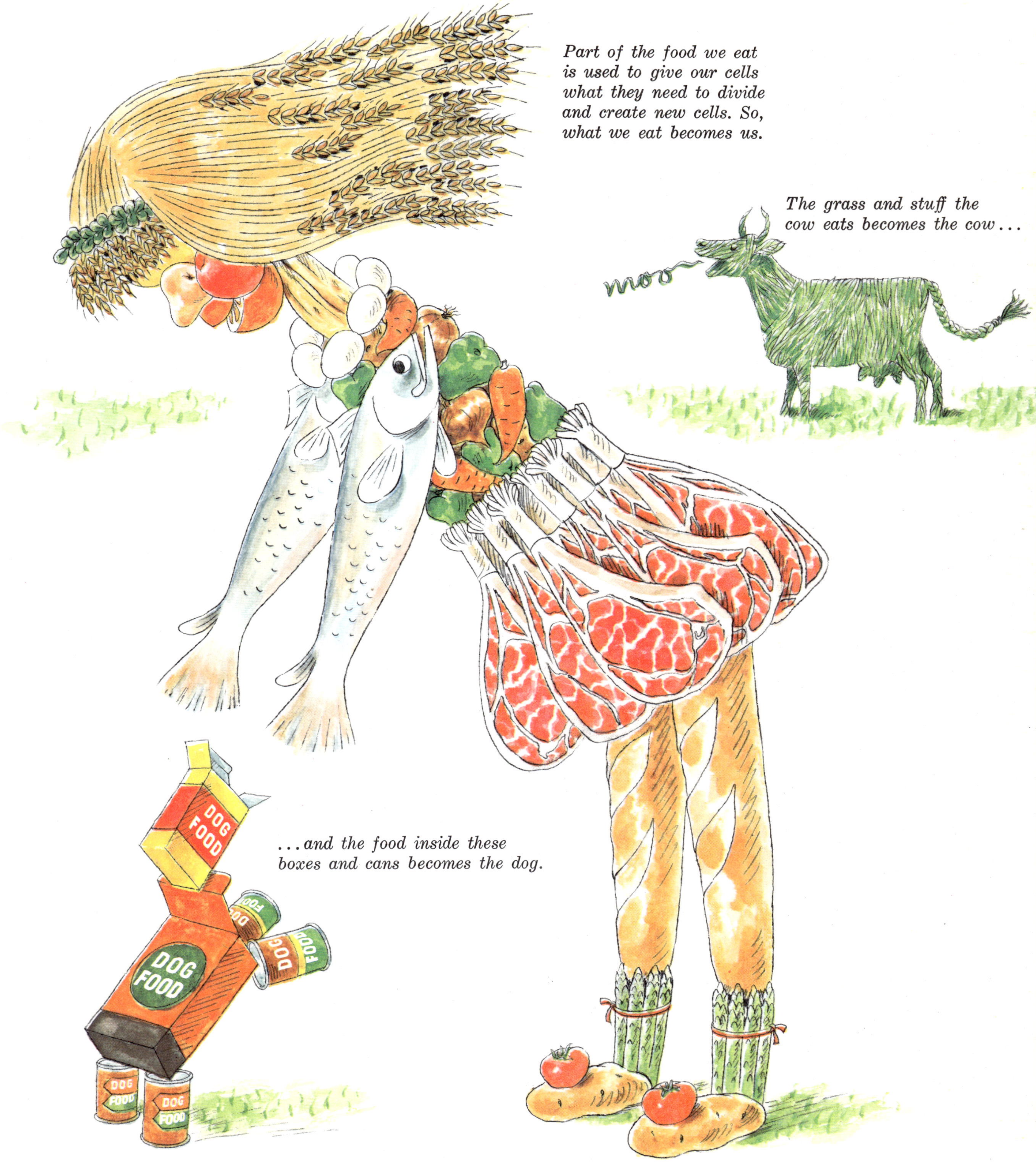

. . . and the food inside these boxes and cans becomes the dog.

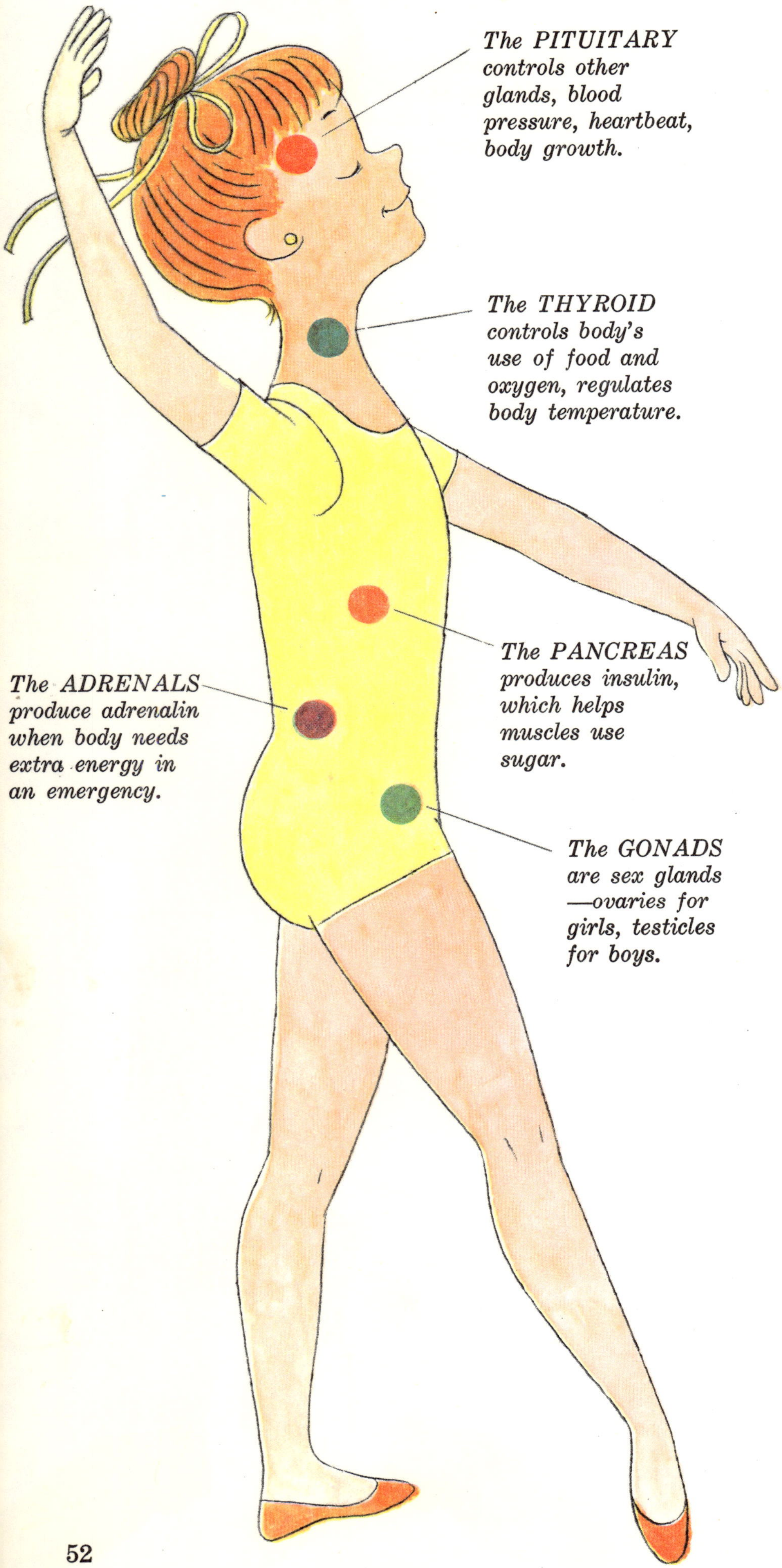

The DUCTLESS GLANDS make chemical substances called hormones, which regulate the work of organs in other parts of the body. The glands release their hormones into the bloodstream, to travel to their destinations.

The pituitary is the master ductless gland. It is as big as a grape and hangs down from the brain over the nasal cavity. One of its hormones controls the making of hormones in the other ductless glands. Other pituitary hormones control the blood pressure and heartbeat, regulate the speed of body growth, and influence organs—one controls how much urine the kidneys make. The pituitary itself is controlled by a part of the brain just above it, called the hypothalamus.

The thyroid gland is in the front of the neck. Its hormones control how quickly the body uses up food and oxygen, and they regulate body temperature.

The pancreas produces the hormone insulin which helps the muscles convert sugar into energy.

The two adrenal glands, one on top of each kidney, produce adrenalin. When you are frightened enough to run away from something or angry enough to fight, adrenalin is there to help you. It makes your heart beat faster, sending more blood with food and oxygen to the muscles that will need it. It makes you breathe more air. You suddenly have more energy.

Boys' sex glands are called testicles, and girls' sex glands are called ovaries. When boys and girls reach their teens their sex glands begin to produce hormones. A boy's hormones make his shoulders get broader than his hips, his beard and new body hair grow, and his voice get deeper. A girl's hormones make her hips get broader than her shoulders, her breasts grow bigger, and her voice get a little fuller. She begins to grow new body hair, too, but she doesn't get a beard.

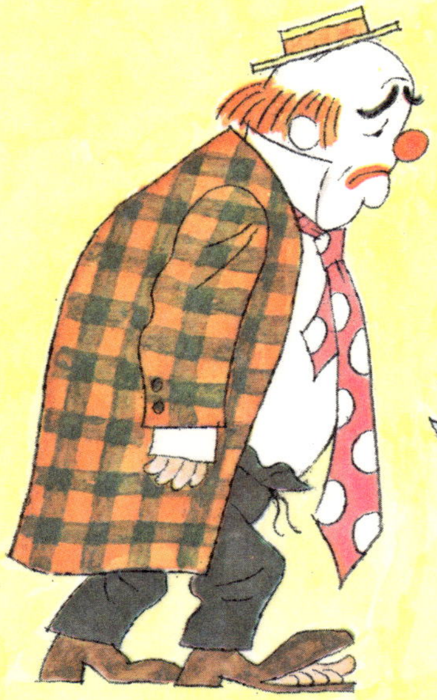

underactive thyroid

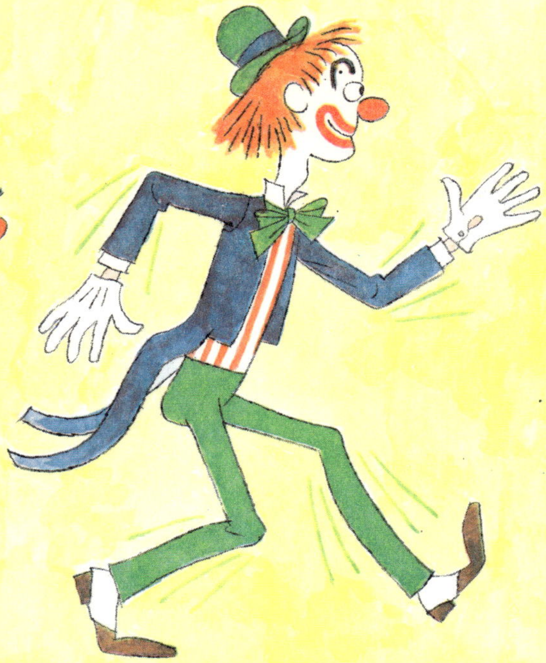

overactive thyroid

Adrenal glands are useful in dangerous situations.

adrenalin to the rescue

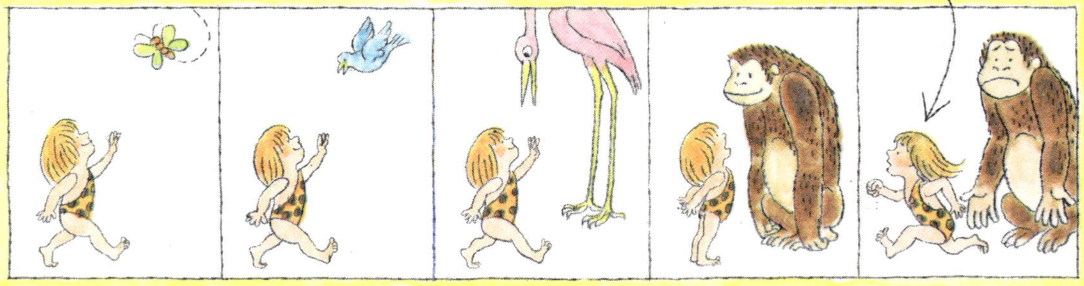

If young boys and girls wear their hair alike and dress alike, it's hard to tell them apart.

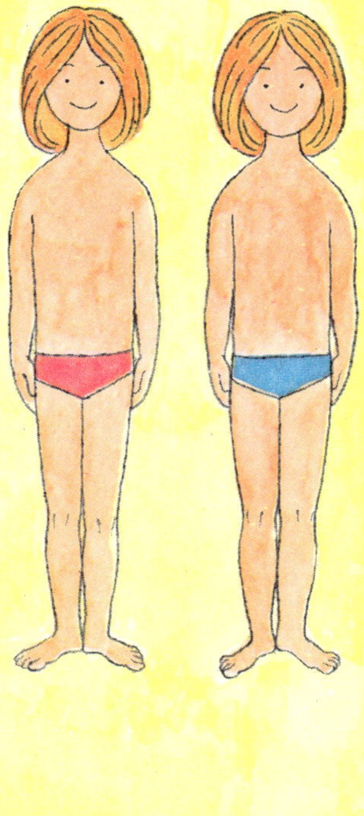

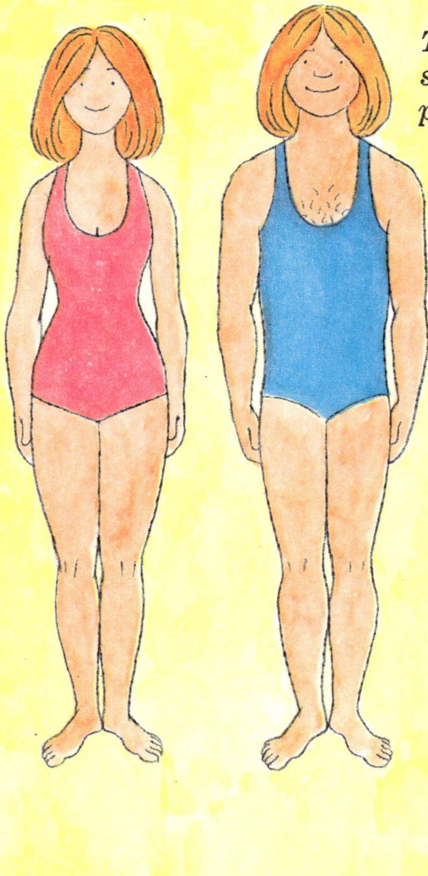

The pituitary and sex glands change people's bodies as they grow older. Now it's easy to tell them apart.

An overactive pituitary gland produces a giant.

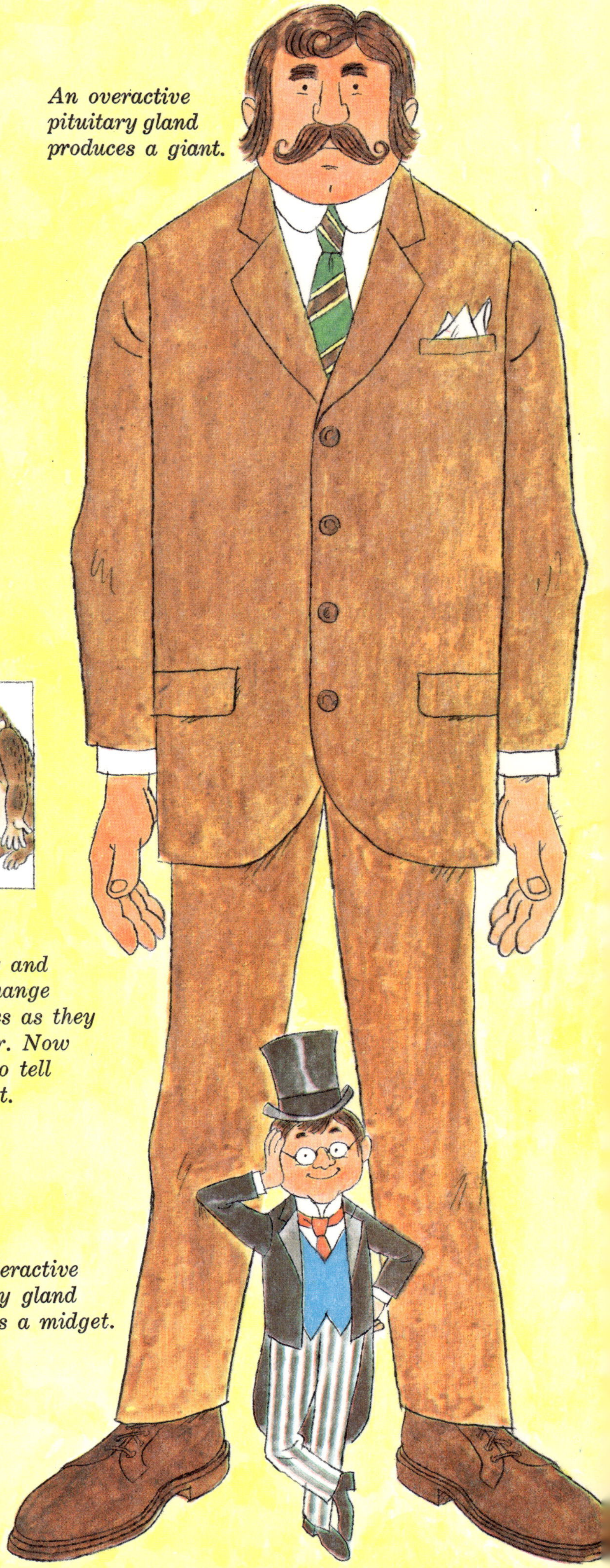

An underactive pituitary gland produces a midget.

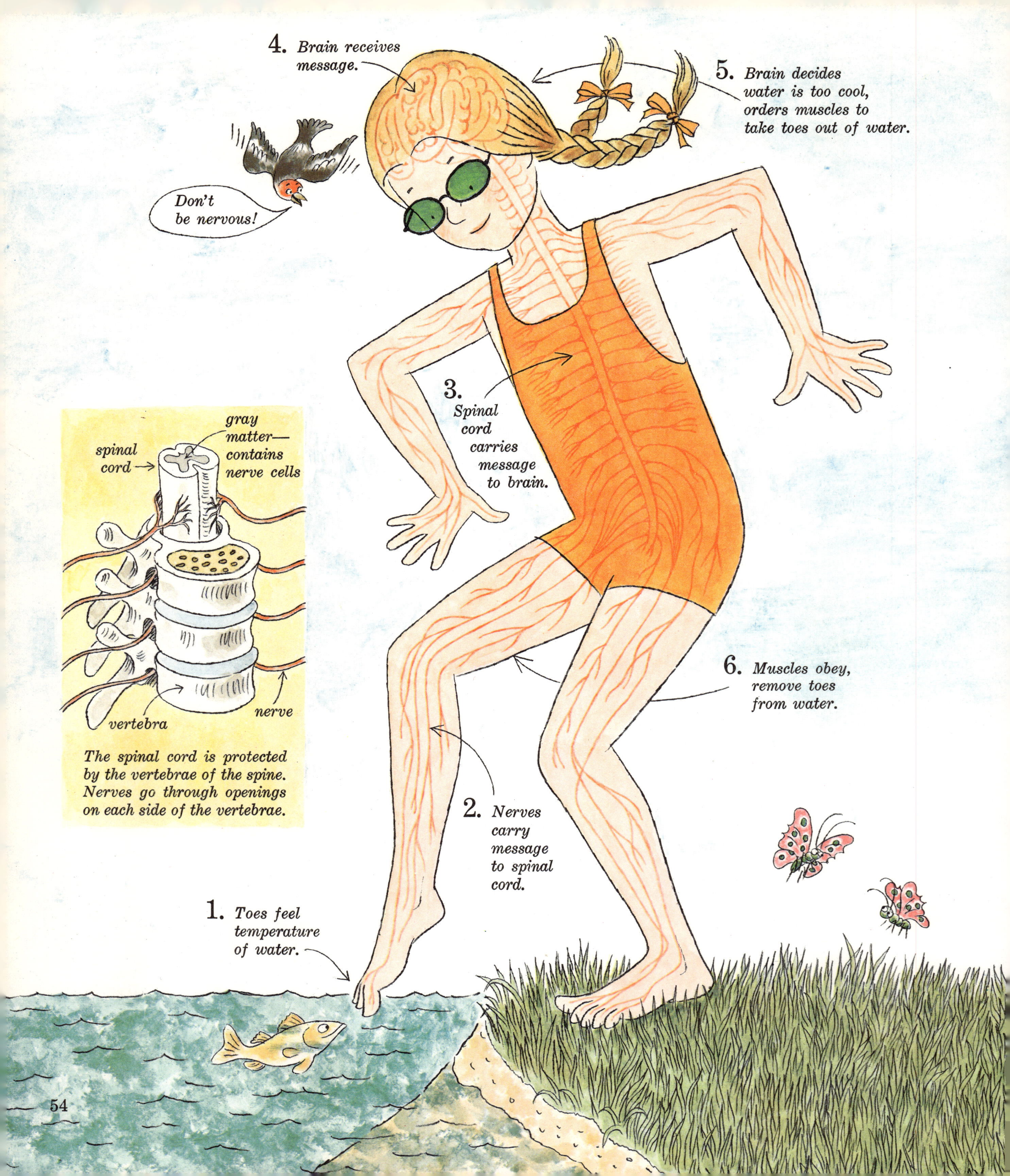

The spinal cord is protected by the vertebrae of the spine. Nerves go through openings on each side of the vertebrae.

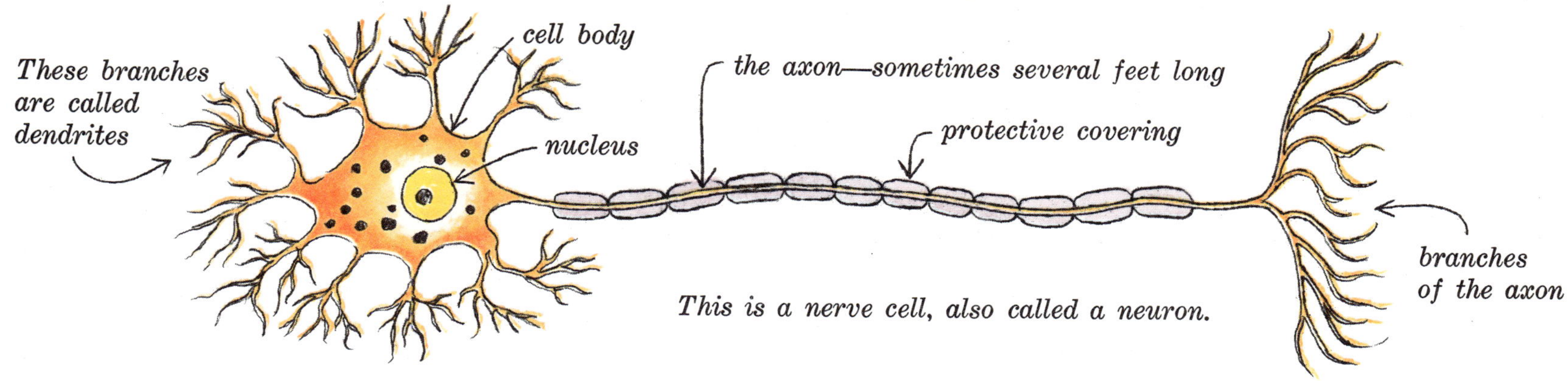

This is a nerve cell, also called a neuron.

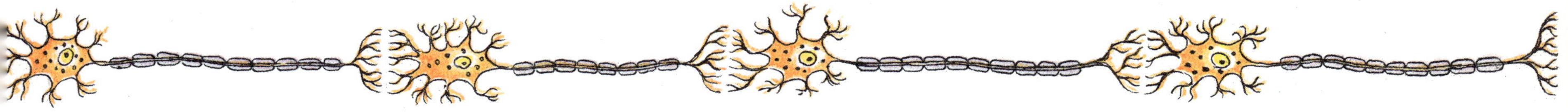

How a message is passed along from one nerve cell to another until it reaches the brain

The NERVOUS SYSTEM has three main parts—the brain, the spinal cord, and the nerves. The brain is the center of this amazing communication system. It receives information through the nerves and either stores it away or sends out orders to the body to do something about it.

The spinal cord is a half-inch-thick cable that runs down from the brain through the channel of holes in the vertebrae of the spine. Nerves lead from the spinal cord to most parts of the body. Other nerves go directly from the brain to the eyes, ears, and other parts of the head.

There are two kinds of nerves—those that carry messages to the spinal cord and brain and those that carry orders away from the spinal cord and brain. A message from the skin of your toe to your brain might be, "This water feels chilly." The message travels from your toe through a nerve to the spinal cord, then up through the cord to the brain. The brain sends an order, "Pull the toe out of the water," down through the spinal cord, along a nerve to the proper leg muscle, which pulls out the toe.

Each nerve cell has branching nerve ends leading into it, and a thin extension called the axon leading out. The axon branches out at its far end. A message is received by the cell from its branching nerve ends, and is sent out through the axon. The message jumps from the branches of the axon across a tiny gap to the branching nerve ends of the next nerve cell. The message is relayed from one nerve cell to the next until it reaches its destination.

Sometimes quick action is needed. If you touch a hot pot, that message only goes to the spinal cord, which immediately sends an order to an arm muscle to pull away quickly from the pot. This is called a reflex action. If the message had to go all the way to the brain, and the order to let go had to make the long trip back, you might burn your hand. Other reflex actions are blinking, and kicking your leg when the doctor taps you below the knee.

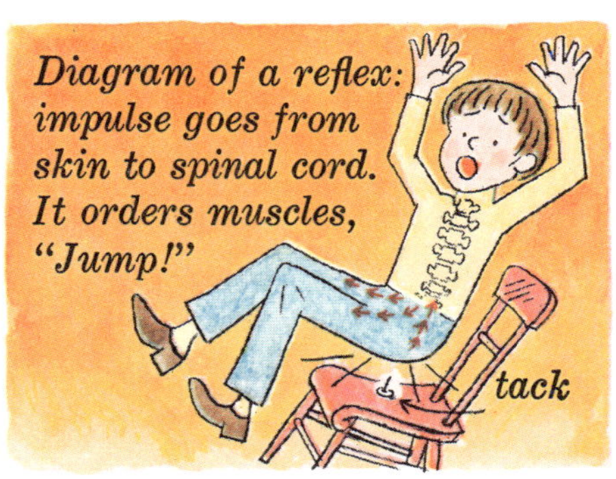

These are some other examples of reflex actions—actions without thought.

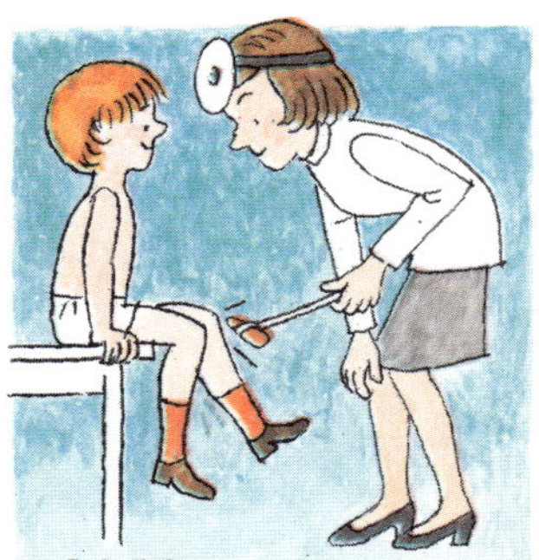

kicking your foot

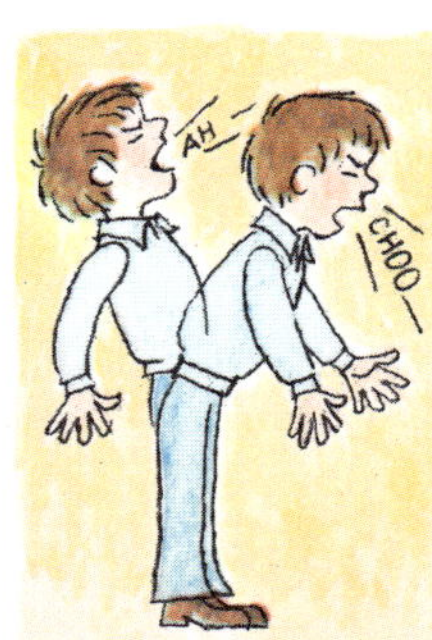

sneezing

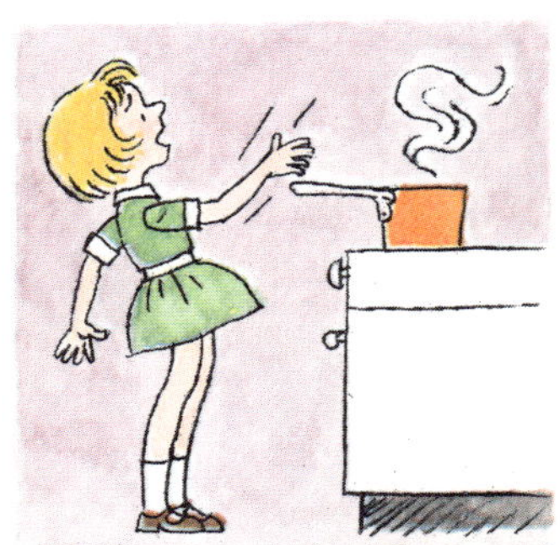

letting go of a hot pot

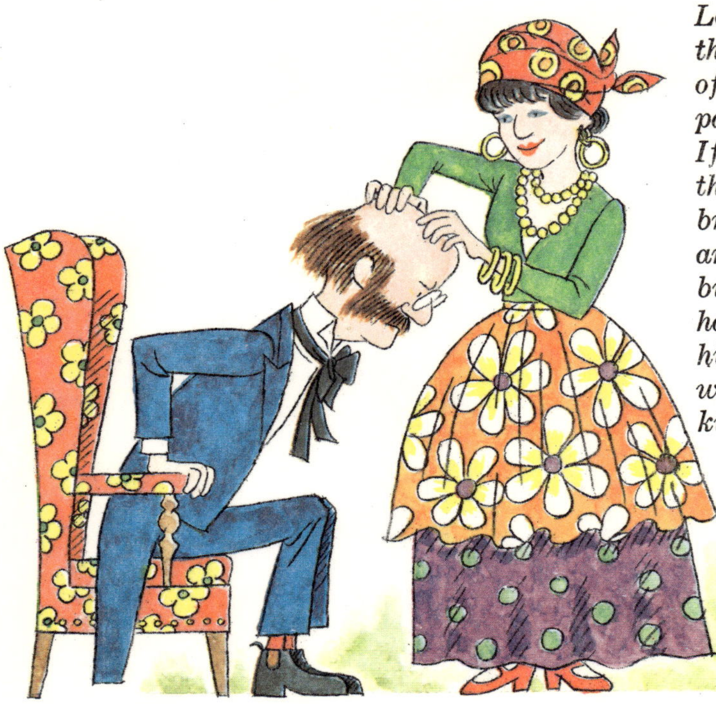

Long ago, people thought they knew just which part of the brain controlled each part of someone's character. If a man was funny, people thought the fun-part of his brain would be bigger and make his skull bump out. All you had to do was feel his bumps and you would know just what kind of person he was.

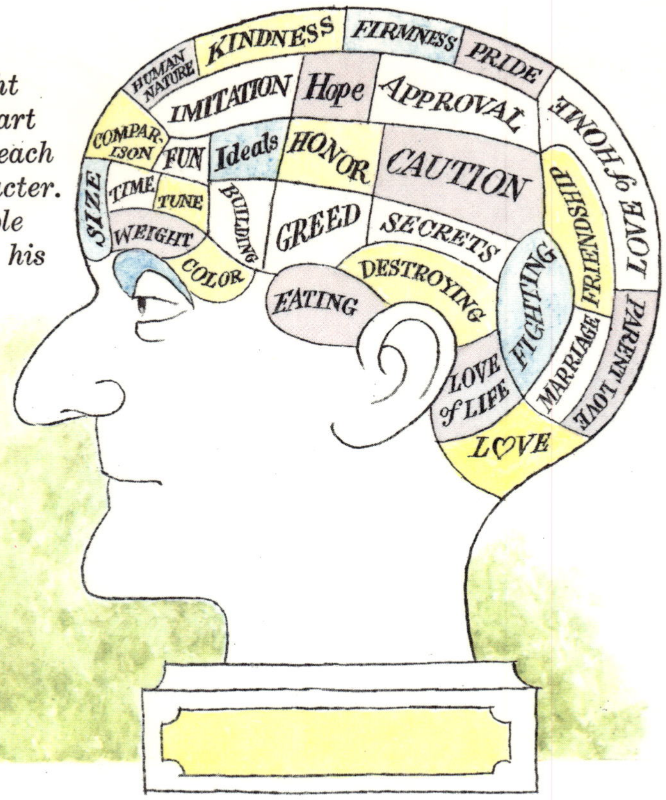

The BRAIN fits into and is protected by the skull. Yet, small as it is, it is more complicated and can do more than the biggest computer ever built. The brain is made up of billions of nerve cells and is divided into three main parts. Each part has its own work but they also work together.

The cerebrum (se-REE-brum) is the largest and most important part of the brain. All of your ideas, and all your feelings, such as anger, happiness, and sadness, come from the cerebrum. What you remember is stored there. The information your senses gather goes there and the cerebrum tells the body what to do about it. The cerebrum is divided into two halves. Strangely enough, the right half controls the left side of the body and the left half controls the right side.

The cerebellum (ser-uh-BEL-um) sits under the back part of the cerebrum. It controls the body actions that go on without your being aware of them. Walking is a good example. Learning how to do it was difficult and you fell often. Now, without even thinking, you can balance and make all those complicated muscle movements. Your cerebellum has your balance and coordination under control.

The brain stem, which connects the cerebrum to the spinal cord, is made up of several small but important parts. The thalamus (THAL-a-mus) receives such messages as pain, heat, and cold and passes them on. The hypothalamus (HY-po-THAL-a-mus) controls such things as body temperature, hunger, and thirst. The midbrain controls movements of the eyes and certain other parts of the body. The pons relays messages between the main parts of the brain. The medulla (meh-DULL-uh) controls such automatic body functions as breathing and heartbeat.

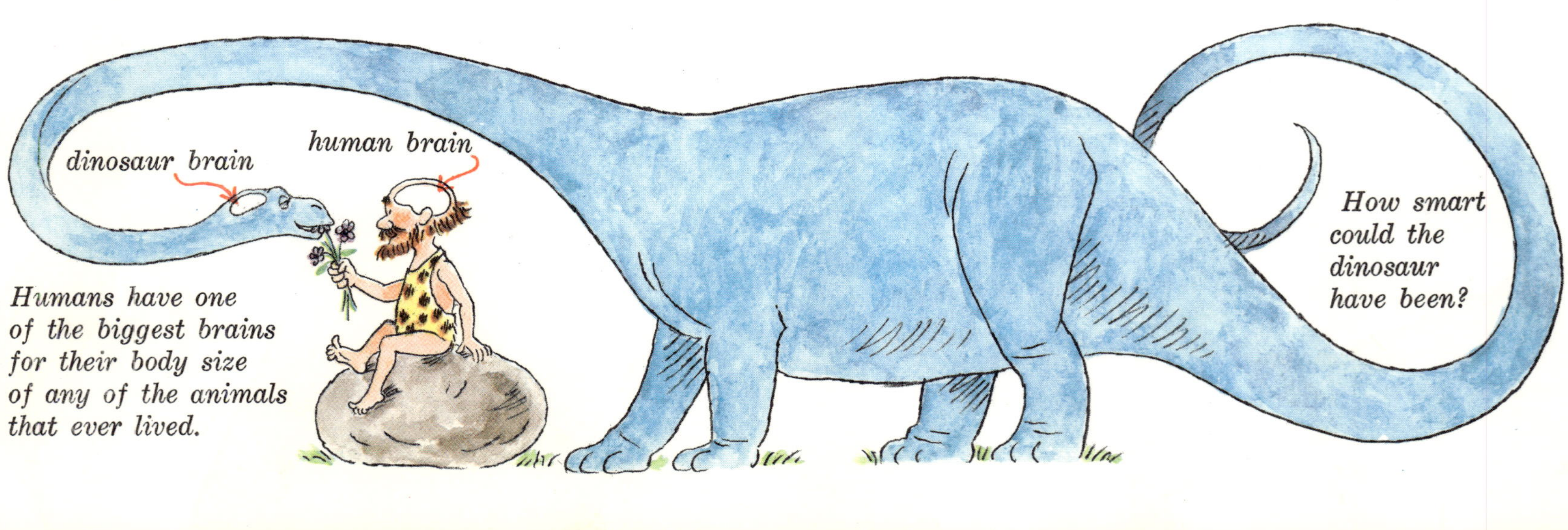

Humans have one of the biggest brains for their body size of any of the animals that ever lived.

How smart could the dinosaur have been?

While we no longer believe that you can tell someone's character by bumps on the head, we now know that certain areas of the brain really do control different parts of our thoughts and actions. This is a rough idea of the sections of the brain and their different jobs.

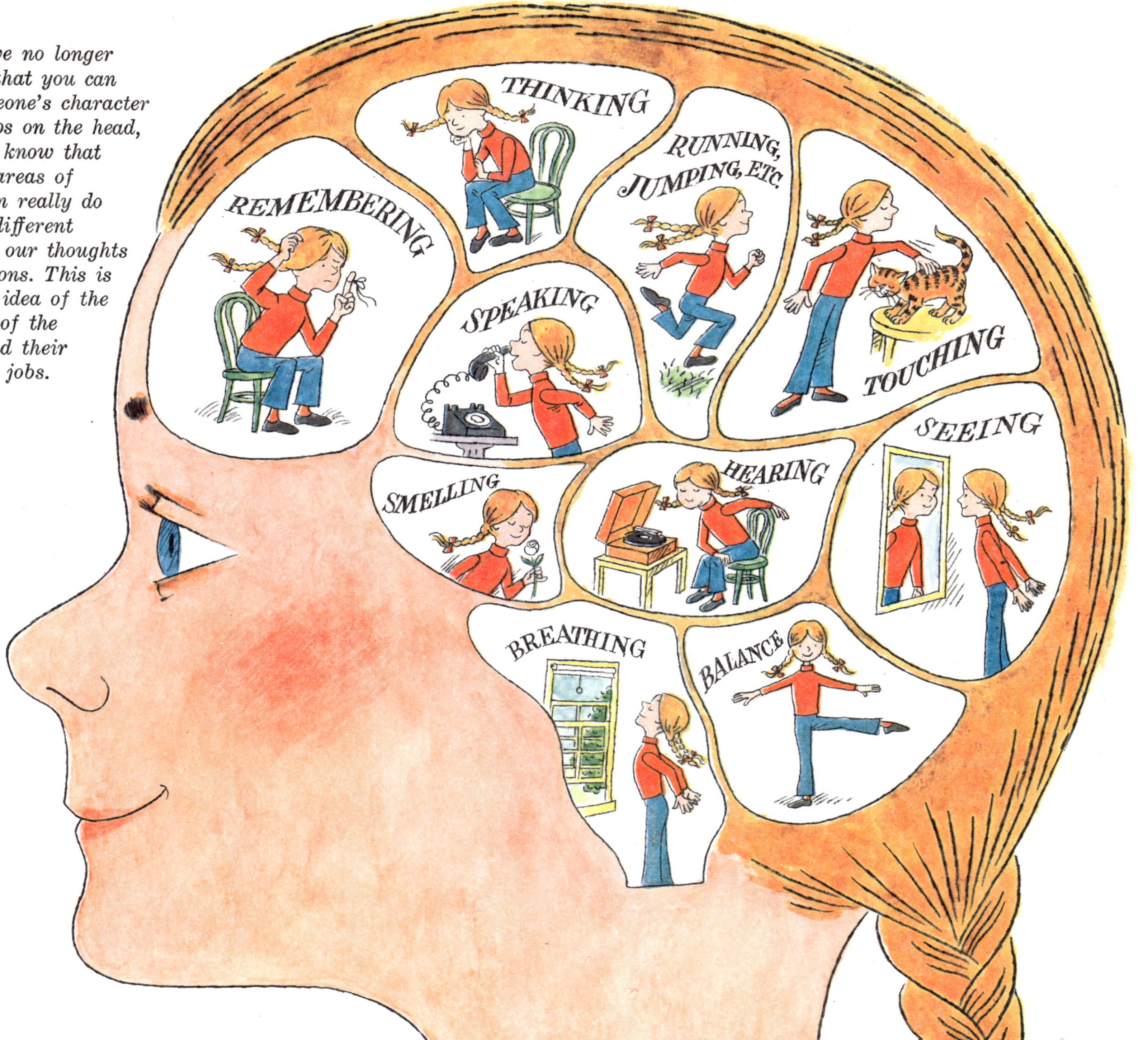

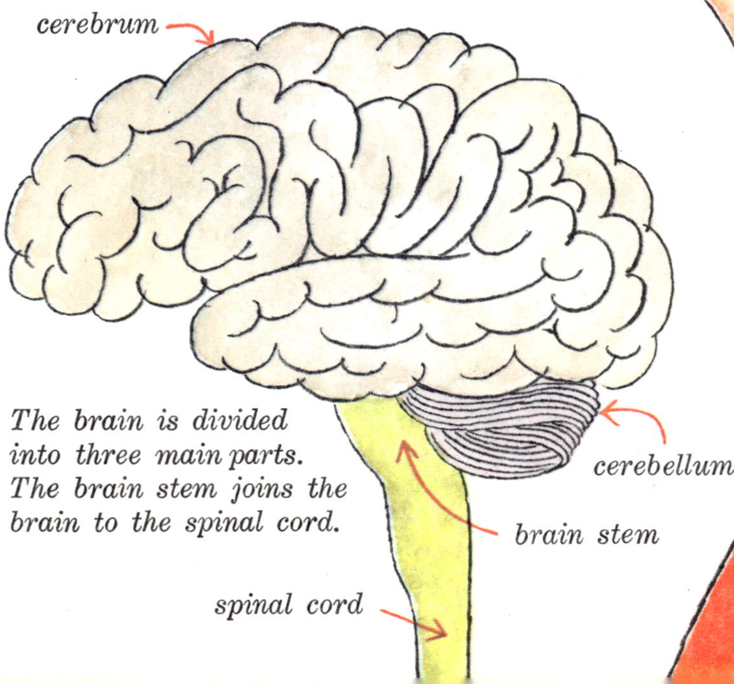

The brain is divided into three main parts. The brain stem joins the brain to the spinal cord.

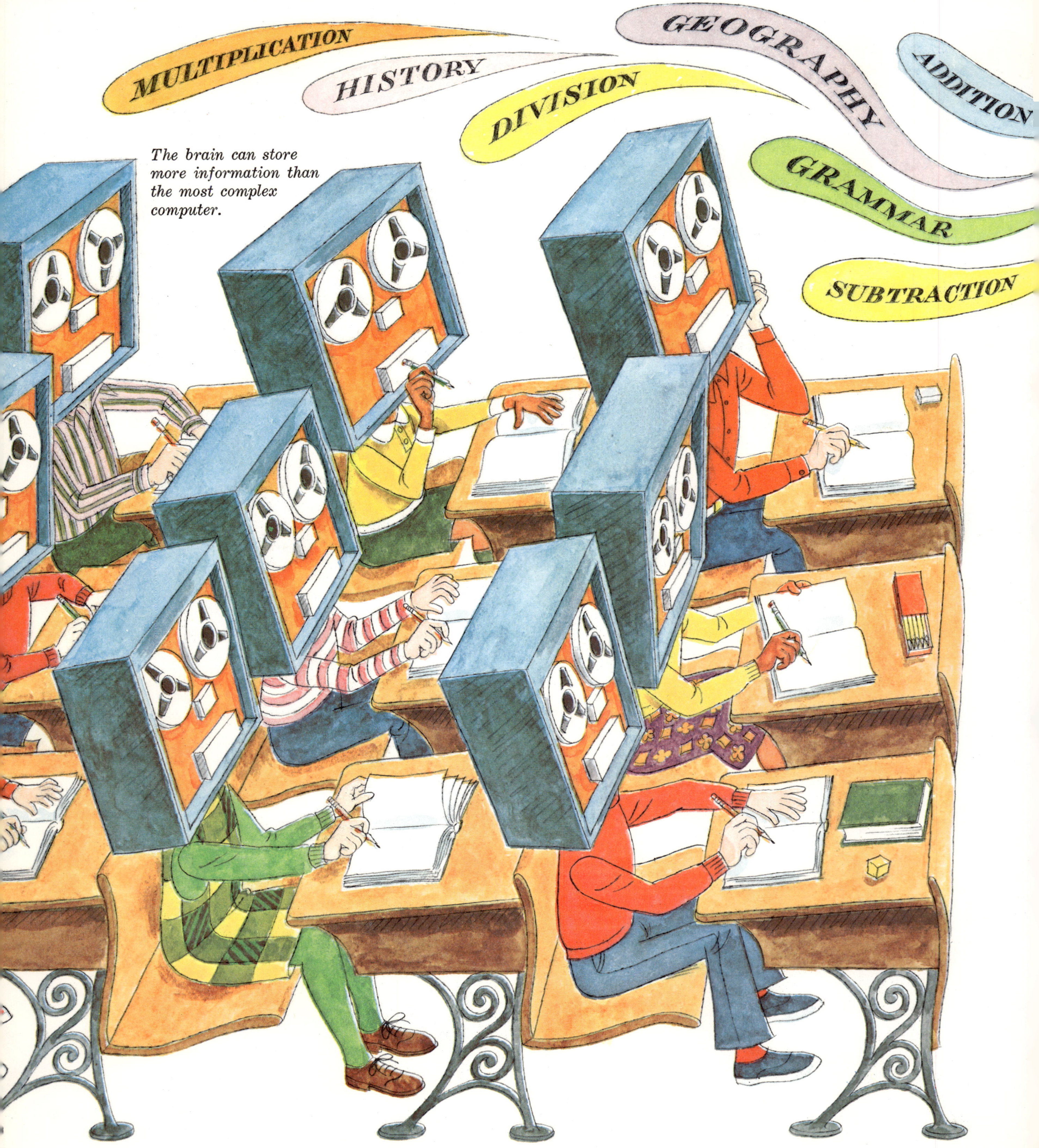

The brain can store more information than the most complex computer.

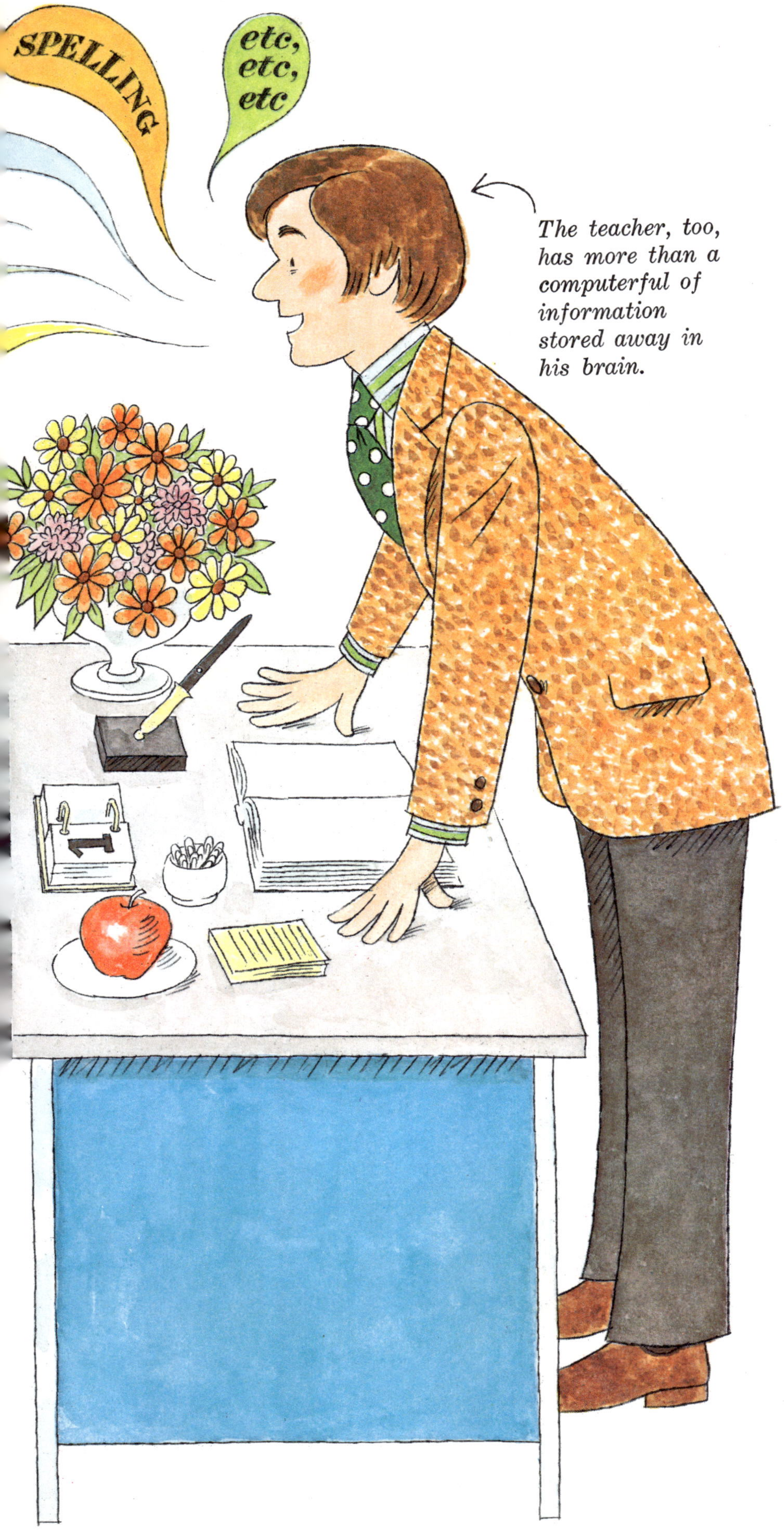

The teacher, too, has more than a computerful of information stored away in his brain.

LEARNING is the process of getting new information through the senses (sight, hearing, touch, sound, and taste) and storing that information in the brain. The information may be about how to do something (playing the flute), or how to behave (saying "thank you"), or it may be factual information (your new friend's name and address).

Everything we know is stored in the brain. But we don't know exactly what happens in the brain when someone learns. A newborn baby can't speak or understand words. It doesn't "know" anything. Yet somehow the baby learns so quickly that by the end of its first year it is beginning to walk, talk, recognize people, and play simple games.

As they grow, children learn how to read and write, how to play baseball, how to bake a cake. Their brains have soon gathered great amounts of information ready to be used at a moment's notice. This learning process goes on throughout life. Even grown-ups are still learning new things every day.

Scientists have many theories about how the millions of brain cells store all this information, and about how they take it out of storage when we want to use it or "remember" it. Some compare the brain to a tape recorder, recording and playing back all our sense experiences. The brain has also been thought of as an incredibly complex computer, because so many millions of facts and impressions are stored in it.

Research into how we learn shows: we learn best when what we are learning is interesting and important to us; frequent rests are helpful while learning, perhaps a five- or ten-minute break each hour; and people often learn well together because they benefit from each other's mistakes.

And research shows how well children learn by imitation. They learn their language by imitating the sounds made by older children and adults. By the age of three or four, children have learned a lot of language by imitation, although they still cannot read a word and certainly have no notion of grammar.

EXPERIMENTS with animals to find out what they are able to learn and how they learn help scientists understand how people learn. These are some of the experiments:

A DOG salivates (that is, his mouth waters) when he is fed or when he sees food that he likes. The same thing happens to people when they see or even think of food that they like.

The Russian scientist Ivan Pavlov tried the following experiment. He began to feed a dog in his laboratory. The dog would respond in the usual way at each mealtime—his mouth would water as the food was brought to him. Pavlov then began to ring a bell each time he brought the dog's food into the laboratory. Eventually the dog would salivate at the sound of the bell, even if no food came with it. Pavlov had taught the dog to salivate at the sound of a bell.

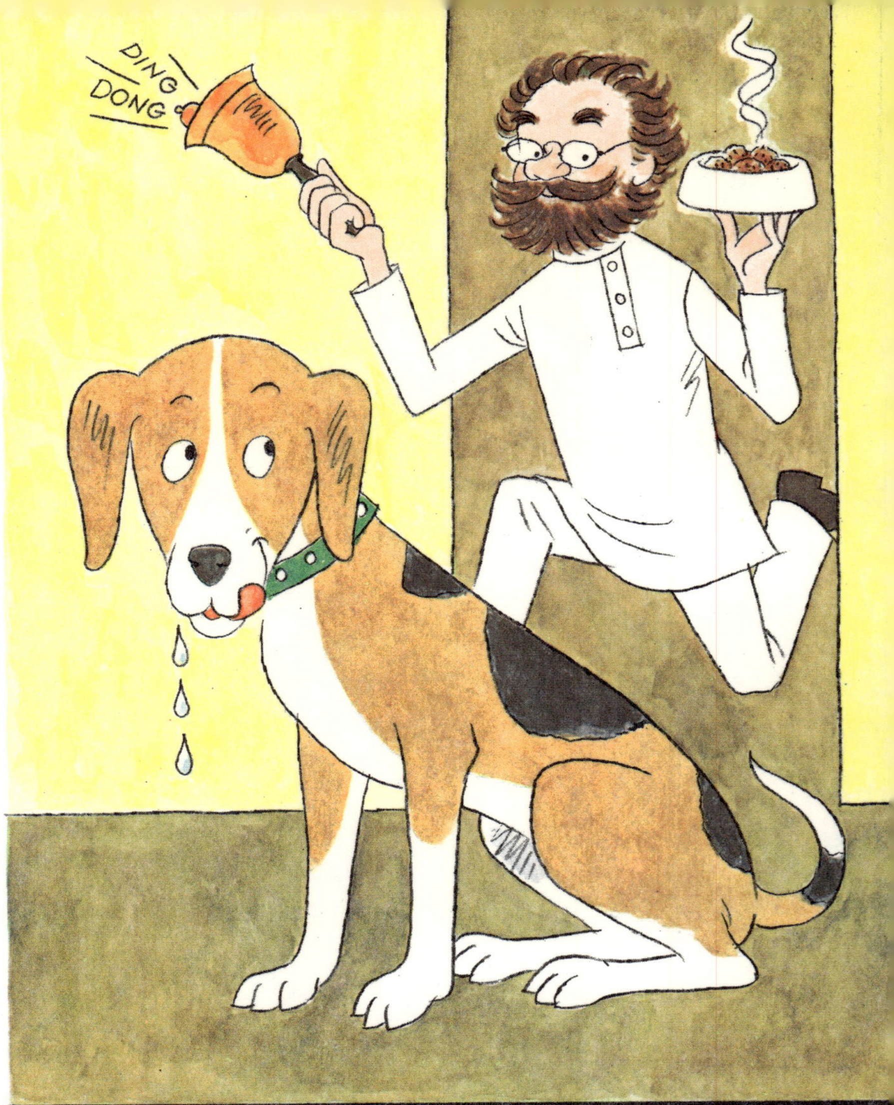

A WHITE RAT isn't the kind of animal you might expect to be able to learn circus tricks. Yet the psychologist Loh Seng Tsai has taught his laboratory rats to do some very difficult tricks. This is one of them.

Loh Seng Tsai fastened a shelf on a wall too high for a white rat to reach by jumping. On the opposite wall he fastened another shelf and put some cheese on it. Between the shelves he hung a basket from the ceiling, like a swing. The basket could be pulled to the first shelf by a string fastened to it.

Soon a white rat learned to climb a ladder to the first shelf, pull the basket to itself, get into the basket, and swing over to the other shelf to get to its reward—the cheese!

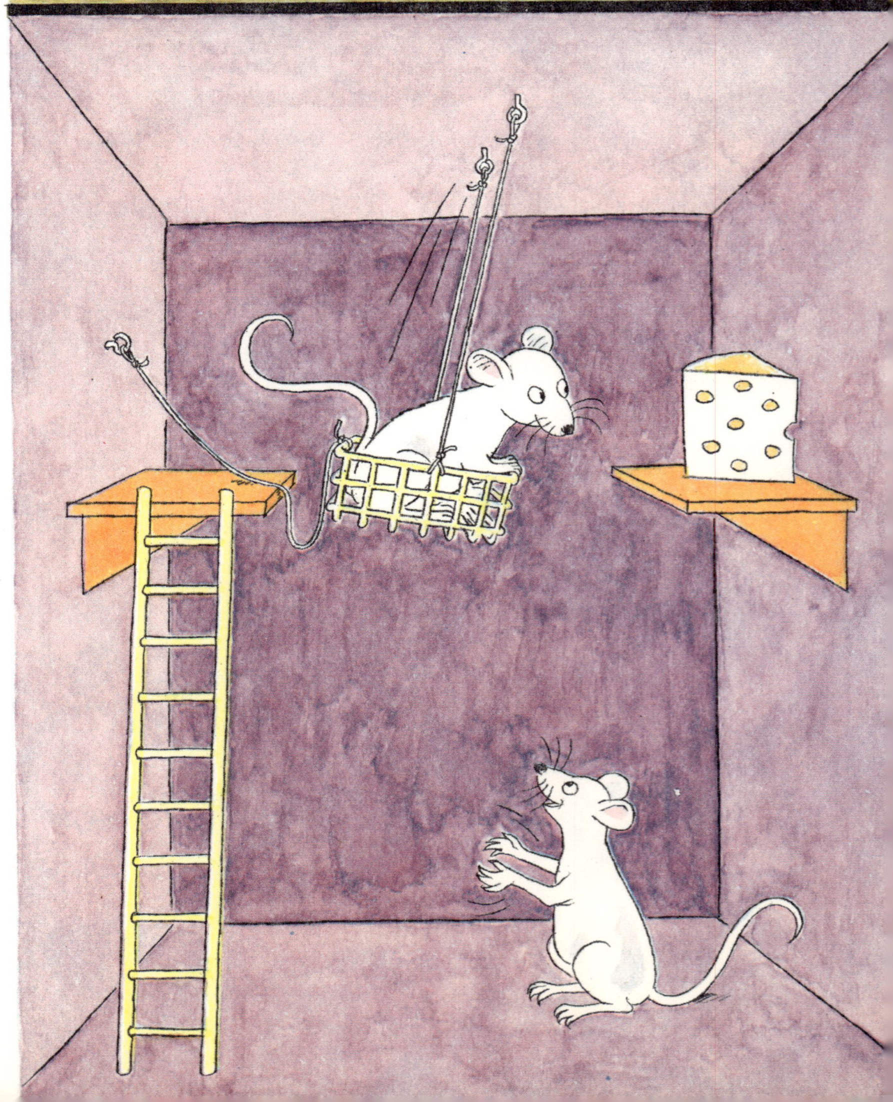

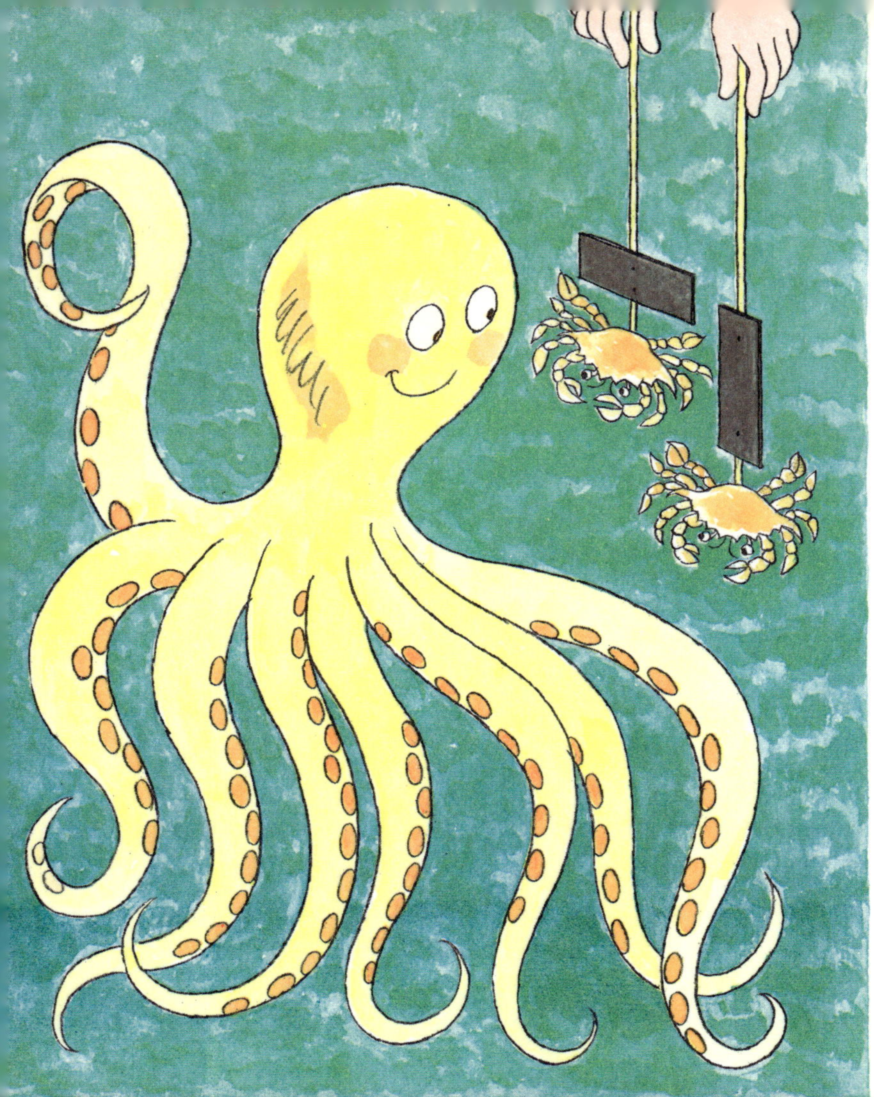

An OCTOPUS can learn to tell the difference between a horizontal shape and a vertical shape. This is how it is taught:

Two crabs, a favorite octopus food, are fastened to two sticks. A horizontal shape is also fastened to one of the sticks and a vertical shape to the other. The octopus learns that different shapes come with the food, but it eats crabs attached to both shapes.

Then a wire carrying a weak electric current is fastened to the stick and crab with the vertical shape, so that each time the octopus tries to eat *that* crab it gets a mild shock. Soon the octopus learns to avoid vertical shapes and to eat only crabs attached to horizontal shapes.

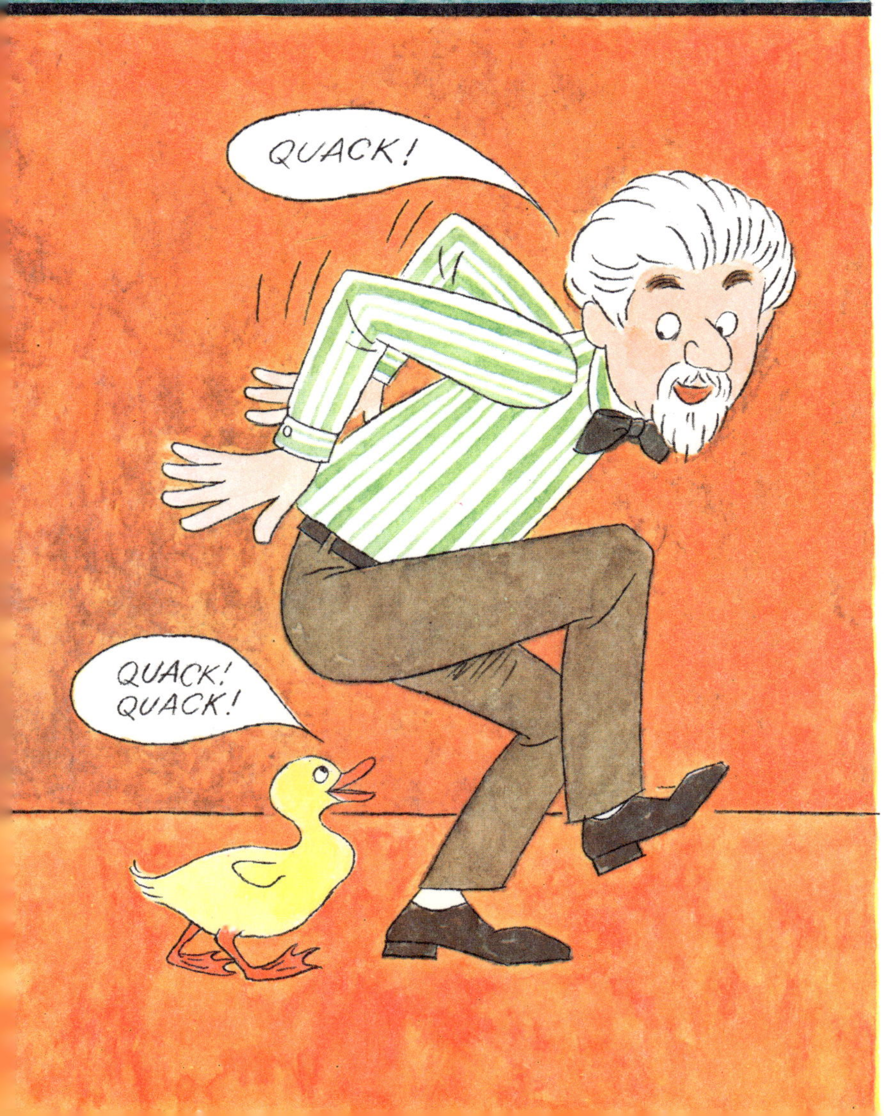

A DUCKLING, when it is newly hatched, can learn to follow a person making quacking sounds instead of following its own mother. The duckling will also follow a box if some sound is coming out of it, or any other sound-making object if it is not too big or too small. As a matter of fact it will continue to follow that person or object for the rest of its life.

It is very important, though, that the duckling be newly hatched. A few days after it is born the duckling can no longer be taught to follow anyone or anything other than its own mother.

We know this about ducklings from the research of Konrad Lorenz, who studies and experiments with animals in their natural environment.

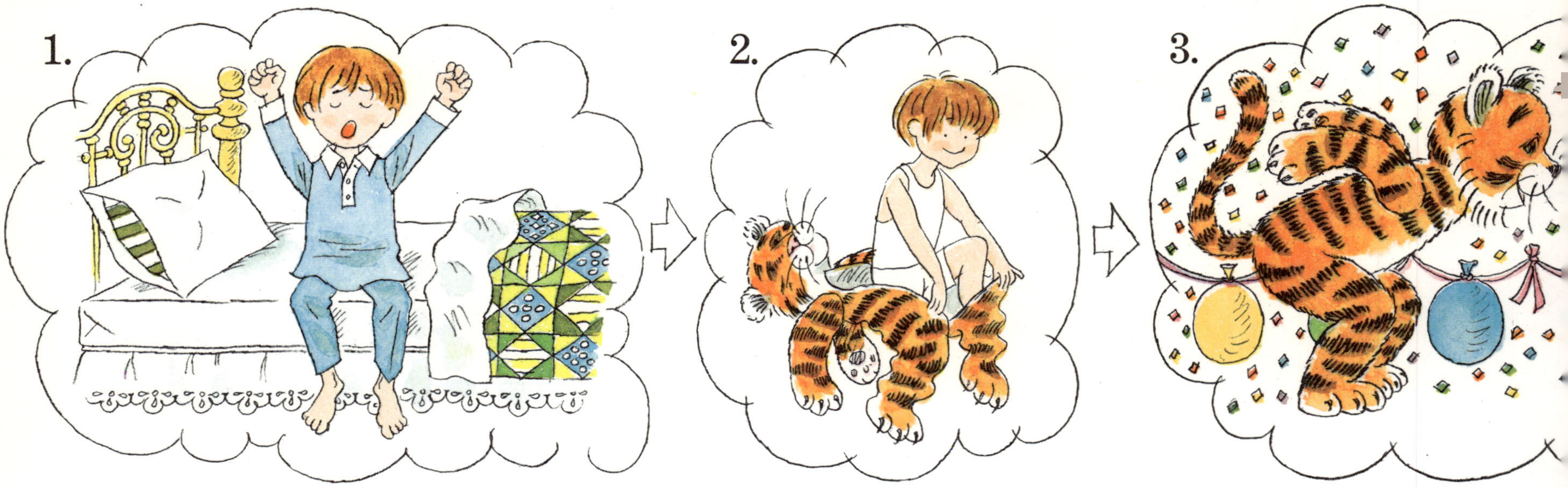

SLEEP is necessary for good health. People who stay awake for a long time as an experiment become confused and can't think clearly.

A new baby sleeps about eighteen hours out of twenty-four. As the baby gets older, it needs less and less sleep. A child usually needs ten to twelve hours a night, and a grown-up, about eight.

When you sleep, your muscles relax and your heartbeat and breathing slow down. Your whole body is at rest. But it keeps on growing, and continues to replace and repair worn-out or damaged tissues.

While you sleep, you change position (about thirty times a night) so you don't lie all night on any one part of your body. The moving lets your muscles rest evenly and helps your blood circulate freely.

Yawning often happens when we are relaxed and bedtime is near. It is a reflex action we can't control and usually means we need sleep. Possibly we yawn to keep awake—to take in more oxygen, increase circulation, and stretch our muscles.

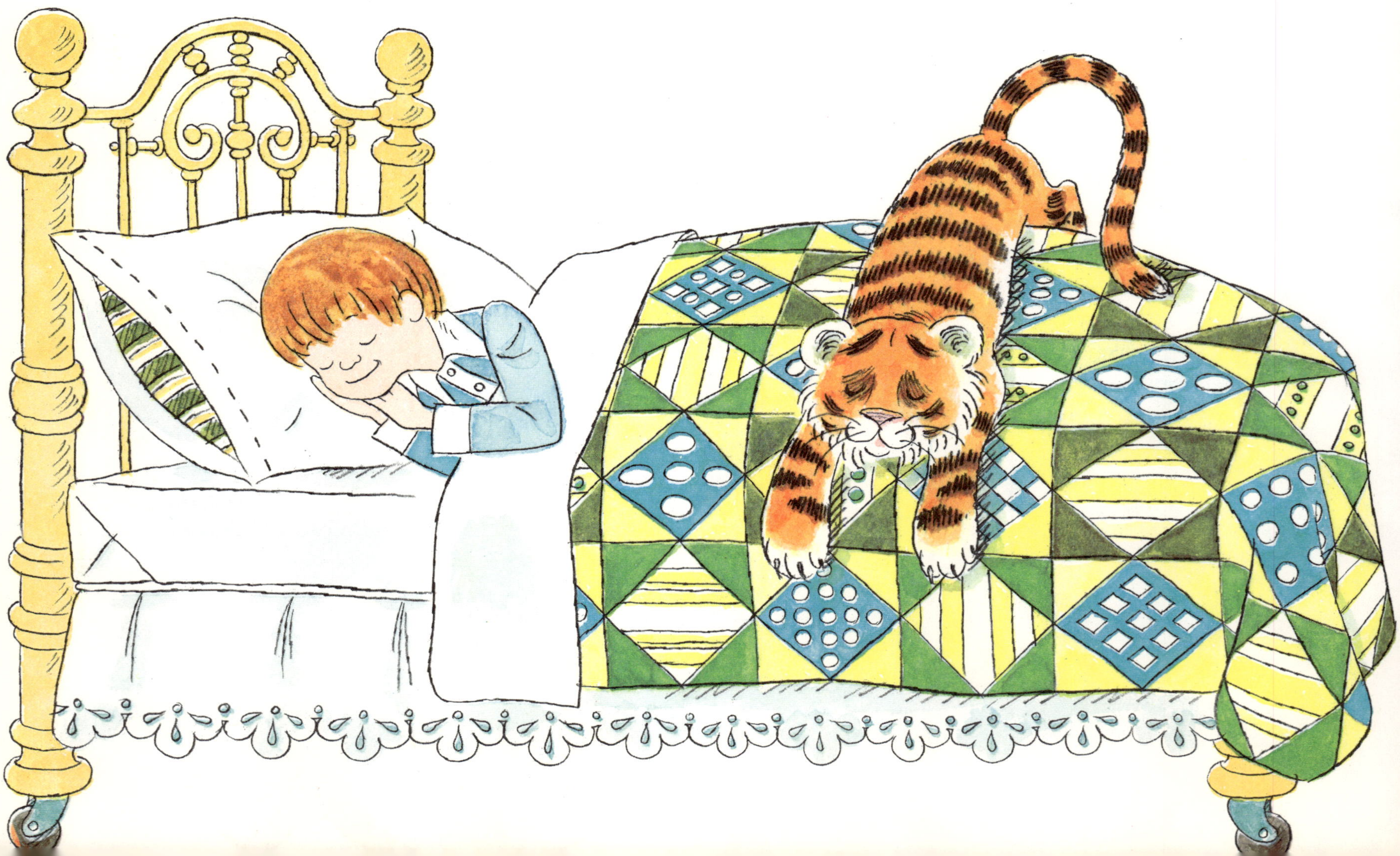

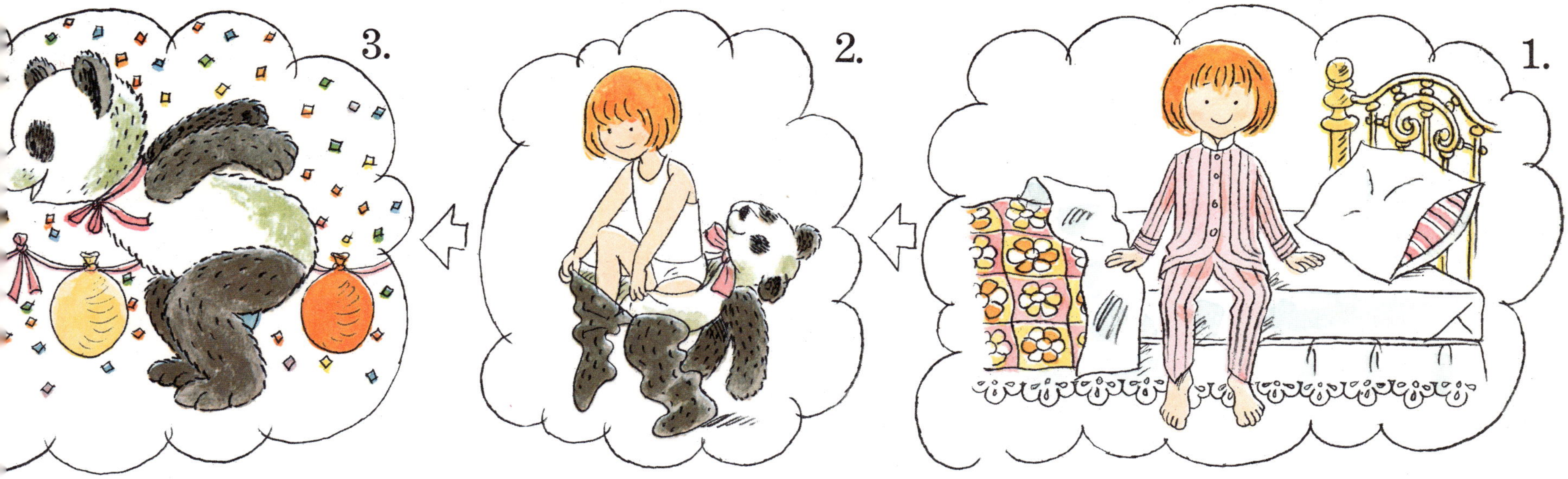

You DREAM every night, even though you may not remember anything when you wake up. And, you have more than one dream each night. Scientists have learned this from experiments. They have learned that quick eye movement under a sleeping person's closed eyelids means that the person is dreaming. From watching these eye movements, scientists have learned that people dream about four to six times a night; that the dreams keep getting longer (the first is about ten minutes long and the last about forty); and that women dream more than men, and children dream more than adults. Also, more people dream in black and white than in color.

Some dreams are happy, some are funny and make you laugh in your sleep, and some are sad. When they are very scary they are called nightmares. When you have a nightmare it is good to remember that dreams are just dreams, and even though they may seem to have real things and people in them, what happens in them is not real.

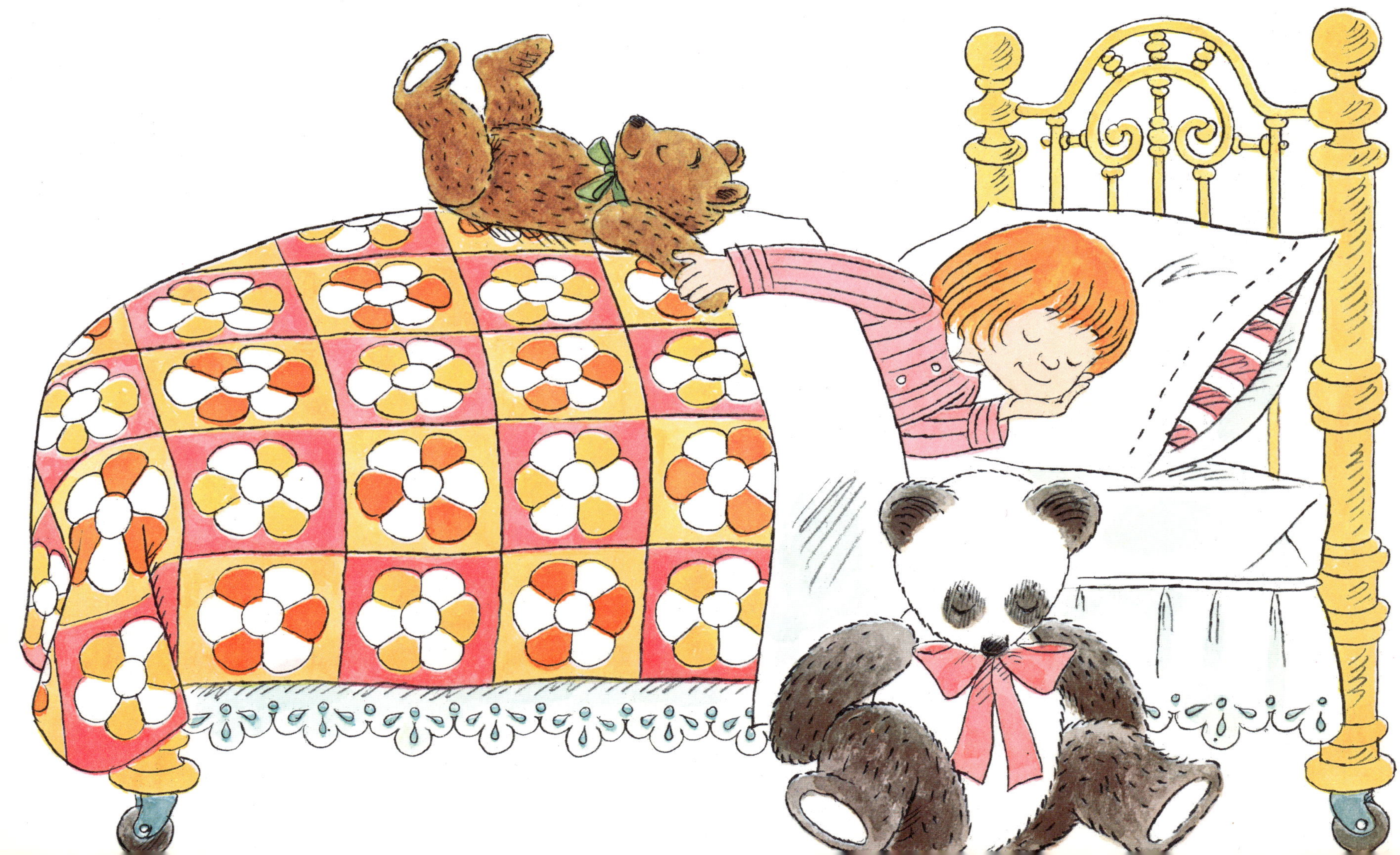

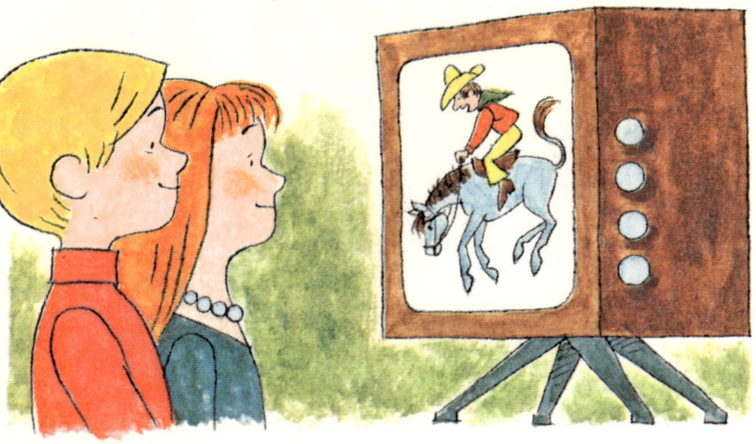

SIGHT tells you about distance, color, light, and dark.

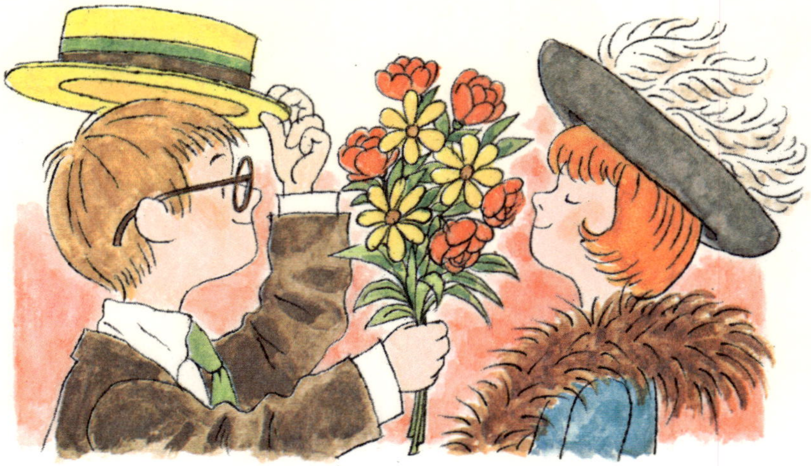

SMELL lets you enjoy nice things, say "phooey" to others.

Through our SENSES we are aware of ourselves and everything around us. Through our senses we can see, smell, taste, hear, touch, balance, and feel pain, and heat or cold.

It would be hard to get along without our senses. Sight makes it possible to read, recognize our friends, catch a ball, and cross streets safely. Smell and taste make it fun to eat food we like, and help warn us to stay away from things that may be bad for us. Hearing allows us to enjoy music and listening to other people's ideas. Touch lets us enjoy patting a soft, fuzzy kitten or giving a hug to someone we love. If we had no sense of balance, we would fall every time we moved. We need the senses of pain, heat, and cold for safety—to warn us if something is too hot or too cold or to tell us if we have been hurt or are getting sick.

It would be hard to get along without all of the senses, but there are people who do very well without one or two of them. The human brain can almost always learn to get along with the senses it has available. Blind people can use their hearing and sense of touch to recognize people and to get around. Deaf people can use their eyes to understand people talking with hand signals or to read people's lips.

Your brain almost always makes a selection from among the sensations coming to it—choosing the ones that are important for the moment. If you are on a crowded city street you will certainly be paying more attention to the cars and people than to the sun shining overhead. Here your brain acts to help you pay attention to the things that affect your safety. If you are reading and someone else is watching television, your brain can help you concentrate by blotting out noises from the television.

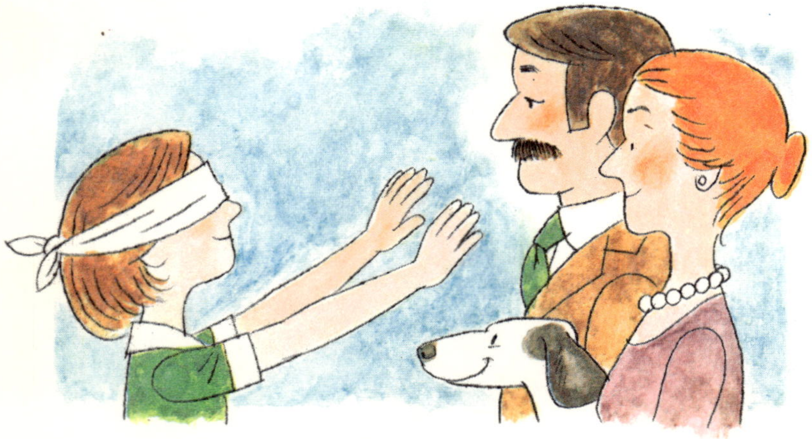

The blindfold TOUCH test. Will she know who is who?

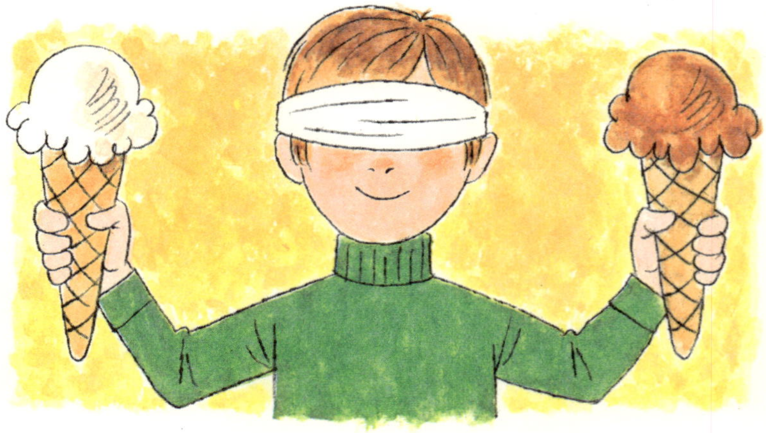

Blindfold test #2. Will TASTE tell him which is which?

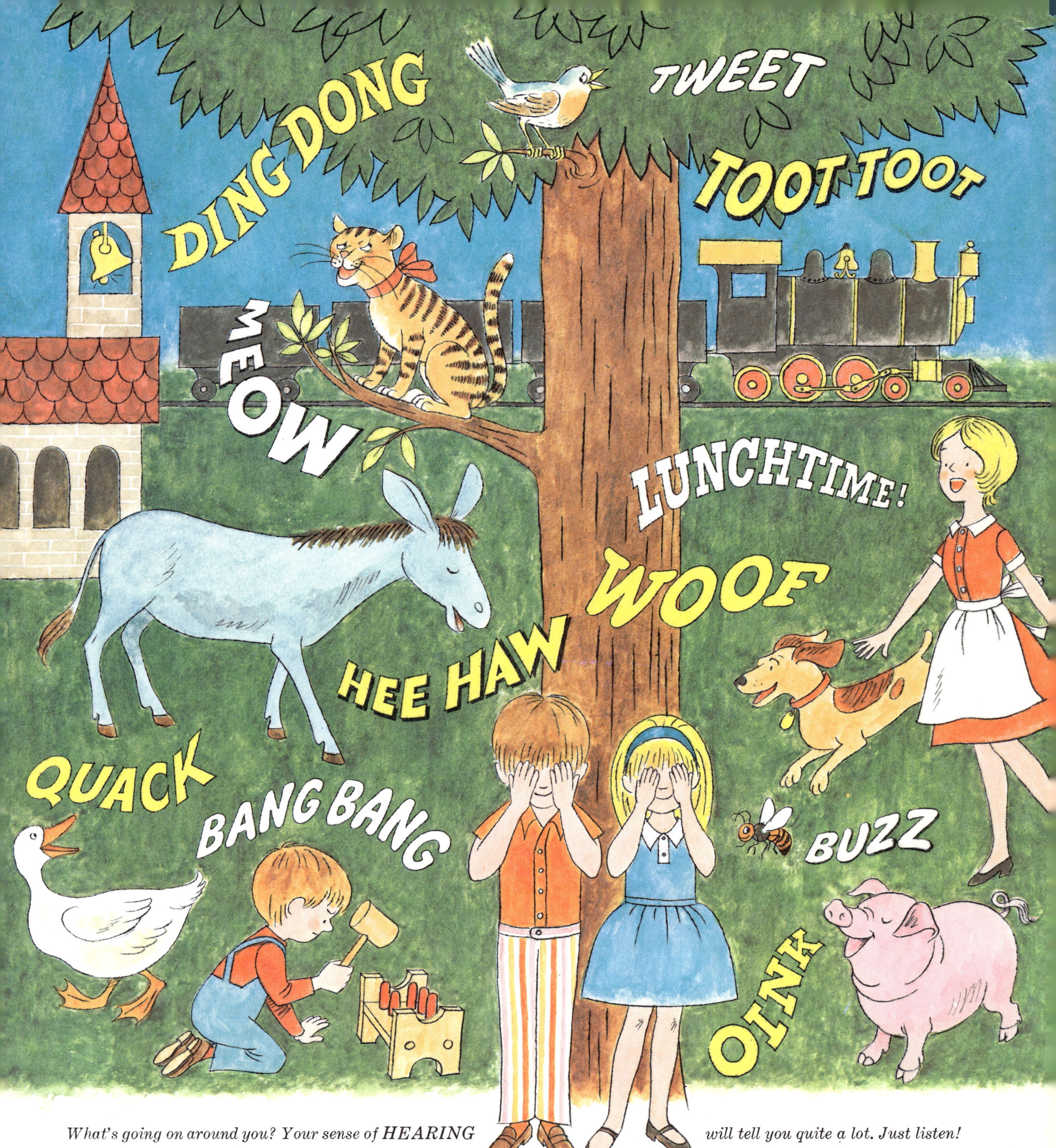

What's going on around you? Your sense of HEARING will tell you quite a lot. Just listen!

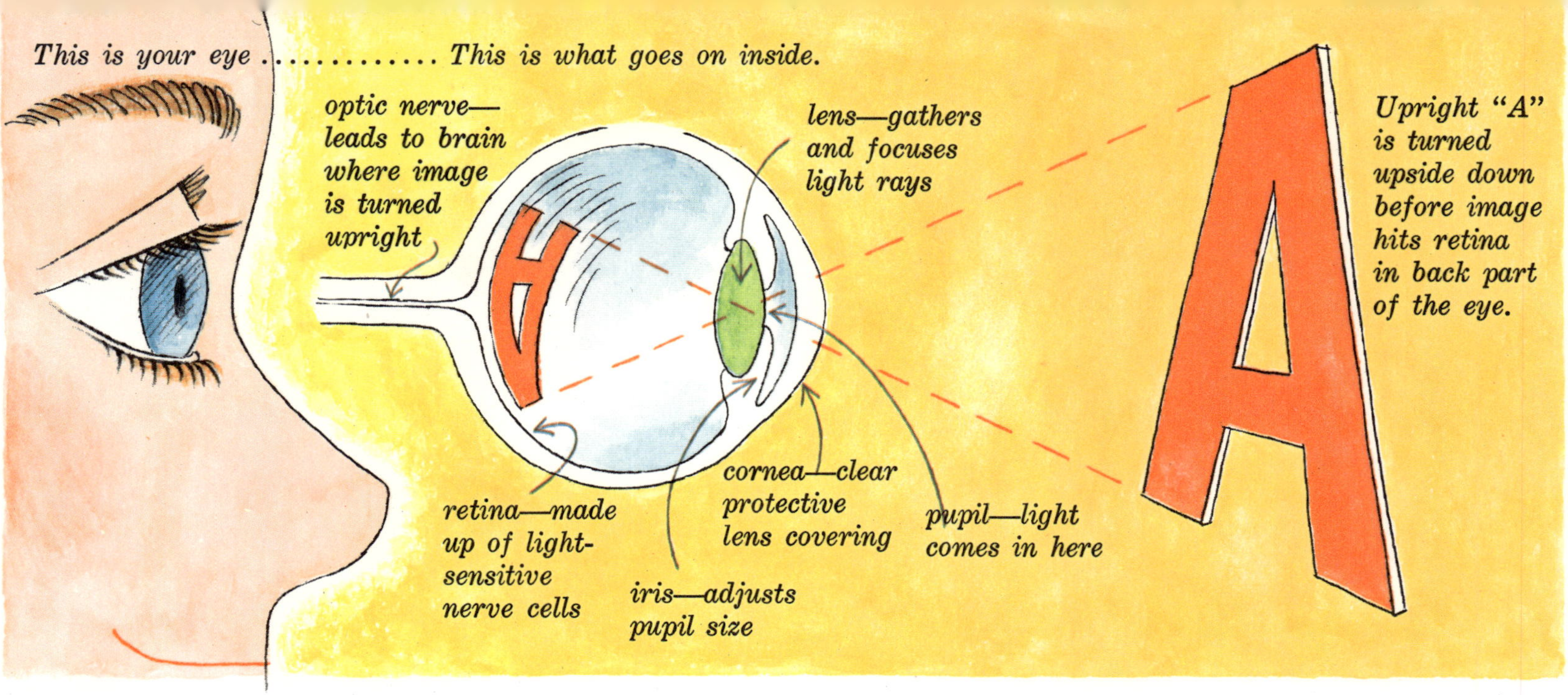

SIGHT happens when light rays come into the eyes and stimulate nerves to send signals to the brain.

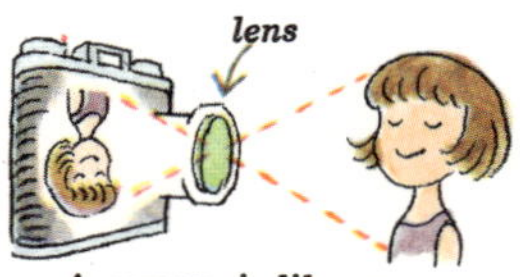

A camera is like an eye

Light rays come into the eye through the lens, which gathers them and focuses them in one bright image on the retina at the back of the eye. The retina is a layer of very fine nerve cells which are sensitive to light. They react to the light and send signals along the optic nerve, which runs from the back of the eye to the brain. The brain receives the information, and understands it as a picture.

When you look at your eyes, you see only part of them. The complete eye is shaped like a ball, which is why it is called an eyeball. It is protected by the skull, and by an outer layer of tough white tissue. The clear cornea, in front, is part of this layer. It protects the lens.

The second layer of the eyeball is dark and full of blood vessels. The front part of the layer, the iris, is between the cornea and the lens. The iris has a hole in the middle called the pupil, and muscles that can make the pupil smaller or larger, controlling how much light gets to the lens and into the eye. The color of the iris—blue, gray, brown, etc.—is what we call the color of our eyes.

Behind the pupil is the lens. Muscles running from the lens to the tough outer layer of eyeball tissue can adjust the thickness of the lens, so it can focus

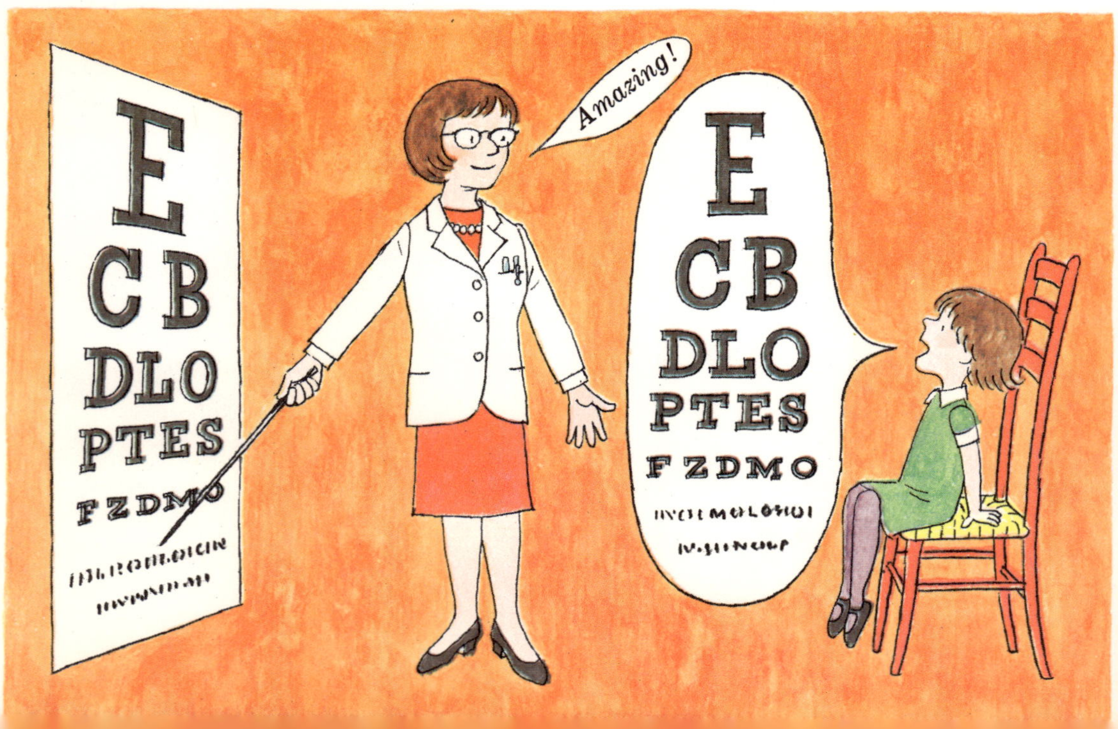

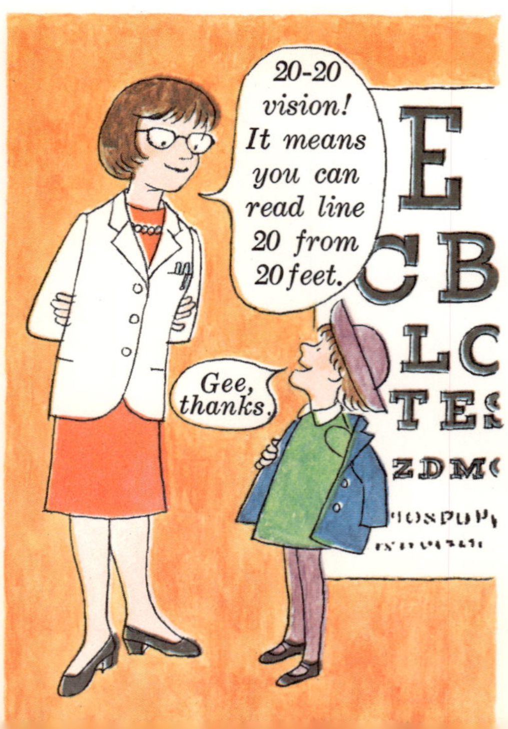

This is line 20.

20-20 vision is normal.

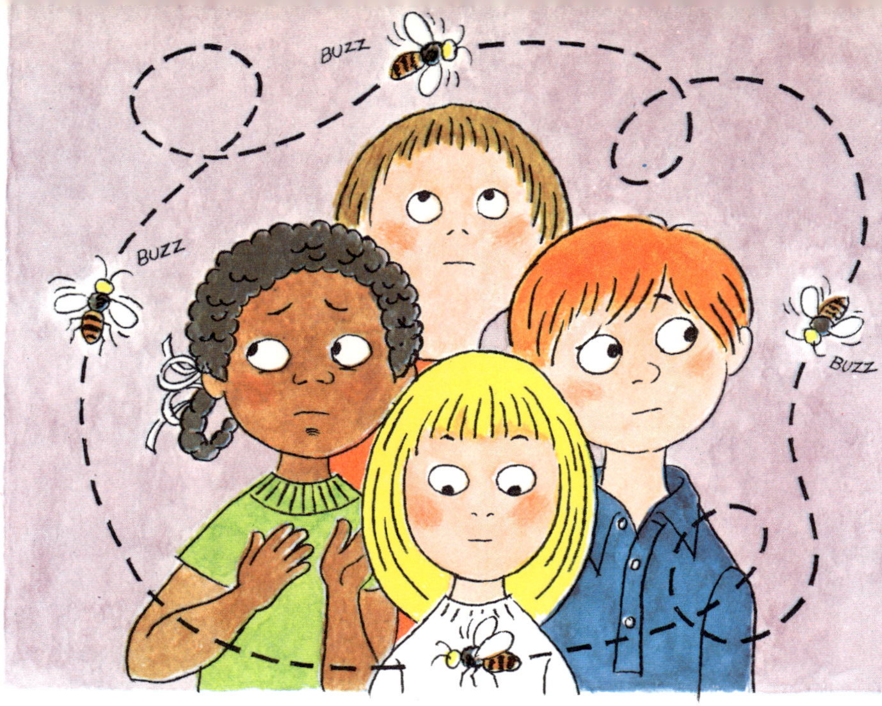

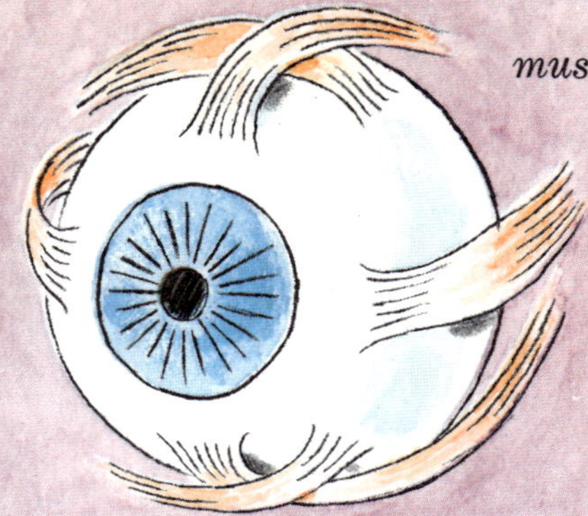

You can move your eyes up or down, left or right, and even roll them around. Six little muscles attached to each eye do all the work.

the light rays on the retina, whether they come from faraway or nearby objects.

The third layer, the inside of the eyeball, is the retina, the layer of light-sensitive nerve cells.

The eye is filled with a clear jelly-like substance which helps focus the light rays even more, and which helps the eyeball keep its shape.

The eyes have upper and lower eyelids to protect them. Behind each upper eyelid there is a tear gland. This is where your tears come from. Tears are not only for crying—they also keep your eyes moist and clean. Your eyelids blink about twenty times a minute—to help keep dust out of your eyes, and to keep them moistened with tears.

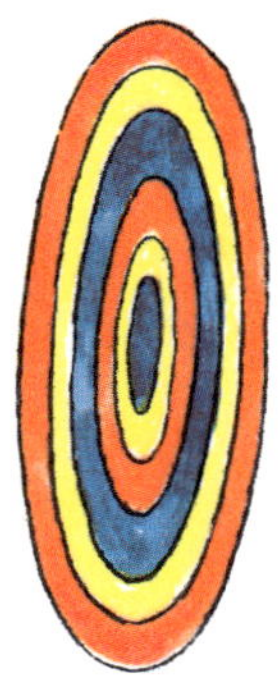

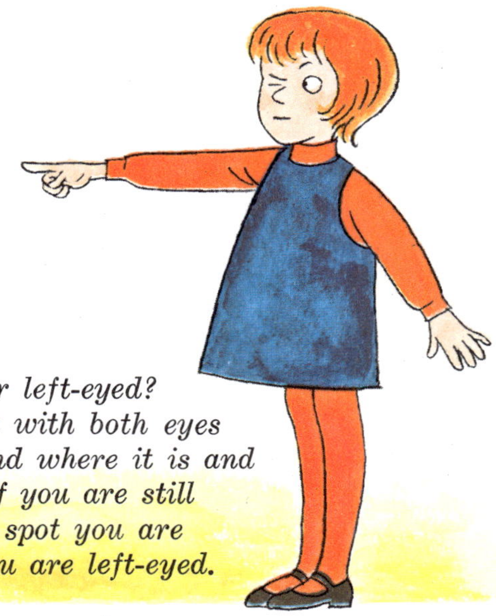

Are you right-eyed or left-eyed? Point to a small spot with both eyes open. Leave your hand where it is and close your left eye. If you are still pointing to the same spot you are right-eyed. If not, you are left-eyed.

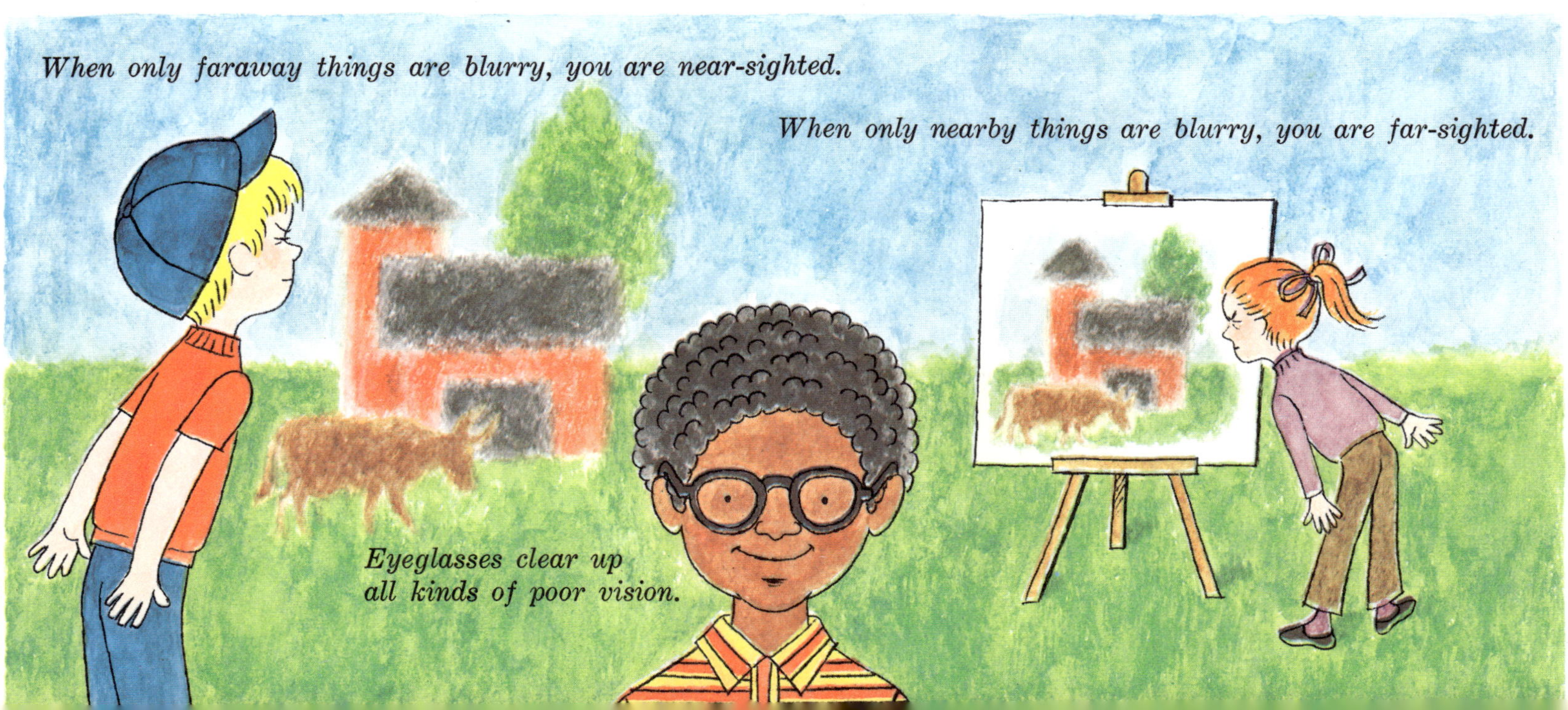

When only faraway things are blurry, you are near-sighted.

When only nearby things are blurry, you are far-sighted.

Eyeglasses clear up all kinds of poor vision.

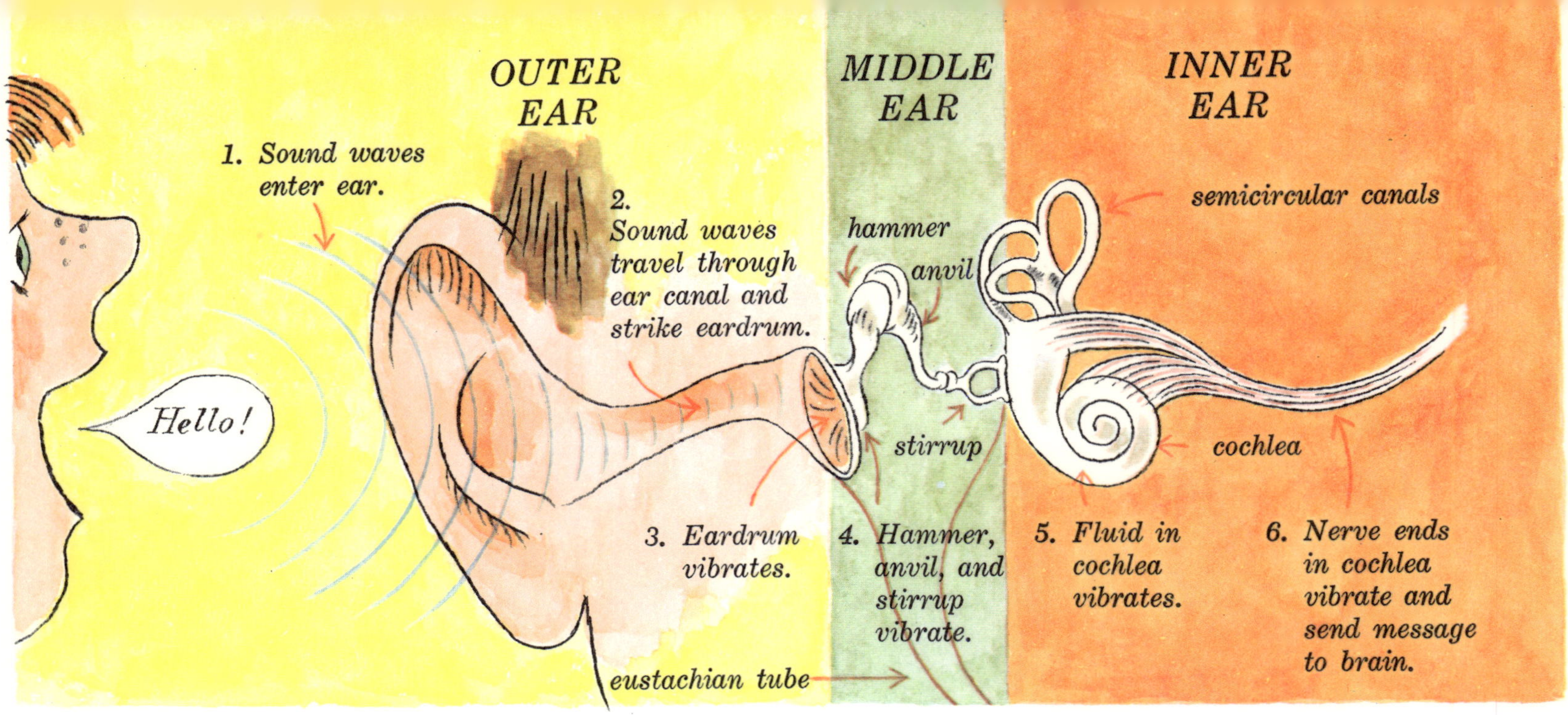

Your **HEARING** depends on the three parts of the ear: the *outer ear*, which includes the ear that you see, the ear canal, and the eardrum; the *middle ear*, which contains three tiny bones called the hammer, the anvil, and the stirrup; and part of the *inner ear*, the snail-shaped cochlea (KOK-lee-uh).

When someone talks, their vocal cords vibrate, making the air around them vibrate. When someone plays a piano, the strings vibrate, making the air around them vibrate. All sounds cause the air to vibrate in waves that spread out in circles like the waves in water when you throw a stone into it. Depending on what makes the sound, the waves will be shorter or longer. A high sound makes shorter waves. A low sound makes longer waves.

When the sound waves are gathered in by your ear and go into your ear canal, they strike your eardrum, making it vibrate back and forth, faster for high notes, and slower for low notes. When the eardrum vibrates, it shakes the hammer. The hammer shakes the anvil, the anvil shakes the stirrup, and the stirrup passes the vibrations on to the cochlea.

The cochlea is filled with liquid and in this liquid there are thousands of hair-like nerve ends. Some pick up the faster vibrations of high sounds and some pick up the slower vibrations of low sounds. These messages travel along the nerves to the brain, which understands them as different sounds.

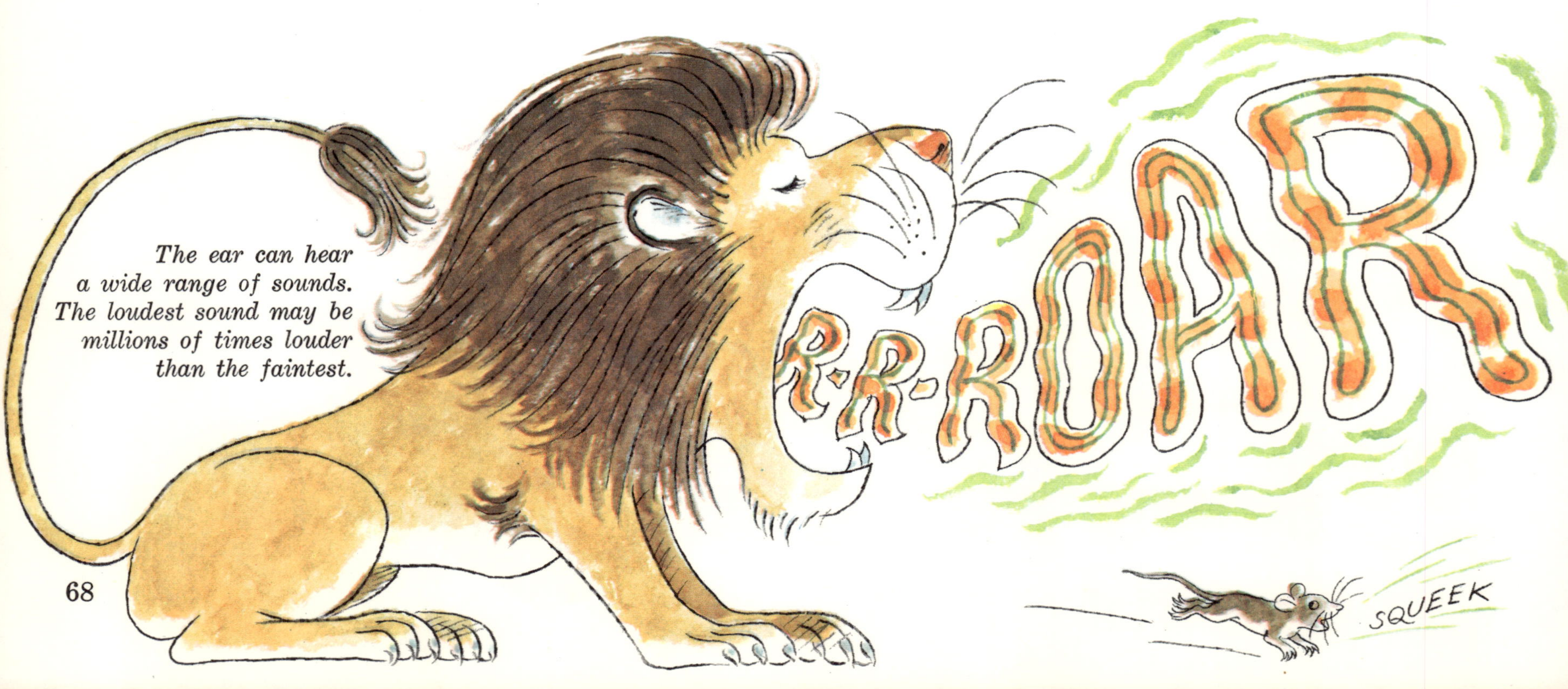

The ear can hear a wide range of sounds. The loudest sound may be millions of times louder than the faintest.

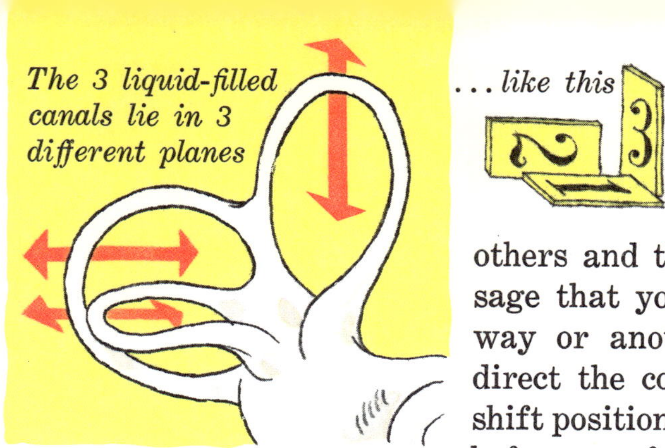

Your BALANCE is controlled by three tiny curved tubes of bone called the semicircular canals. They are deep in your inner ear. Each tube is filled with liquid and has many nerve ends at its base. The three tubes are in different positions, one upright, one resting on its side, and one lying down flat. When you are standing or sitting up straight, the nerve ends in the tubes send messages to the brain that your body is in balance. When you bend forward, backward, or to the side, the liquid in the tubes moves and disturbs the nerve ends, which send messages about their movement to the brain. Depending on which way you move, nerve ends in one tube will be disturbed more than those in the others and the brain will get the message that you are leaning too far one way or another. The brain can then direct the correct part of the body to shift position to get you back in balance, before you fall.

Sometimes the semicircular canals get too much stimulation. If you spin around and around, and the liquid in the tubes sloshes and sloshes against the nerve ends too long, the canals get overworked and you get dizzy. Something like this happens to people who get seasick. As a ship tosses and rocks, the passengers' position is changed so often that their semicircular canals may get over-stimulated. People who are sensitive to this motion may feel sick.

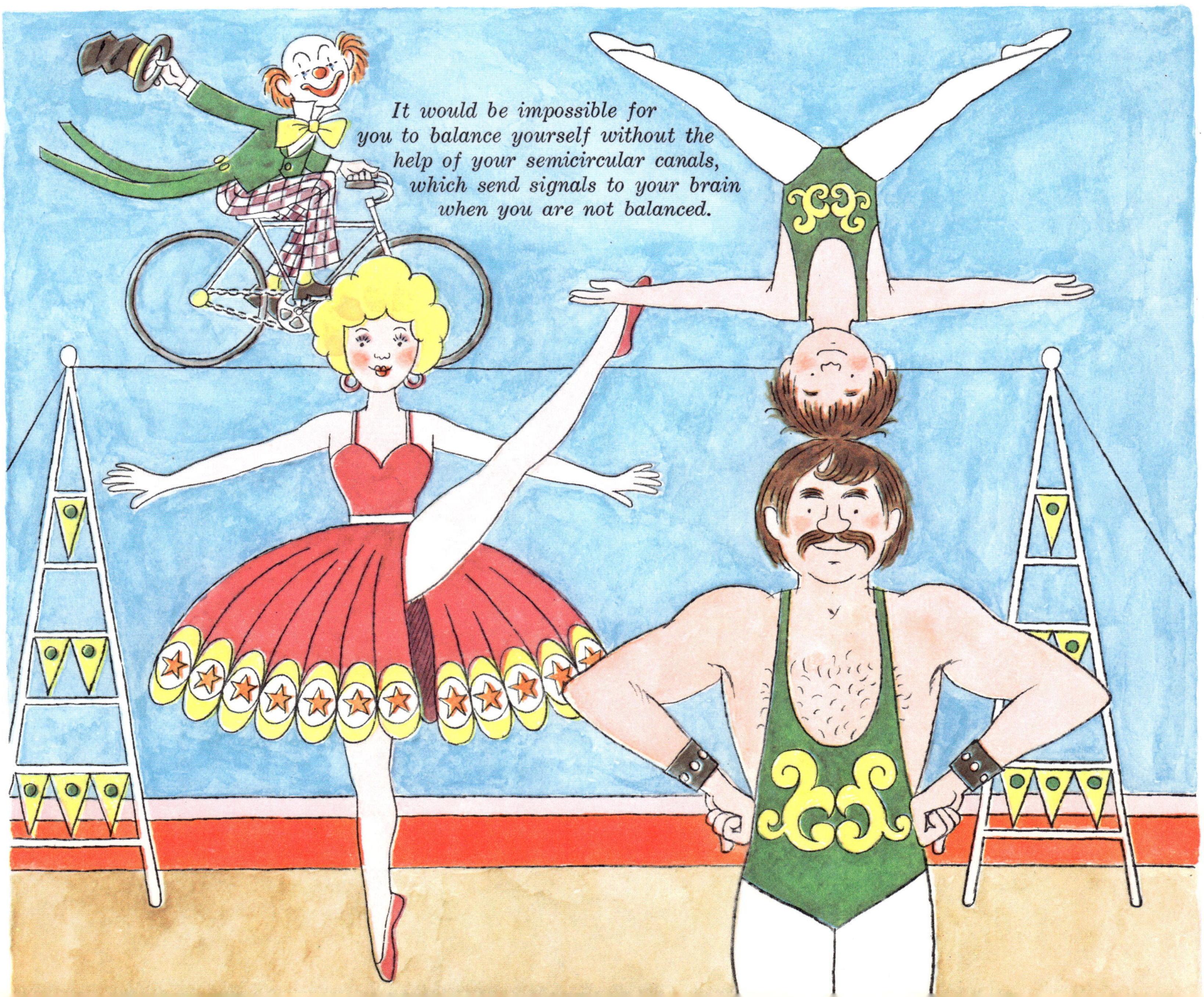
It would be impossible for you to balance yourself without the help of your semicircular canals, which send signals to your brain when you are not balanced.

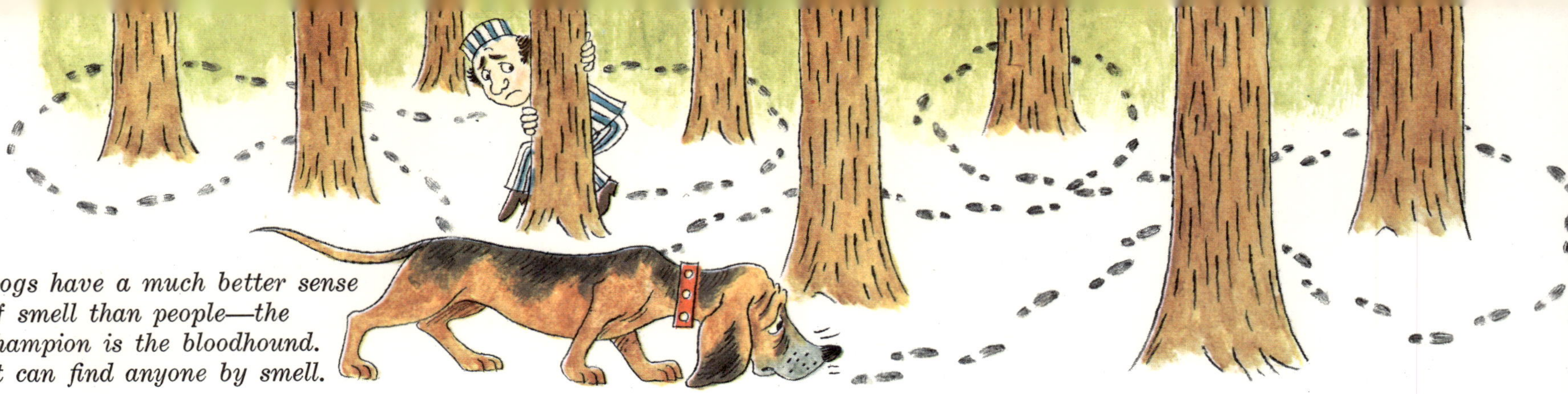

Dogs have a much better sense of smell than people—the champion is the bloodhound. It can find anyone by smell.

Your sense of SMELL begins to work when tiny particles of what you are smelling strike two sensitive areas inside your nose. These areas are on the roof of the passage that leads from your nostrils to your throat. Each area is about one inch square. Thousands of very short hair-like nerve ends stick down from these areas into the air passages. Some of these nerve ends react to certain kinds of particles and some to others.

At mealtime particles of cooking food, too small to be seen, come floating out of the kitchen. Maybe they are particles of soup, roast chicken, and apple pie. Into your nose they go and certain nerve ends get the message. They send it on to the smell center of the brain, "Dinner is ready!" The brain then sends out its own messages, "Wash up and get ready to eat!" and, "Get the digestive juices flowing!"

One thing that makes the sense of smell unlike the other senses is that it gets tired quickly. If you keep smelling one thing, pretty soon you can't smell it any more. When you first come into your home from outside, you may notice a certain smell which will soon seem to disappear, just because you are used to it. This is a good thing for someone who must work where the odor is awful—fortunately, the person will soon become unaware of the smell.

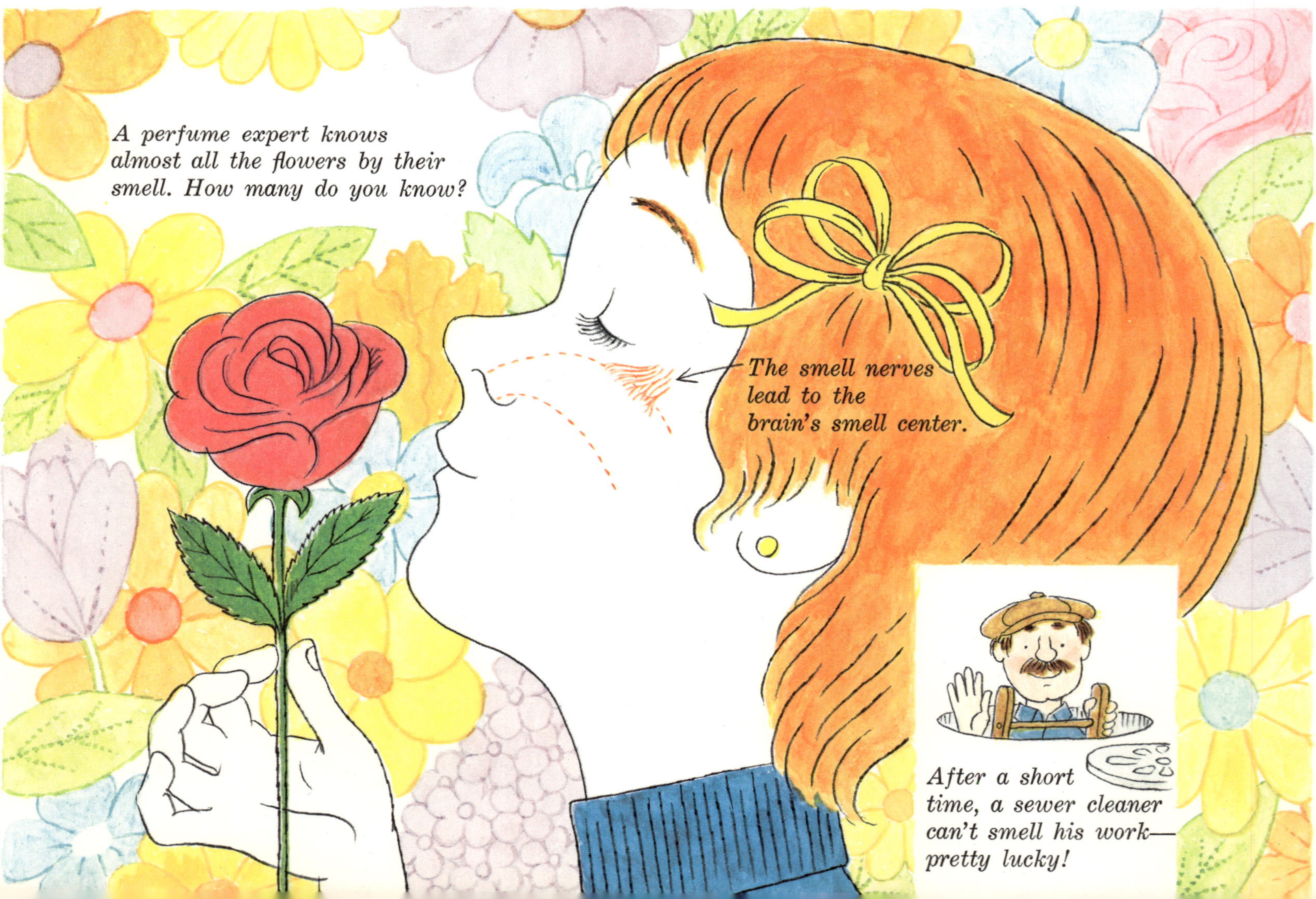

A perfume expert knows almost all the flowers by their smell. How many do you know?

After a short time, a sewer cleaner can't smell his work—pretty lucky!

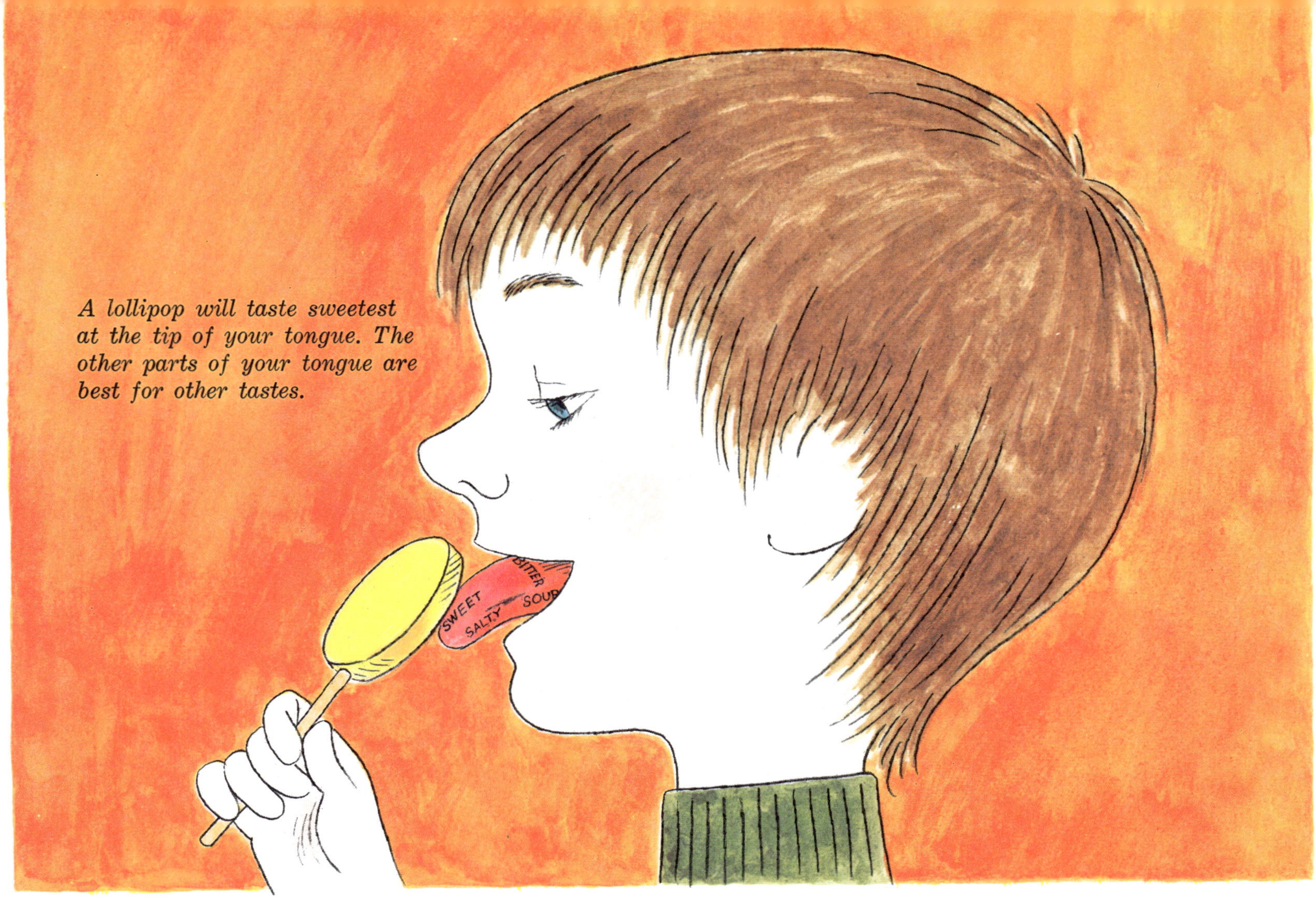

A lollipop will taste sweetest at the tip of your tongue. The other parts of your tongue are best for other tastes.

Your sense of TASTE depends very much on your sense of smell. When you stop the sense of smell by holding your nose, it's hard to taste what you are eating. When you have a bad cold and can't breathe through your nose, food doesn't taste like much because you can't smell it.

But there are four tastes that don't depend on smell: sweet, salty, sour, and bitter. These you taste with the taste buds on the different parts of your tongue. Taste buds are bunches of taste nerves that go from the tongue to the taste part of the brain. Most of the taste buds that recognize sweetness are on the tip of the tongue. The taste buds on the back part of the tongue are sensitive to anything that tastes bitter. The sides of the tongue have most of the salty and sour taste buds, salty toward the front and sour toward the back. You can test these taste areas yourself. Put a little sugar on the tip of your tongue. It will taste sweet. When you put some on the back of your tongue it won't taste so sweet. Saliva is important in tasting—it must mix with the taste chemicals of the food and carry them to the bottoms of the taste buds. Now try tasting salty, sour, and bitter foods. The temperature of food is important, too. You get more of its taste when it isn't too hot or too cold.

These are the four basic tastes—you don't need your nose for these.

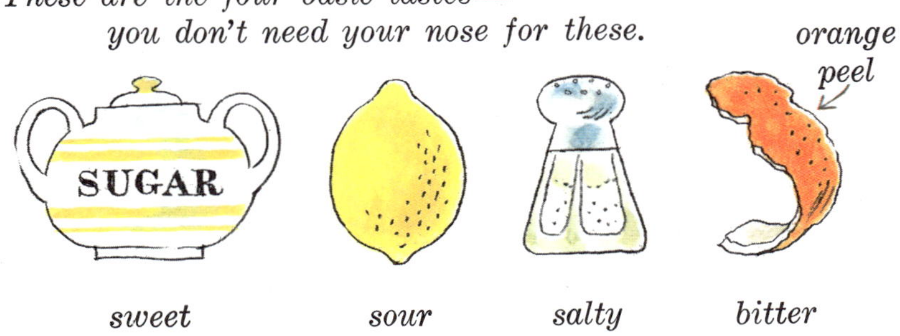

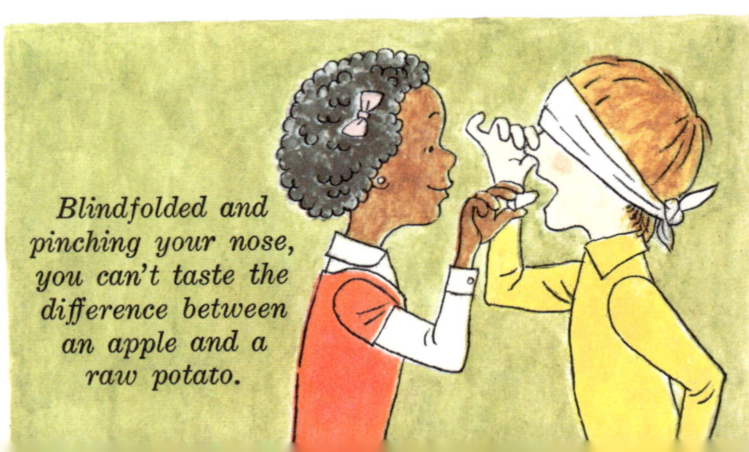

Blindfolded and pinching your nose, you can't taste the difference between an apple and a raw potato.

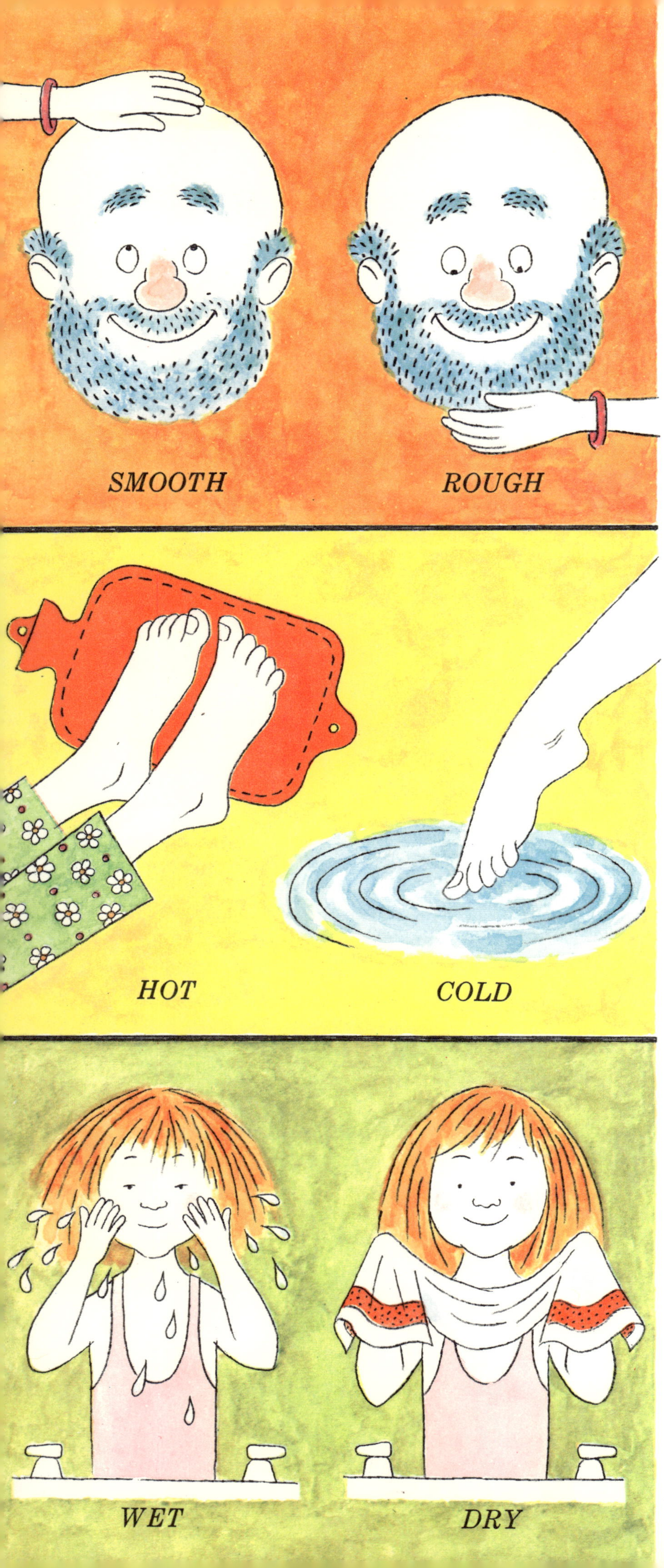

You TOUCH mainly with your skin, although there are other parts of your body such as the inside of your mouth that also have a sense of touch.

Your skin can feel many different sensations. It feels the roughness of a stiff beard or the smoothness of glass. It can tell when something is hot or cold, wet or dry. And, of course, it feels pain.

Every part of your skin has nerve cells to feel these different sensations. Some of the nerve cells feel only the touch of something, some feel only coldness, some feel only heat, and some feel only pain. This is easy to prove to yourself. With the point of a pencil, touch the skin on the back of your hand at spots about an eighth of an inch apart. In some spots there will be just the feel of the touch of the point, in some spots the point will feel cold, and in some spots the point will cause a very slight feeling of pain.

The nerve cells are not distributed evenly throughout the skin. In some places there are only a few, and in other places there are many. They are tightly packed on the fingertips. That's why we use our fingertips when we want to feel something very carefully. Blind people read by using their fingertips to feel tiny bumps on a page. The bumps represent letters. This bump language is called Braille.

The parts of the skin where hair grows have a special kind of sensitivity. Each hair grows out of a hair follicle in the skin. Nerve endings are wound around these follicles. If something is brushed very lightly across a hairy part of the skin, the hairs move. The nerve ends around the follicles pick up this movement, and you feel it as a tickling sensation.

The feeling of PAIN is also a sense. There are many different kinds of pain. The pain of a burn, a cut, a bee sting, or a bruise are some pains felt on the outside of the body. Inside, there's the pain of a stomachache, a headache, or a toothache.

Certain parts of your body are more sensitive to pain than others. The tiniest speck of dirt in your eye, a little cut in your finger, or the tiniest splinter in the bottom of your bare foot is very painful. And you feel the exact location of the pain.

The pain you feel inside you is different. When you have a stomachache you feel the pain somewhere in the area of the stomach, but you usually can't point to a small spot with your finger and say, "This is where it hurts." Sometimes the origin of pain is even harder to locate. Someone with heart pain will often feel it in the left arm, and a liver pain may feel like a pain in the right shoulder.

The reason you know the exact location of a surface pain is that throughout the skin there are nerve cells that are sensitive to pain. The slightest touch of a pin to one of them hurts, and you feel which nerve it is. There are no such pain nerve cells in our inner organs to tell us just exactly where the pain is. But we know there is pain.

Even a baby who has swallowed too much air along with her milk and stretched her stomach knows there is pain. She cries, her mother picks her up, "burps" her to get rid of the air and she feels better. So pain can be a useful sense. It helped the baby get relief, it tells you to let go of a hot pot before you burn yourself, and it may warn you to see a doctor before an illness becomes serious.

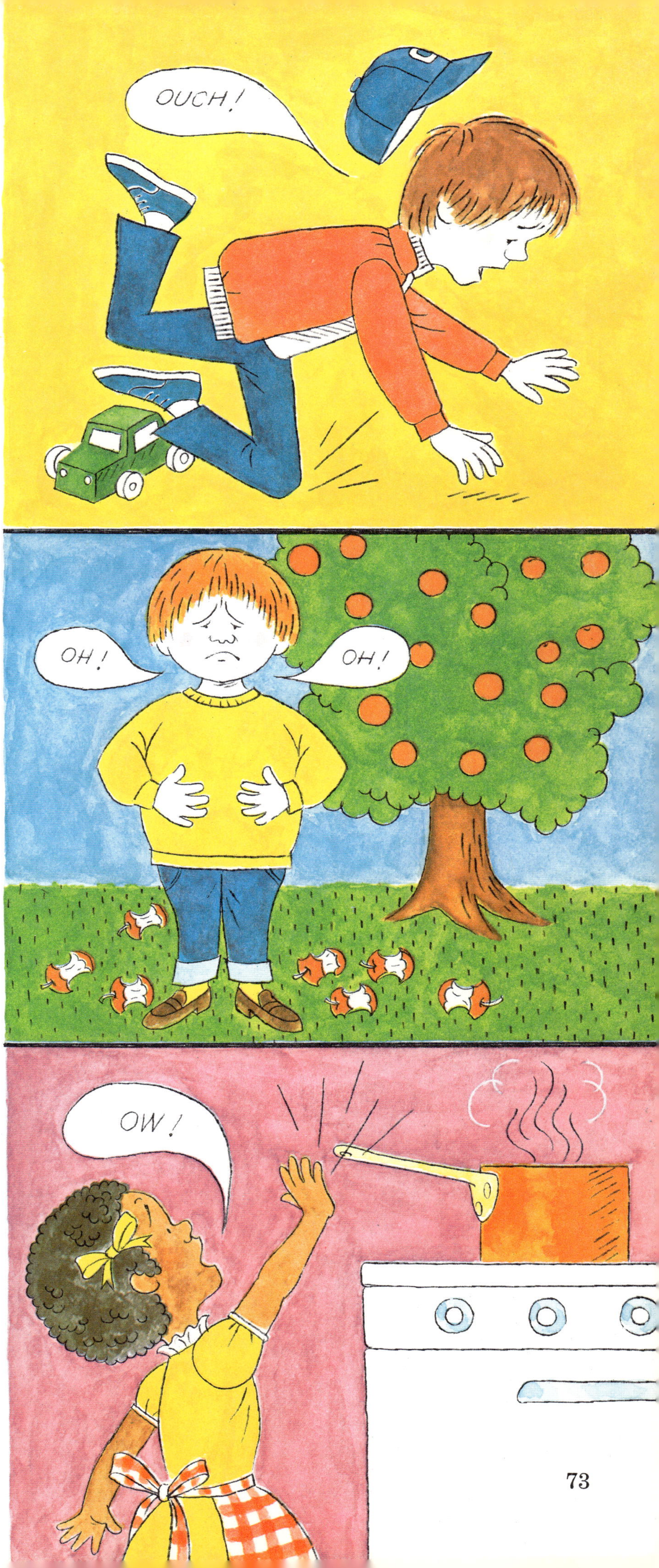

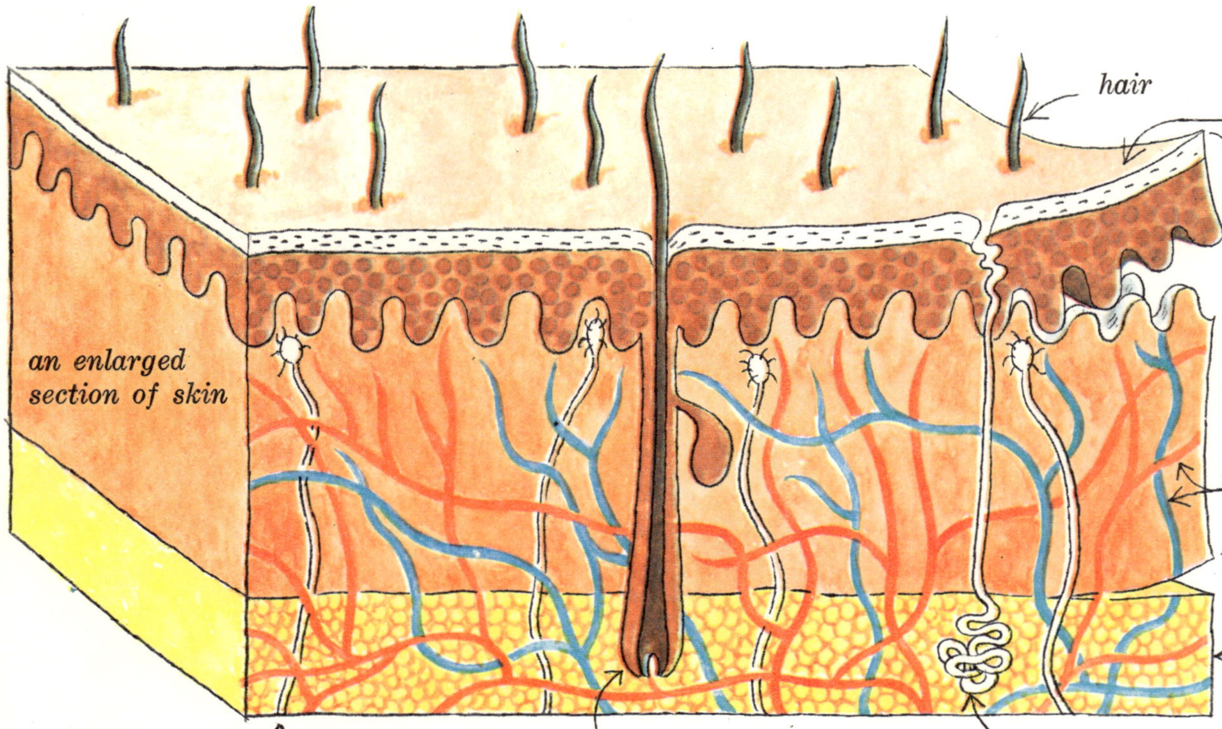

Your SKIN, the largest organ of your body, is like a garment that covers you completely from head to foot. It protects you from germs and dirt and helps to keep your body at the right temperature.

The skin is not the same thickness all over. For example, it is thin on the eyelids and thick on the soles of the feet. But all your skin has two layers.

The thin outer layer, the epidermis, protects your body from the outside world. It is made up of dead skin cells. As they rub off, they are replaced by other cells from underneath. There are no blood vessels in the epidermis, so a cut that bleeds has gone through it. The skin's color is in the epidermis, and the epidermis is what tans to protect light-skinned people from the sun's burning rays.

The thicker inner layer, the dermis, is filled with blood vessels, nerves, hair follicles and sweat glands. The blood vessels feed the skin cells and carry away their wastes. The nerves send messages to the brain about things you touch. The sweat glands take water from your blood and push it out as perspiration onto the surface of your skin, where it evaporates, making you cooler. Under the dermis there is a layer of fat cells which protects you from cold and is the body's extra fuel supply.

When you are embarrassed, blood vessels in the skin of your face and neck dilate (open wider) and fill with extra blood. This makes the skin look red—you are blushing. You can't control the nerves that make blushing happen. Although scientists know *how* we blush, nobody is quite sure *why* we do, or why some people blush more than others.

Fingernails and toenails are a special kind of skin, a clear, stiff material. They have no nerves, so there is no pain when you cut them if you are careful and don't cut the skin around them.

No! Warts do not come from toads. They are rough bumps of skin caused by a virus.

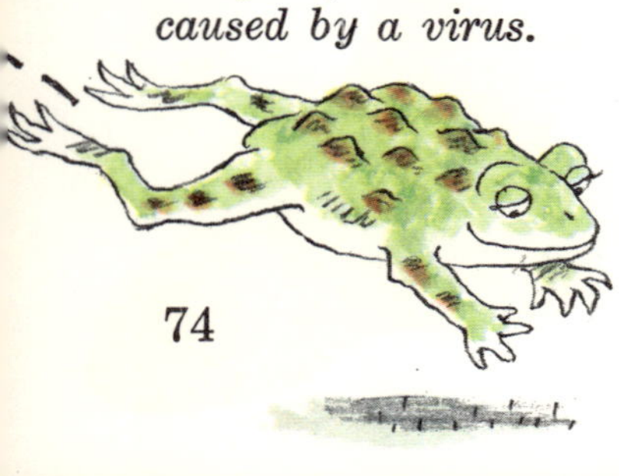

Did you know that fingernails are considered part of the skin?

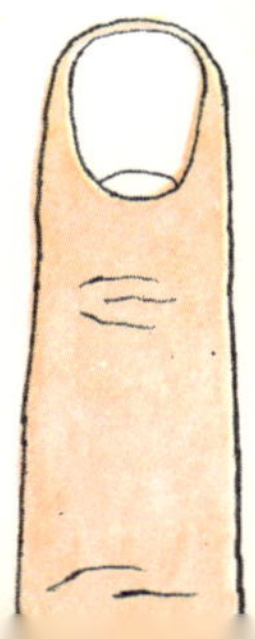

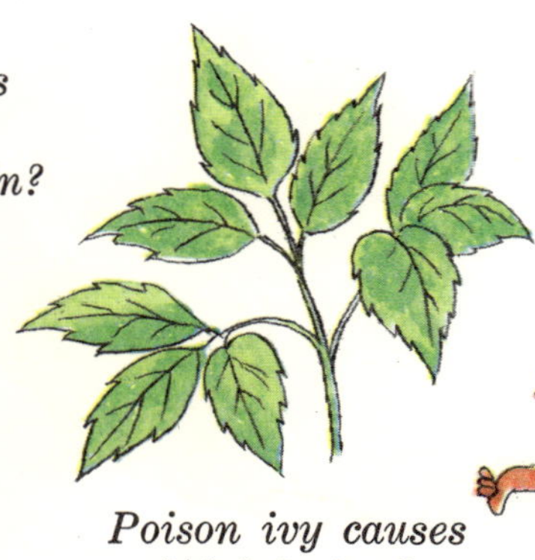

Poison ivy causes painful irritation to the skin. Don't touch!

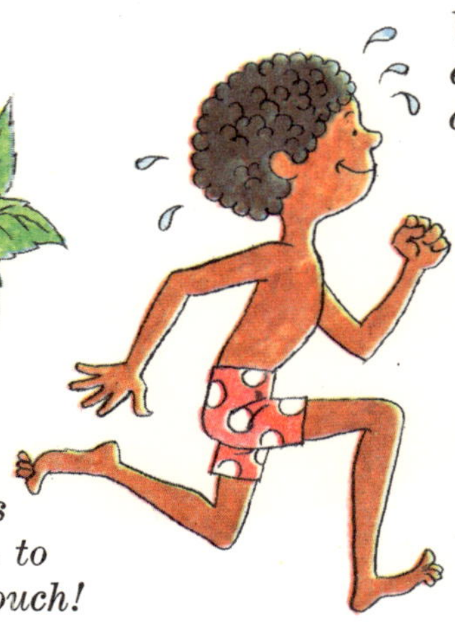

When perspiration evaporates, it cools your body.

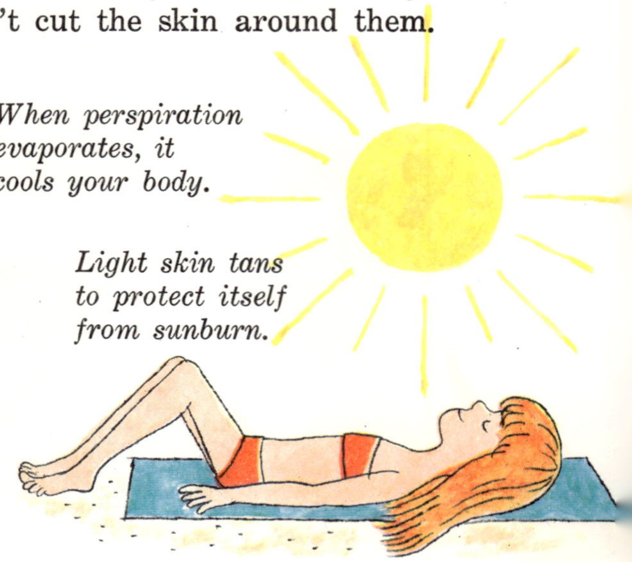

Light skin tans to protect itself from sunburn.

The ridged skin on your fingertips forms a pattern. Everyone has different patterns, even identical twins. Police use fingerprints to help them find out who committed a crime.

Just like fingerprints, everyone's footprints are different. Hospitals take footprints of newborn babies to help keep track of them, since many newborn babies look alike.

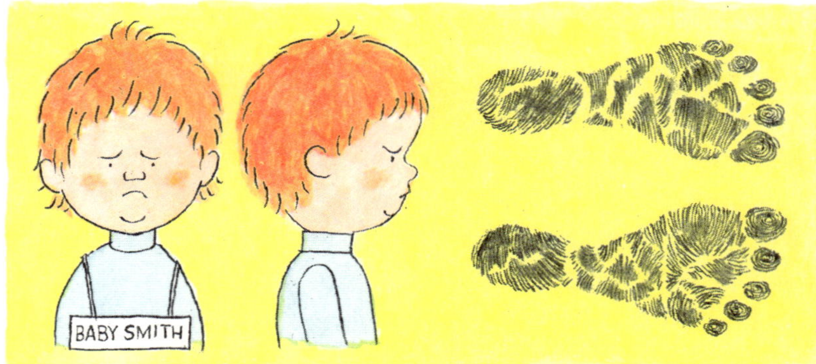

Your skin is like a garment that covers you completely from head to foot.

It protects you from germs and dirt, and helps to control your body temperature.

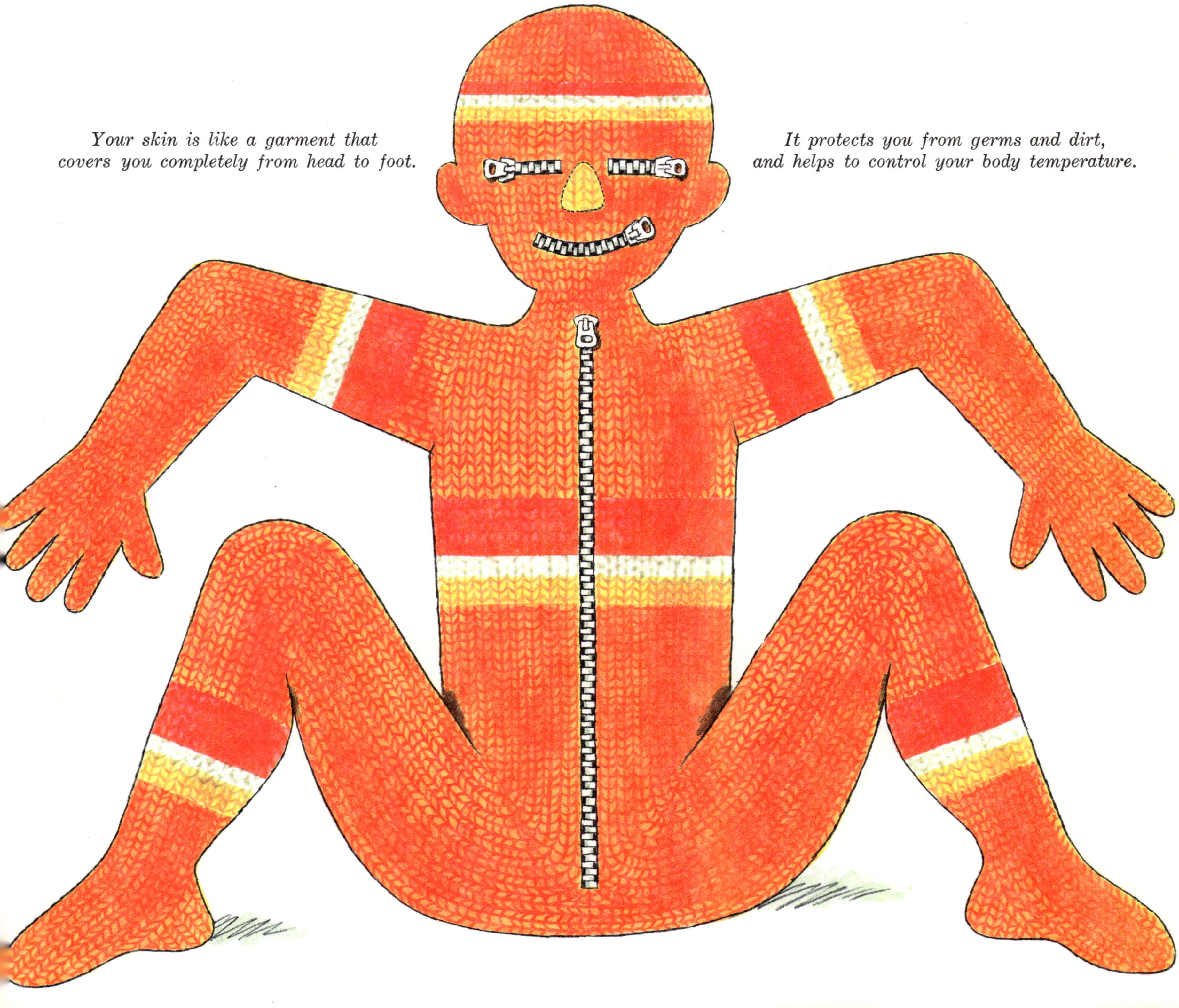

No two people's **SKIN COLOR** is exactly the same. And nobody really has pure black, white, red, or yellow skin. We are all shades of a varying mixture of brown, yellow, and pink. An American Indian's face isn't red at all, it's just a reddish light brown. A white person's skin is really some shade of pink. A black person's skin is some shade of brown. And, of course, yellow skin is really a light combination of yellow and brown.

The color of skin is determined by the amounts of certain chemicals it contains. These chemicals, called melanin and carotene, are pigments—coloring matter. They are found in the outer layer of the skin—the epidermis. The melanin gives the skin brown-black tones, and the carotene gives it yellowish tones. The pink tones in skin come from all the tiny blood vessels near the surface.

All of us have these pigments except albinos—people with no pigment in their skin, hair, or eyes. Only the color of the blood vessels shows, so albinos' skin is very pale pink, their hair is white, and their eyes are light pink.

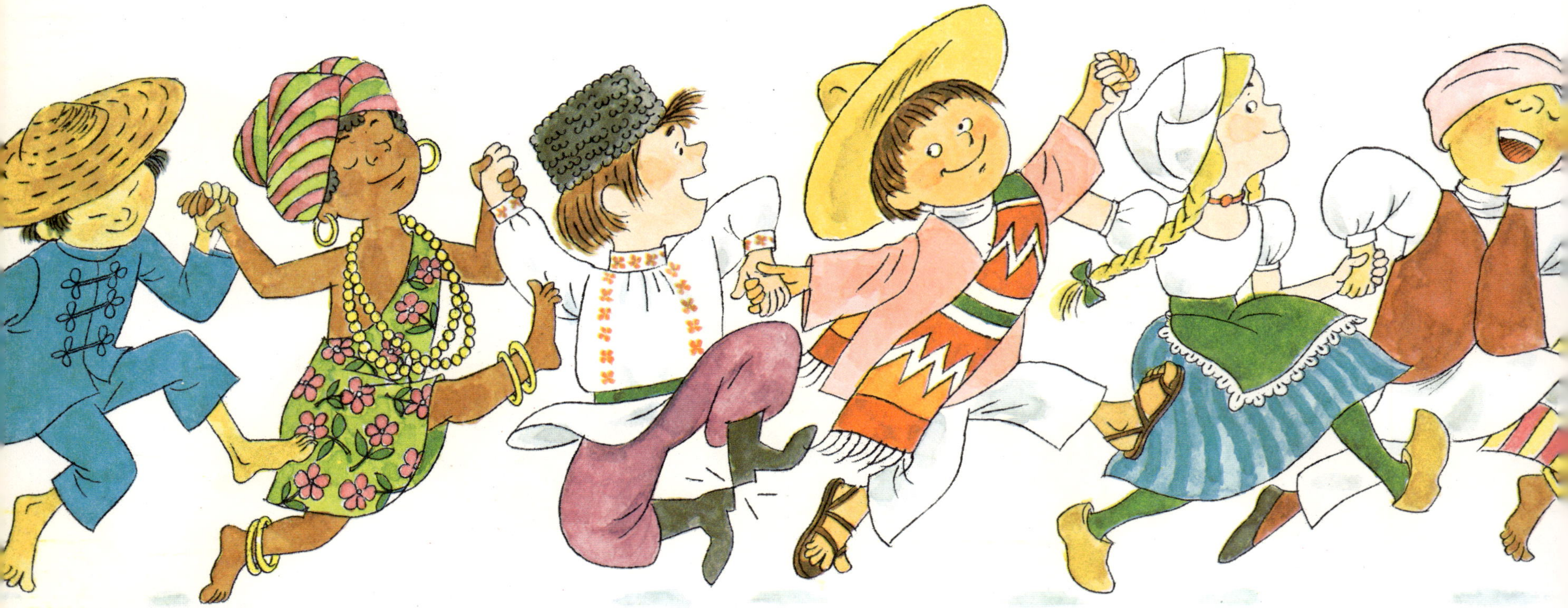

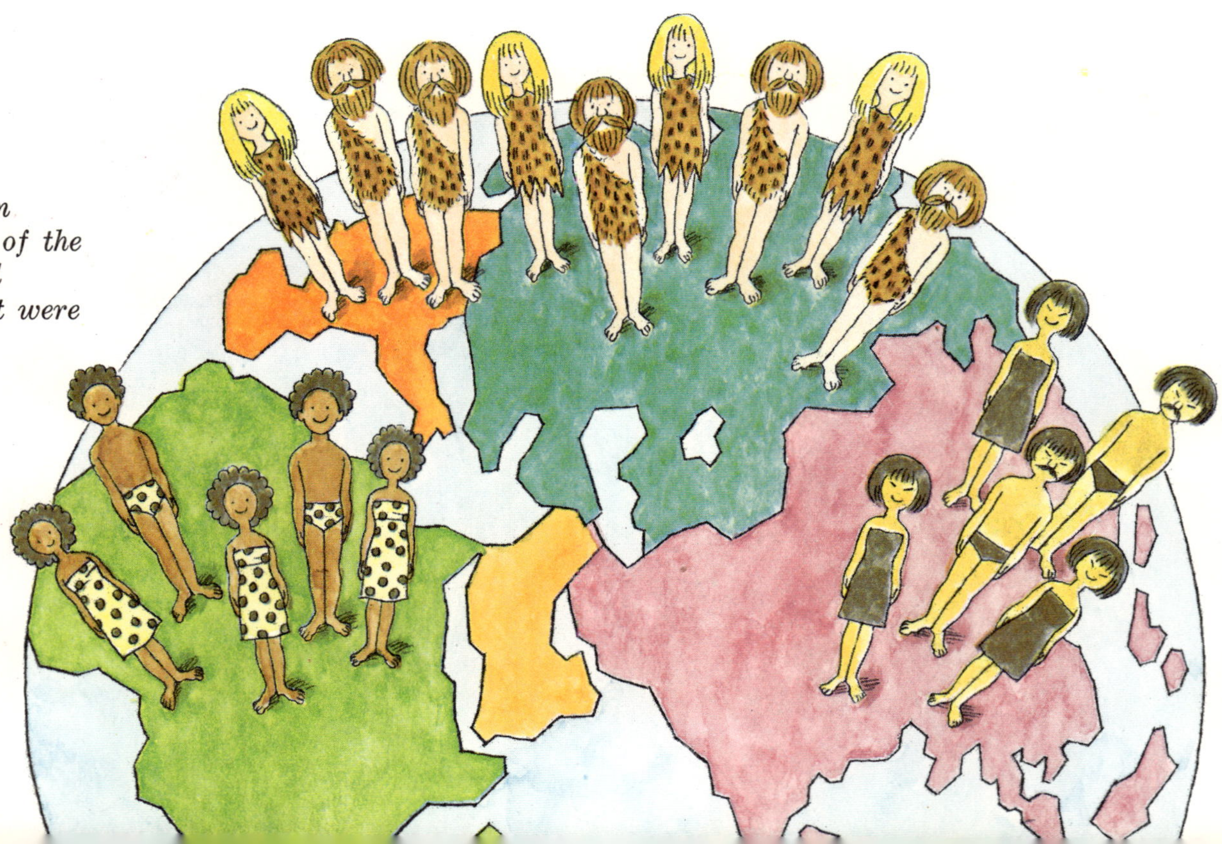

People living in different parts of the earth developed skin colors that were suited to their climate.

We all inherit our skin color from our parents and other ancestors. The skin colors of different groups of people probably developed because of the climates in which they originally lived. Melanin protects skin from sunburn, so in very hot countries, like those in Africa and South America, the people had lots of melanin in their skin, which made their skin dark. People living in countries with less direct sun had less melanin, and so had lighter, pinker skin. Today, it is so easy to move around the world that people of all colors live in all parts of the world.

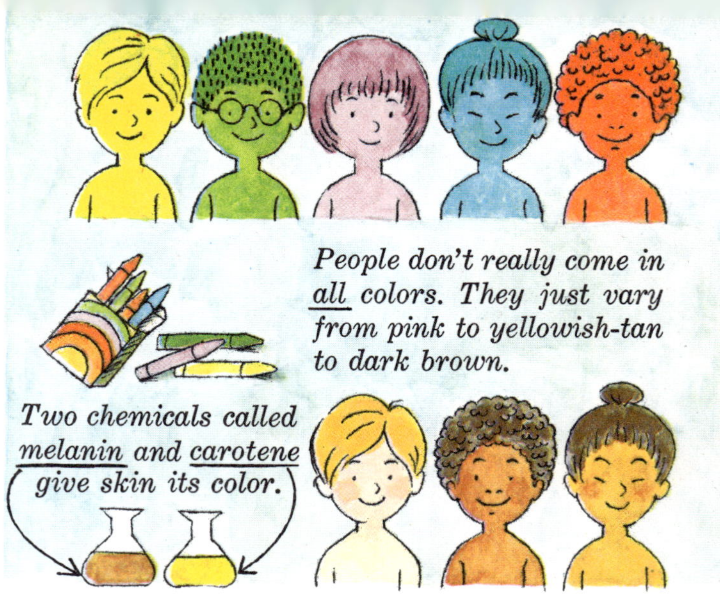
People don't really come in all colors. They just vary from pink to yellowish-tan to dark brown.
Two chemicals called melanin and carotene give skin its color.

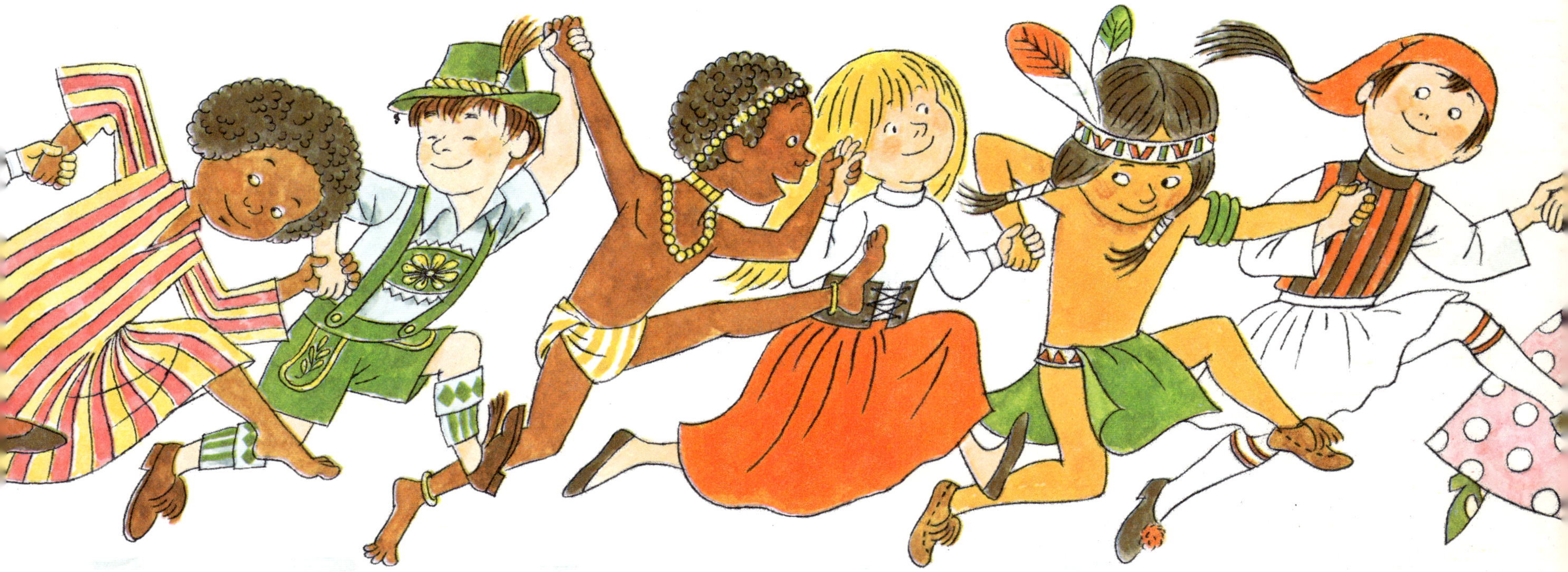

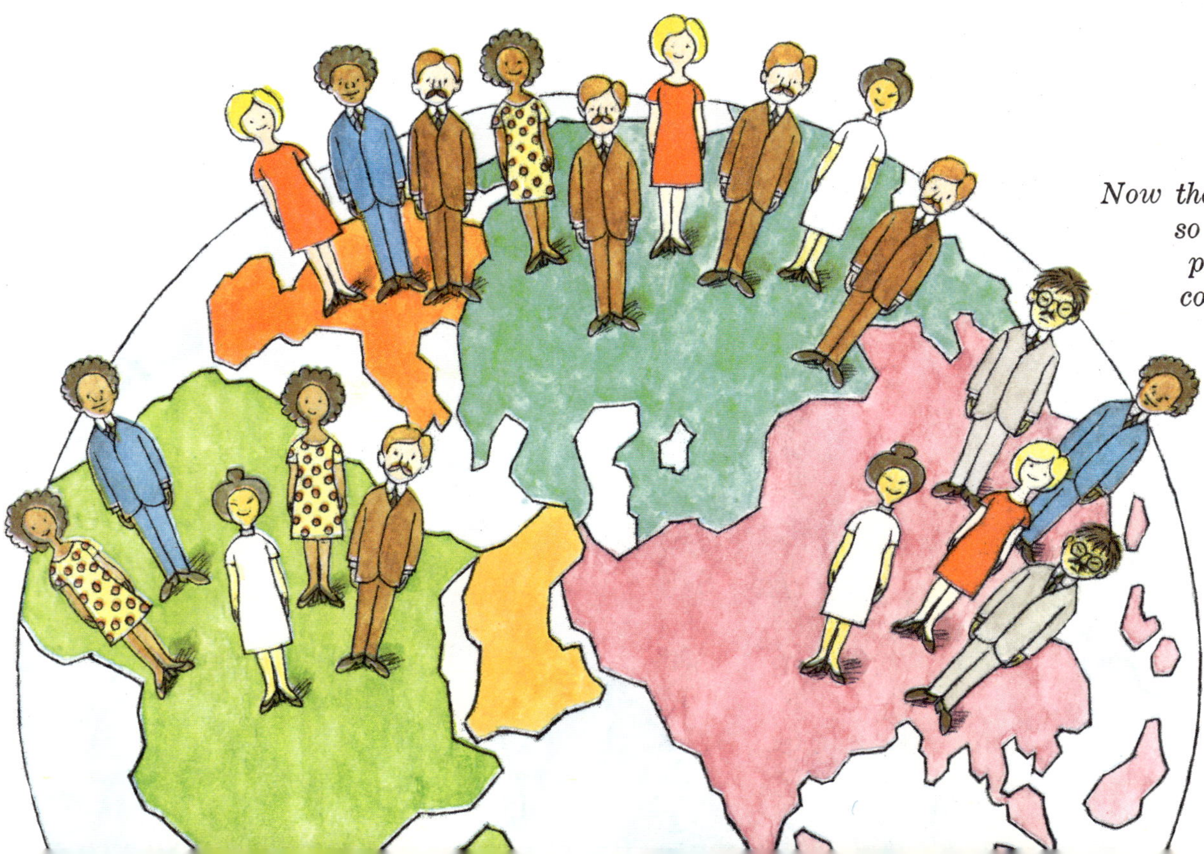

Now that there has been so much migration, people of different colors live together wherever they have settled.

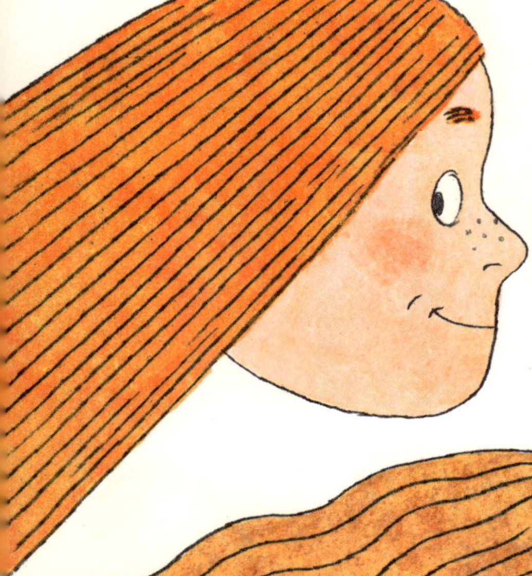

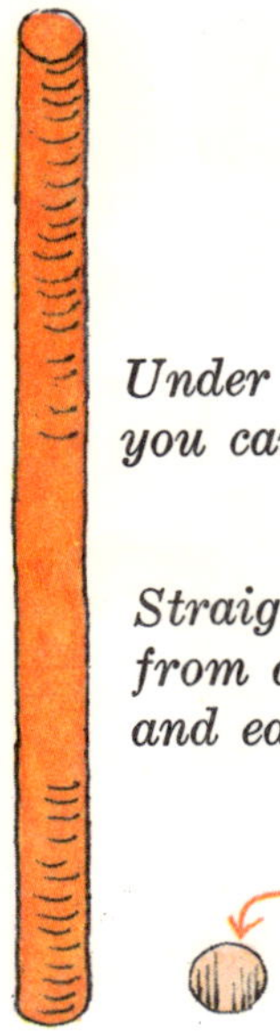

Under a microscope, you can see that:

Straight hair grows from a round follicle and each hair is round.

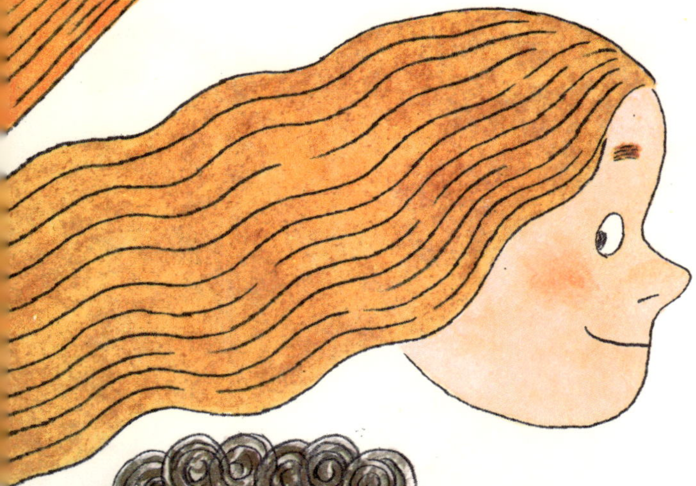

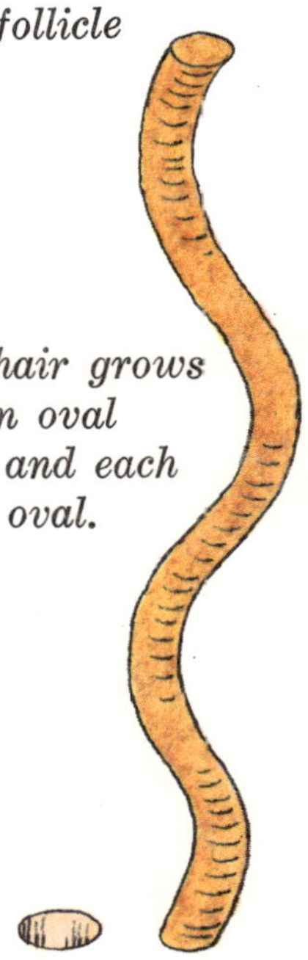

Wavy hair grows from an oval follicle and each hair is oval.

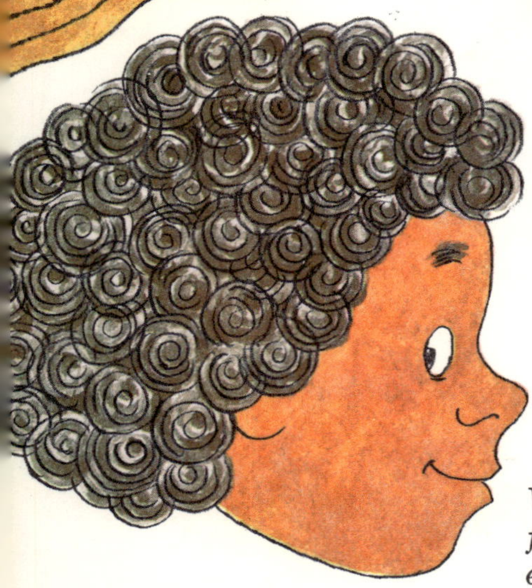

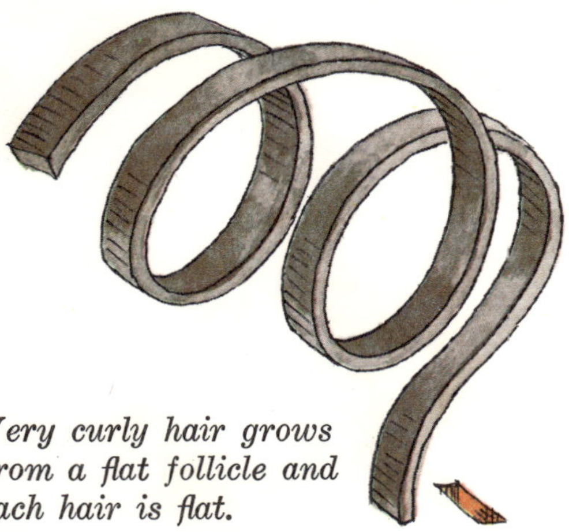

Very curly hair grows from a flat follicle and each hair is flat.

Your own hair color is due to the pigments in your hair cells.

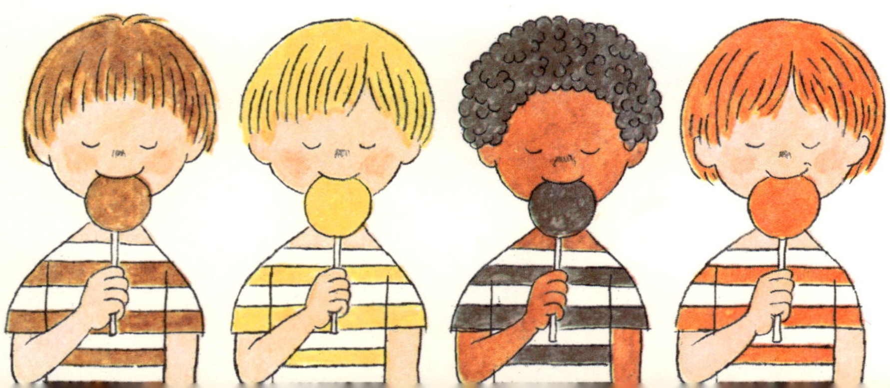

Most of your HAIR may seem to be growing from the top of your head, except for the few hairs of your eyebrows and eyelashes. Actually, you also have hair on most parts of your body, but it's so fine that you can hardly see it. People do get more body hair at about age fourteen, but not all over.

You don't get too much protection from the little crop of body hair you have. In that way, animals are much better off. Think of how well protected from the freezing cold a polar bear is in his permanent, thick fur coat. But your hair does help a bit by keeping the hot sun off your head in the summer, and by keeping your head warmer in the winter. It's a sort of natural hat. Also, eyelashes help keep dust out of your eyes, and the hairs in your nose help keep dust from the lungs.

You have thousands of hairs growing from your scalp. Each hair has a shaft, which is the part you

hair growing through the layers of skin

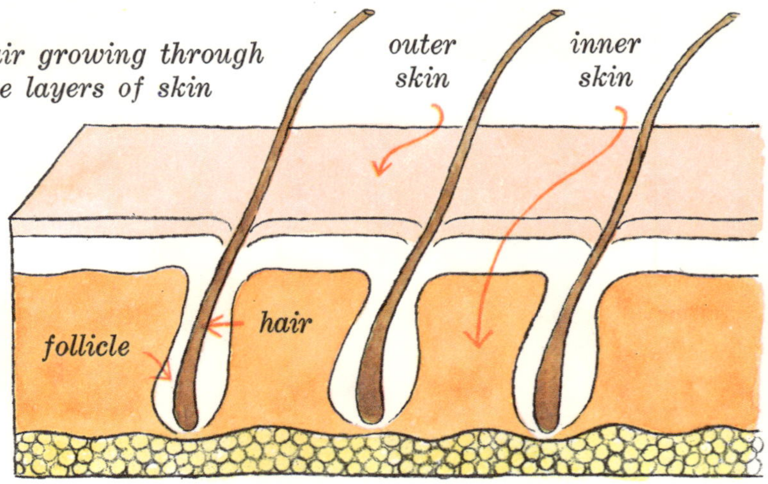

can see, and a root, inside the scalp. The root grows in a follicle, where small blood vessels bring nourishment to it.

Hair grows from the root up. That is why your hair can keep growing after you have a haircut. New cells are added to the bottom all the time. When a new hair first starts to grow, the shaft pushes its way up through the follicle, then up above the surface of the scalp. It keeps growing until it reaches its full length. Then it falls out and a new hair starts to grow in its place.

Each person's scalp hair has its own natural maximum length. Scalp hair grows about a half inch each month, or about six inches a year. So if the full length of *your* scalp hair is twelve inches, it will take about two years for one of your scalp hairs to become full-grown. Then it will fall out. Of course, the hairs are all on slightly different schedules, so you always have a full supply, even though old hairs are falling out and new ones are beginning all the time. (When a man becomes bald, the old hairs keep falling out, but the follicles, for some reason, do not start any new hairs growing to replace them.) The natural length of some people's hair is less than twelve inches, and some have hair that grows much longer. Some people have even been able to grow their hair down to their knees.

Some hair is straight, some is wavy, and some

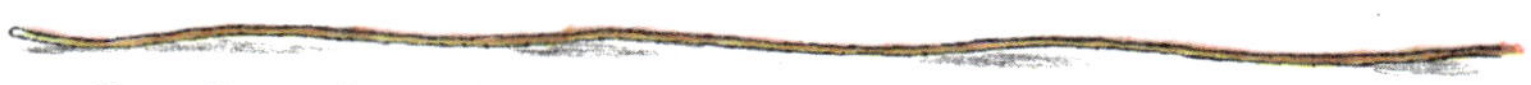

It takes about 7 months for a hair to grow this long.

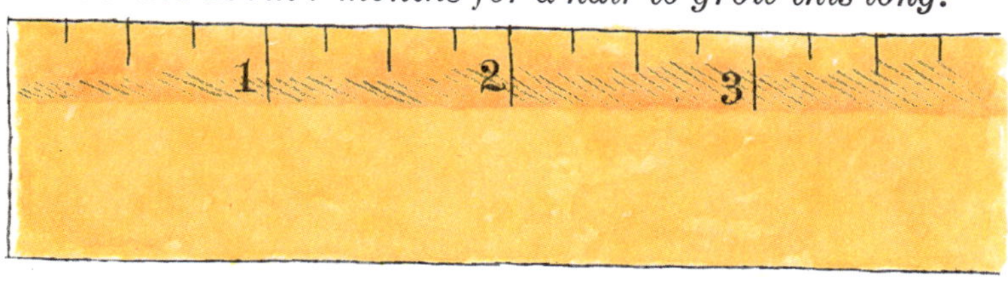

is very curly. The color of people's hair varies, too, from white to the deepest brown-black. The main reason one person's hair is blond, another's is red, and still another's is black is that their hair contains different amounts of brown-black melanin, the same coloring pigment found in the skin. The more you have of it in your hair the darker your hair is. Hair color is something you inherit from your parents and grandparents. Some people change the color of their hair by dyeing it, but the change is only temporary. When new hair grows out above the scalp it will be its natural color. When most people get older their hair gradually turns white. This means that melanin is no longer being added to the new hair cells as they develop in the follicle.

Some people with straight hair try to make it wavy . . .

. . . and some with wavy hair try to make it straight.

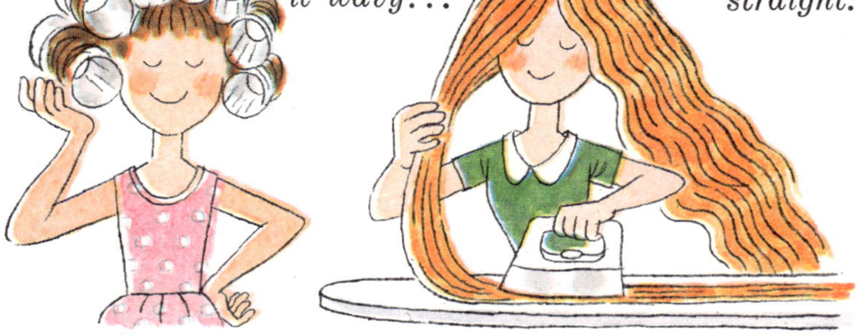

Hair is very strong. A single hair can hold a weight of three ounces.

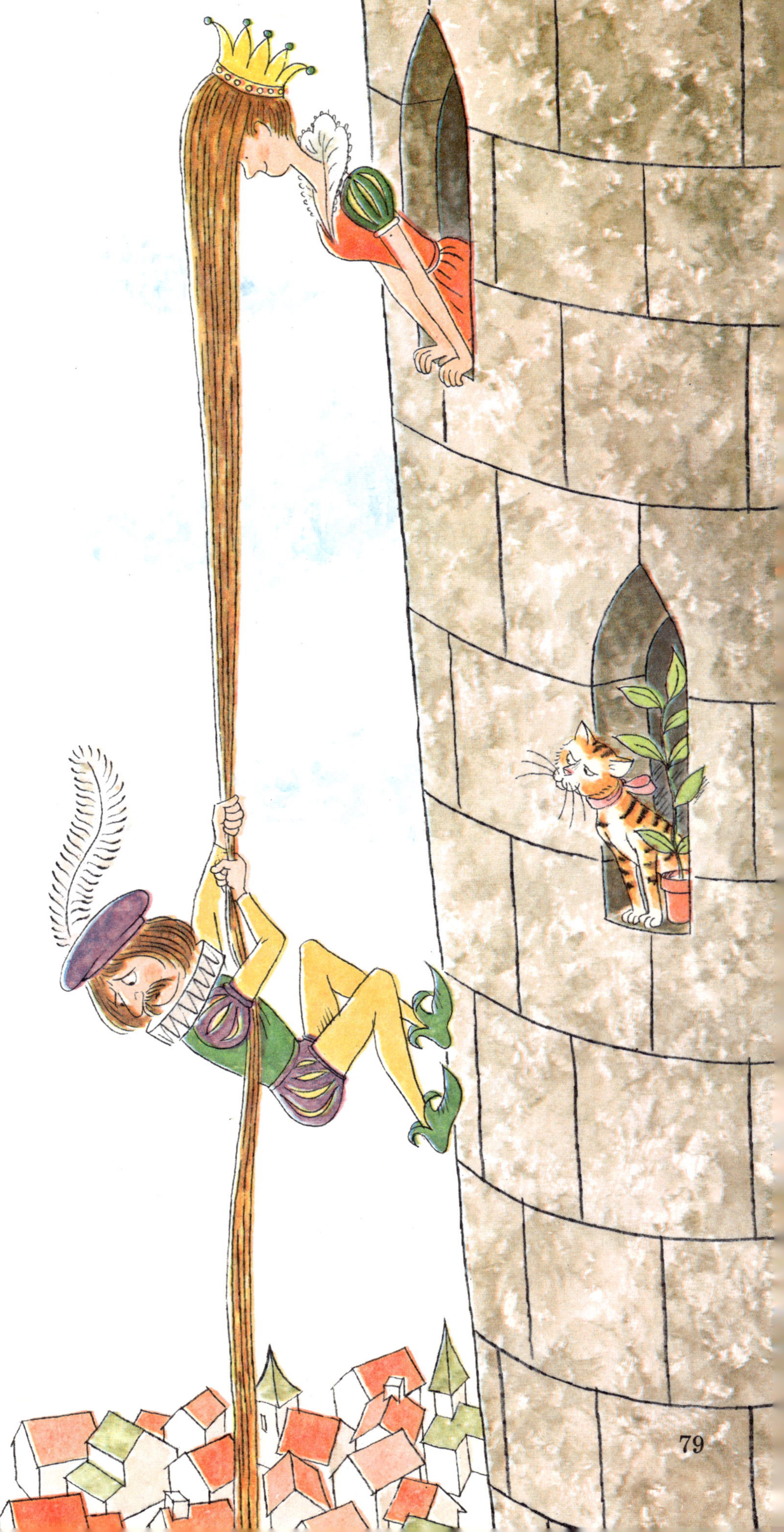

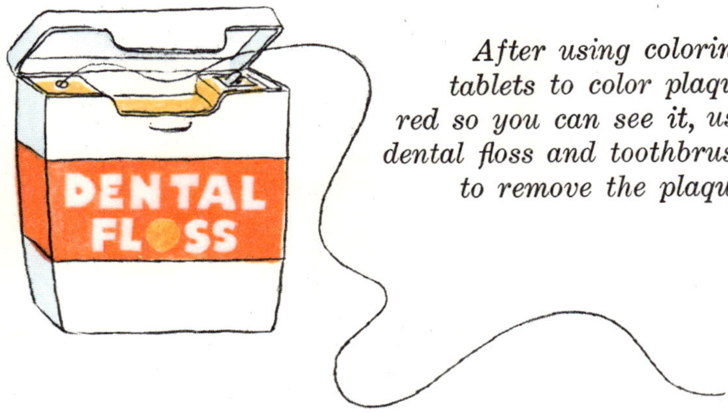

After using coloring tablets to color plaque red so you can see it, use dental floss and toothbrush to remove the plaque.

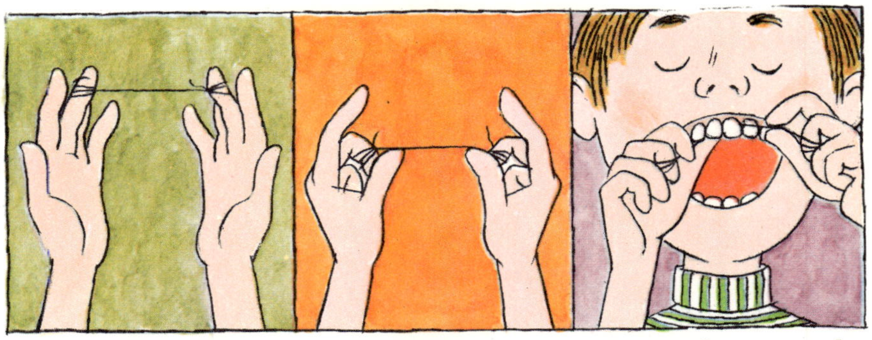

Wrap dental floss around fingers. *Guide with thumbs and forefingers.* *Scrape floss up and down against teeth.*

TOOTH CARE begins with the first baby teeth. At age two or three, when all the baby teeth have grown in, a child should be brushing regularly. This is a good time for a first trip to the dentist.

At each regular visit your dentist usually cleans your teeth—they look better and your gums stay healthy. Then the dentist checks your teeth carefully for any cavities. A cavity begins when a sticky colorless layer called plaque forms on your teeth from the foods you eat. Bacteria stick to the plaque and cause the food to ferment, forming an acid. The acid eats through the hard enamel that protects the outside of the tooth. The acid keeps eating into the tooth, making a hole called a cavity. The dentist fixes a cavity by cleaning away all the damaged tooth material with a tiny electric drill, and filling the hole. If you see the dentist regularly, any new cavities can be found and fixed before they get too large and reach the nerves deep in the tooth.

Your dentist will tell you how to clean your teeth. This is one of the recommended methods:

Pay special attention to removing plaque from your teeth. In addition to providing a place for cavities to start, plaque may pile up and become hard tartar that only a dentist can scrape off. Lots of tartar may cause gum disease and loss of teeth.

To remove plaque you must see where it is. There are tablets you chew or a solution you swish around in your mouth that stains the plaque red. After staining the plaque, tear off eighteen inches of dental floss. Wind an end around each middle finger. Push the floss *gently* between two teeth, using thumbs and forefingers to guide it. Curve the floss around a tooth. Hold it tightly against the tooth, scrape it up and down, and slide it just beneath the gum margin. Do both sides of every tooth, paying particular attention to the red areas.

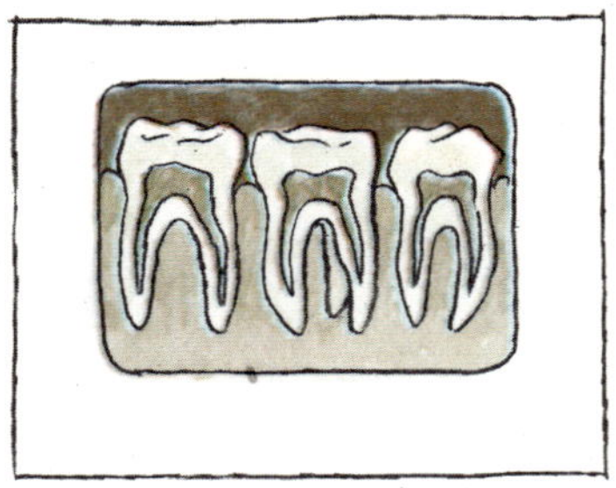

X-ray of teeth and gum

Complete the cleaning with a soft-bristled toothbrush and toothpaste. Place the bristles against your teeth with the tips angled against the gum line. Brush back and forth with a light scrubbing motion. Brush all surfaces of each tooth. Rinse with water.

It is best to brush after every meal, and to avoid eating many sweets, which cause a lot of plaque and decay. Good crunchy foods, like raw carrots, are good for you, and good for your teeth and gums.

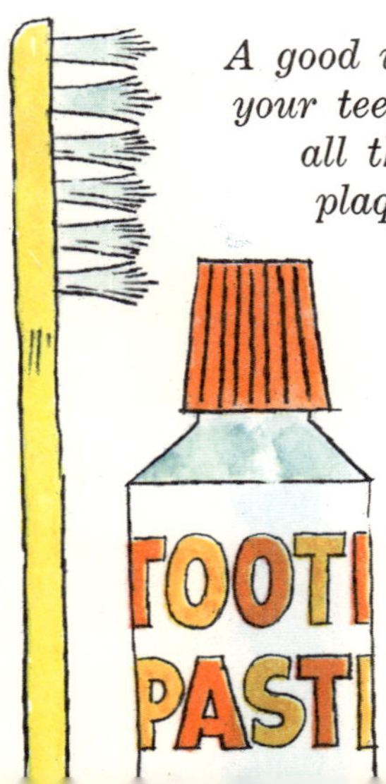

A good way to brush your teeth to remove all the remaining plaque and food:

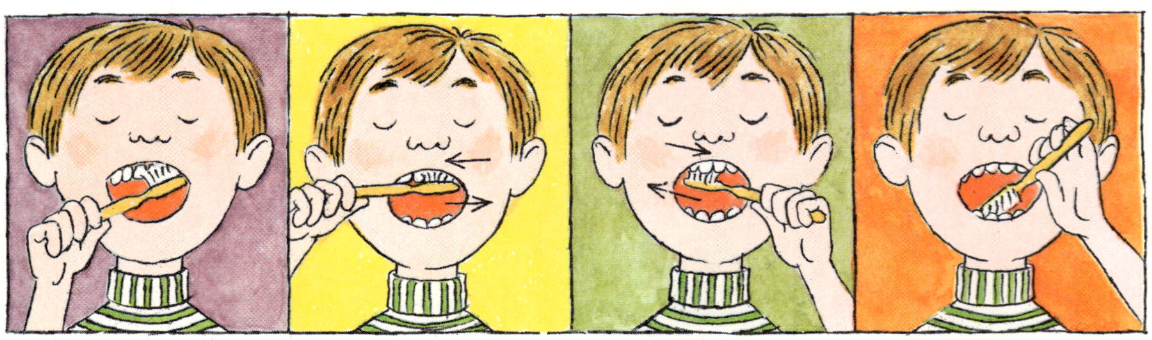

Hold bristle tips angled against gums. *Back and forth with short strokes.* *Brush inside and outside surfaces.* *Brush inside of front teeth with tip.*

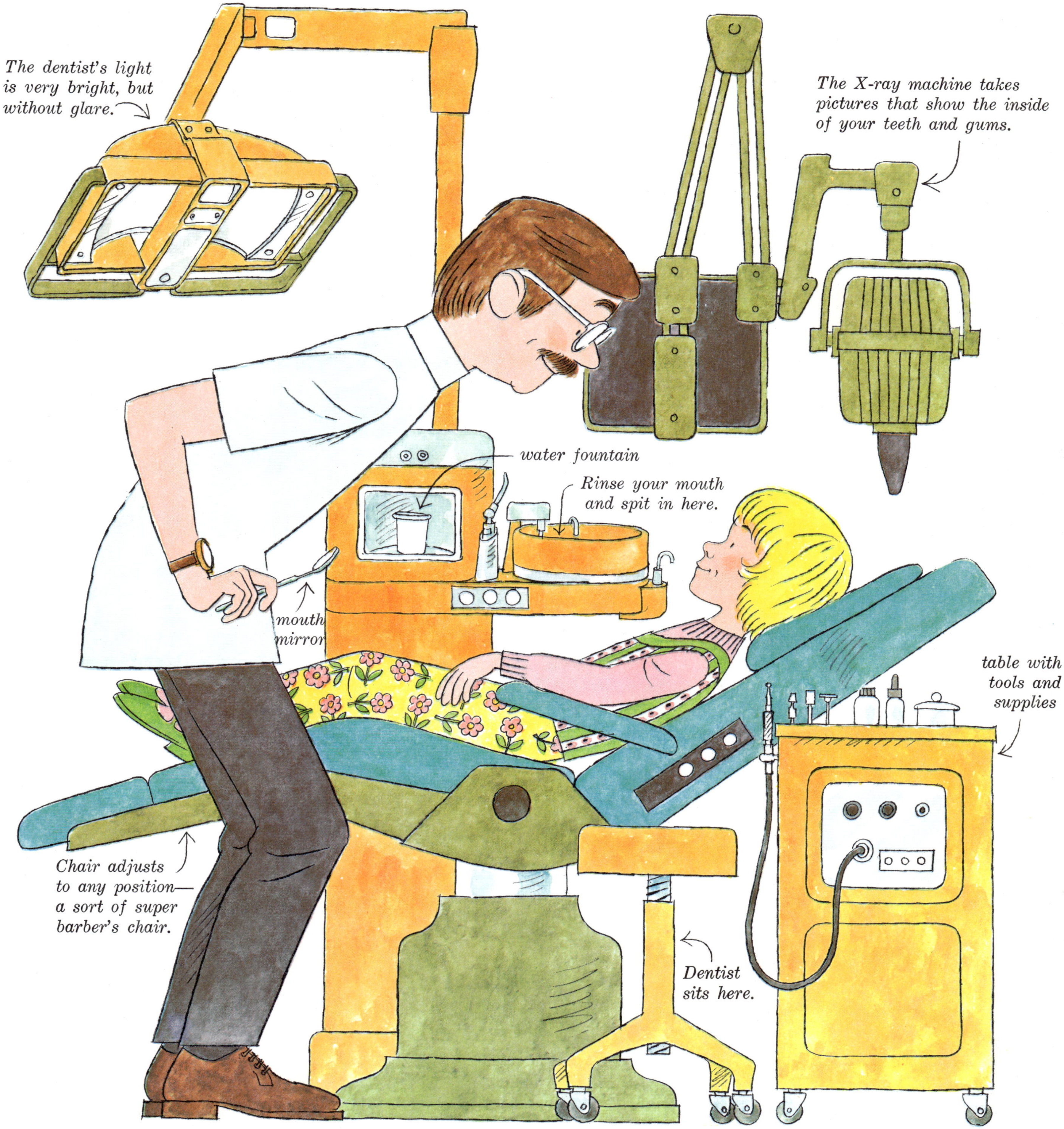
The dentist's light is very bright, but without glare.
The X-ray machine takes pictures that show the inside of your teeth and gums.
water fountain
Rinse your mouth and spit in here.
mouth mirror
table with tools and supplies
Chair adjusts to any position—a sort of super barber's chair.
Dentist sits here.

The modern dentist's office has all kinds of equipment for examining and treating your teeth and gums.

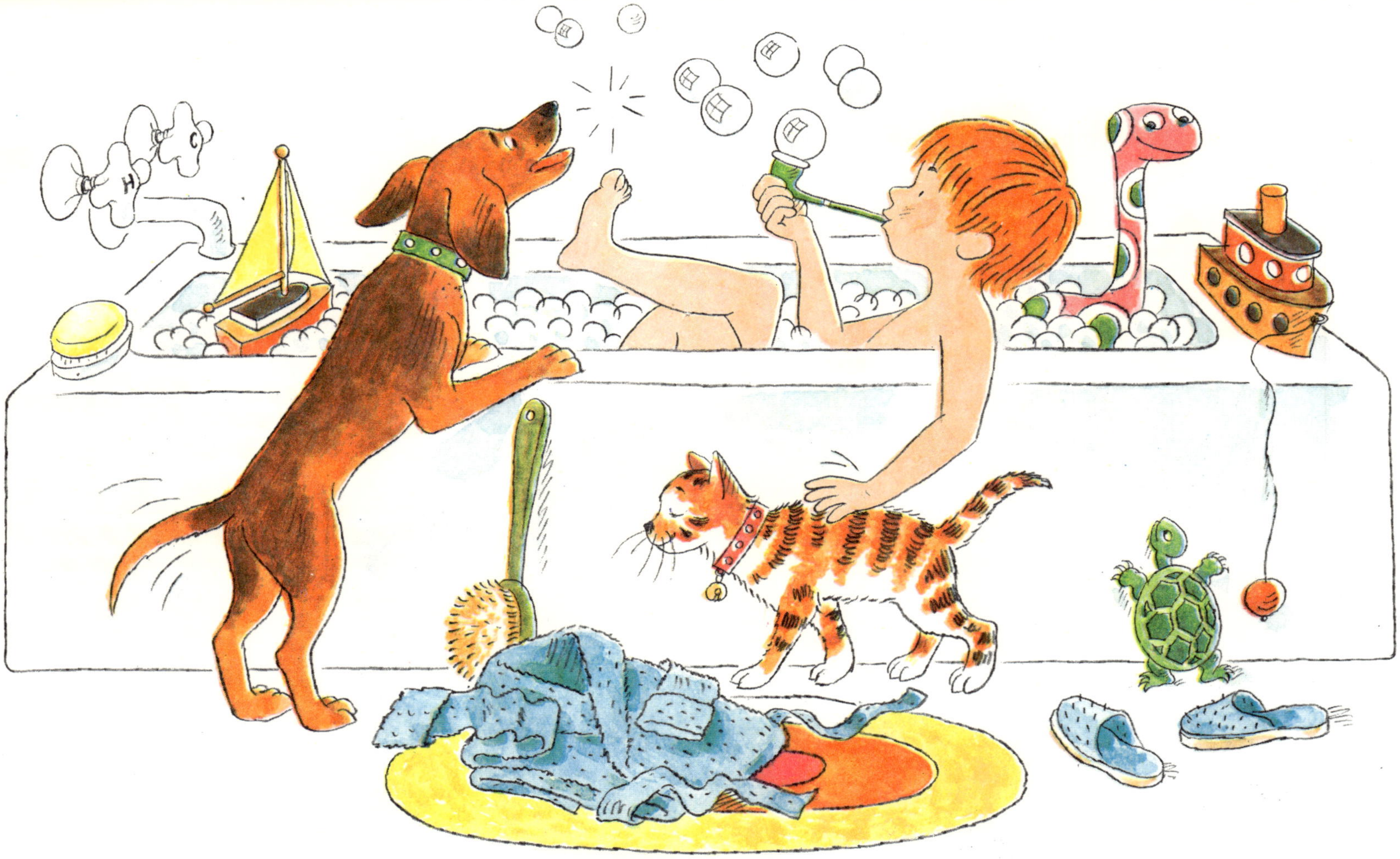

KEEPING CLEAN helps get rid of germs that can cause infections. Some germs can cause disease by entering your body through cuts in your skin. They can also be transferred from unwashed hands to your food and then swallowed. Getting dirt and germs on your hands and other parts of your skin is part of normal living. During the day you handle all sorts of things while you play, outdoors or in. You are bound to touch some that may have infectious germs on them. When you run and play games you may perspire. Dust and dirt stick to the perspiration. Germs grow and multiply on moist, dirty skin. Many diseases of the skin and the rest of the body can start with germs on the skin. Even colds can be spread by accidentally getting cold germs on your hands, and then transferring the cold to yourself by touching the inside of your nose.

Keeping clean means washing your hands and face before eating, and taking a bath and washing your hair regularly. It means cleaning your fingernails and wearing clean clothes.

A century ago Florence Nightingale, the great English wartime nurse, demonstrated the importance of cleanliness. By the use of soap, water, and clean linen in the hospital tents, she was able to keep already-weak wounded soldiers from catching diseases that might kill them. Absolute cleanliness is now the rule in hospitals and other places where there are sick people and many infectious germs.

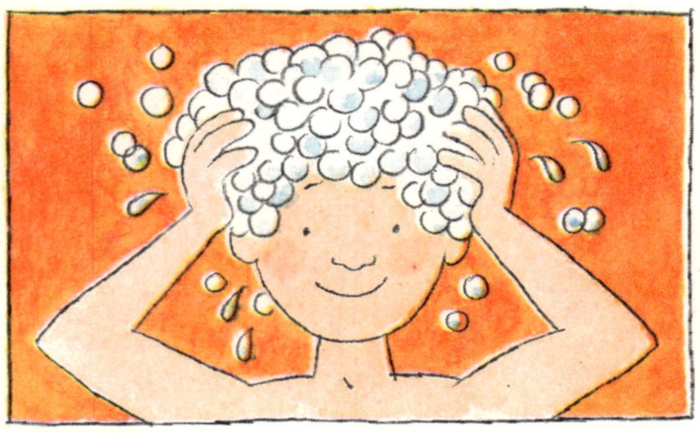

Hair and scalp need regular shampoos.

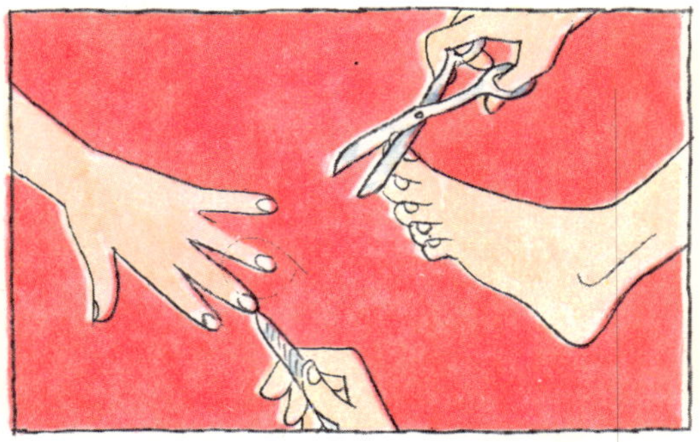

Clean and trim nails and toenails.

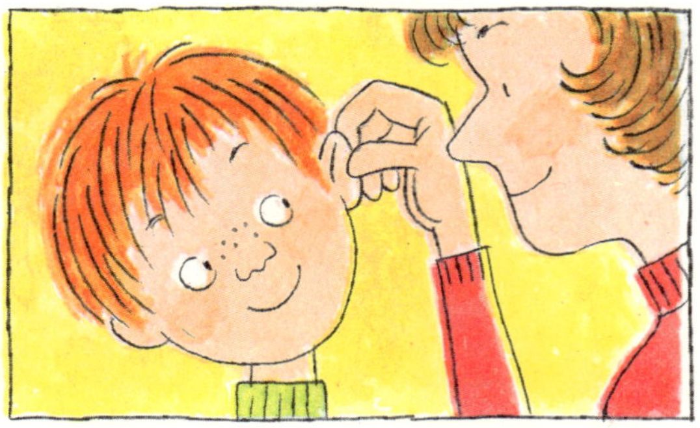

Clean ears gently and with extra care.

All around the world, people have always had many different ways to bathe. Here are just some of them, past and present:

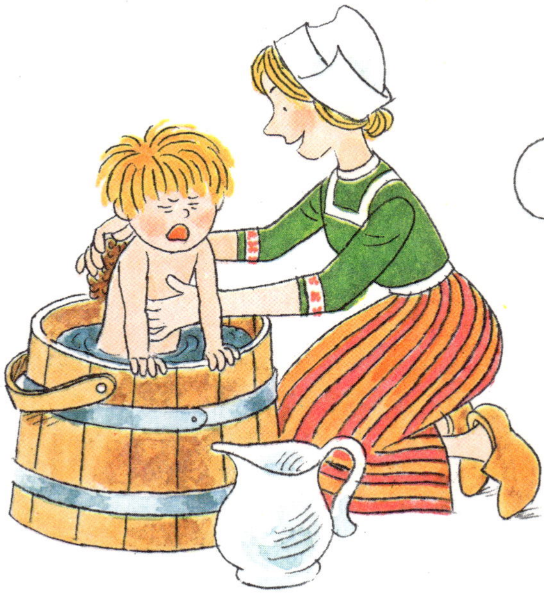

A Dutch child enjoys a bath in long-ago Holland.

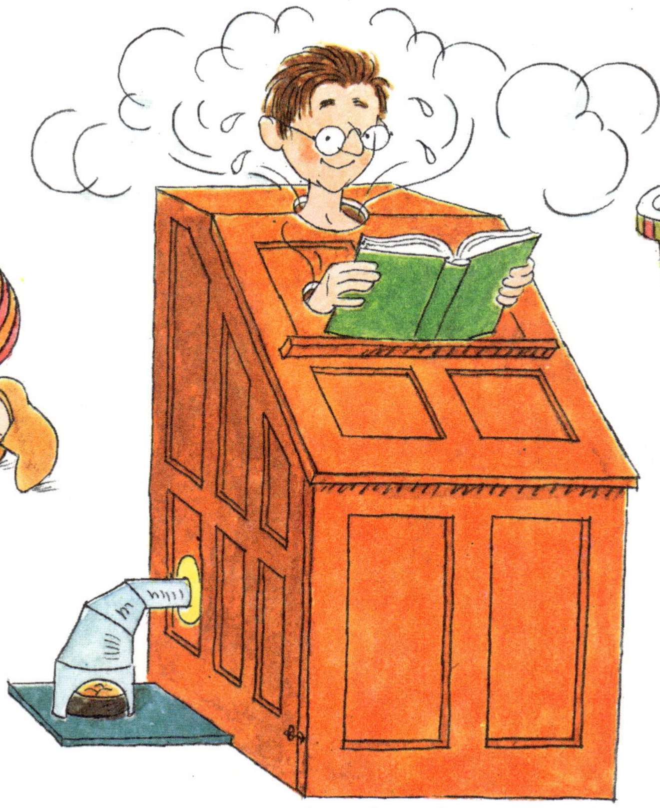

hot-air-and-steam bath Just sit back and relax!

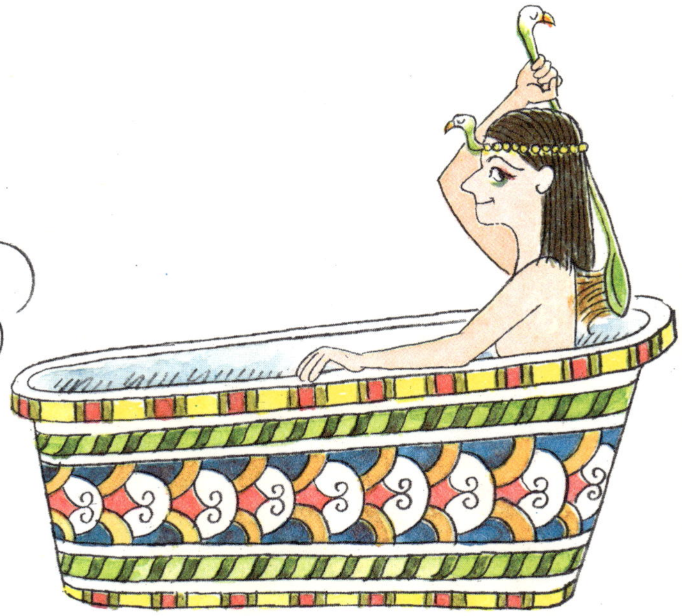

This is the kind of tub Egyptians used 3000 years ago. Looks pretty modern!

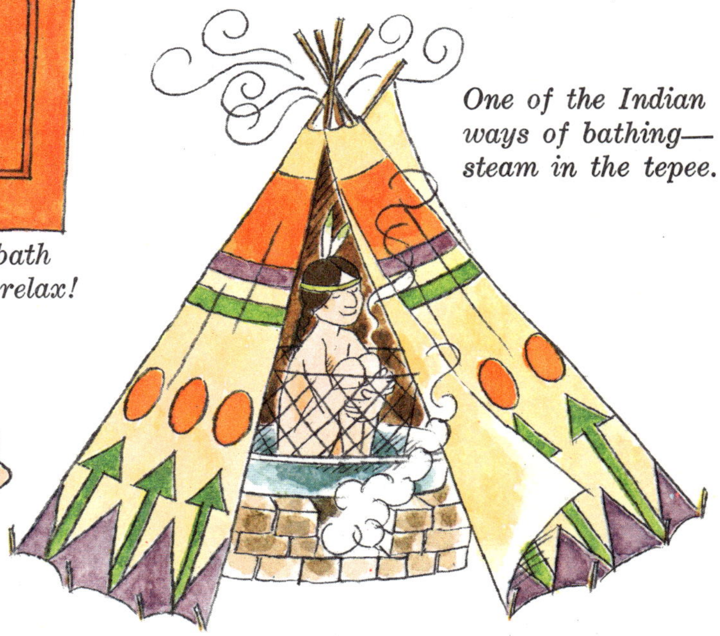

One of the Indian ways of bathing— steam in the tepee.

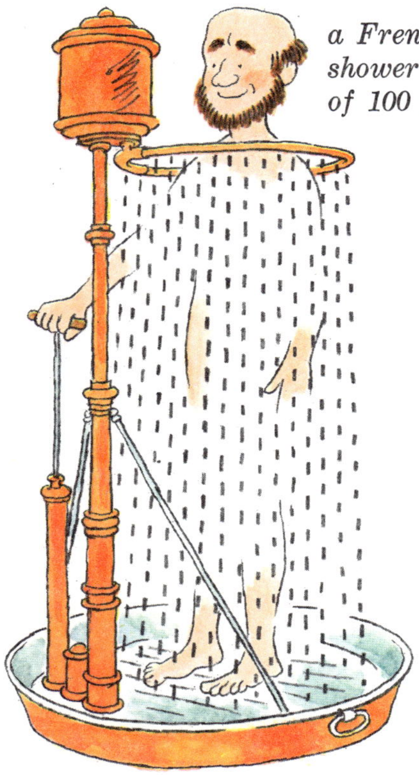

a French shower bath of 100 years ago

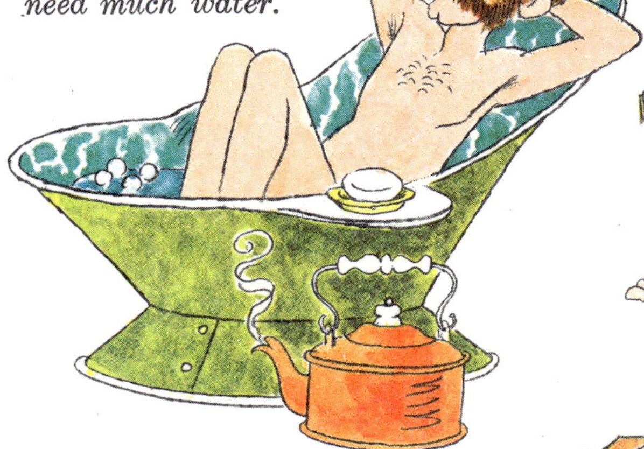

This was called a hip bath. You didn't need much water.

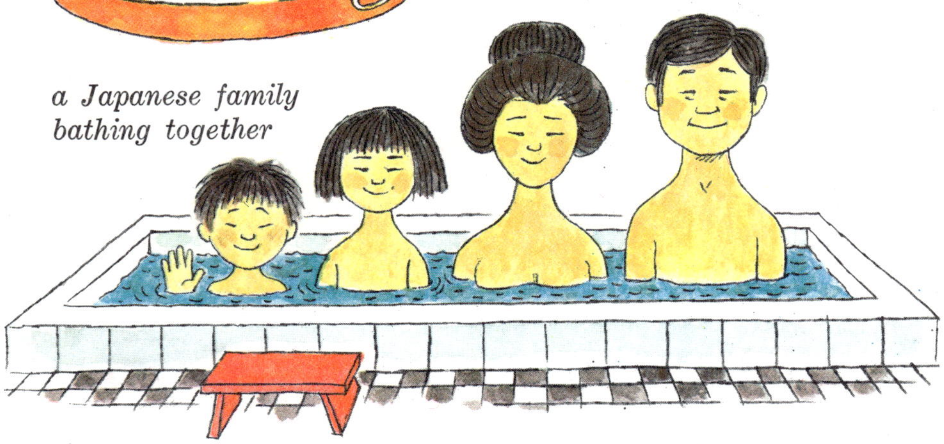

a Japanese family bathing together

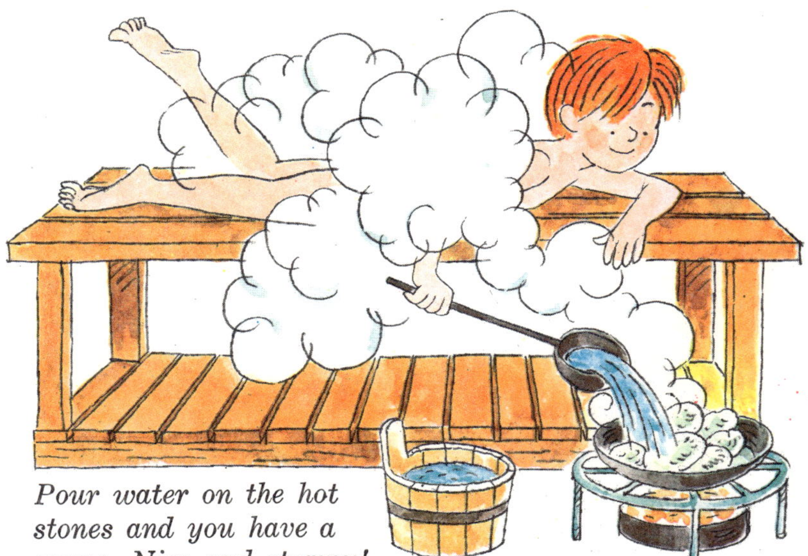

Pour water on the hot stones and you have a sauna. Nice and steamy!

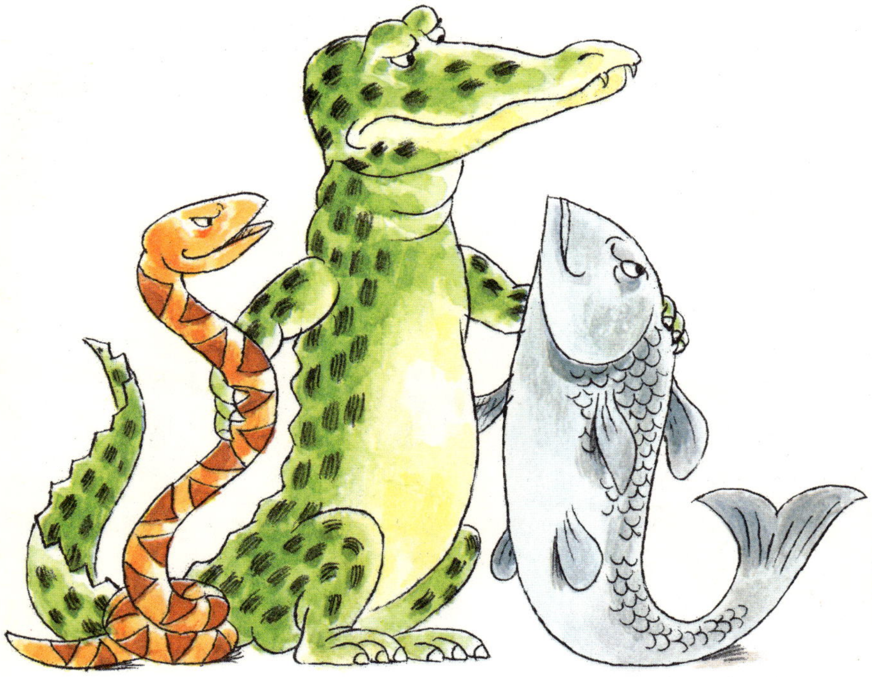

Reptiles, fish, and amphibians are cold-blooded animals. Their body temperature matches that of the surroundings.

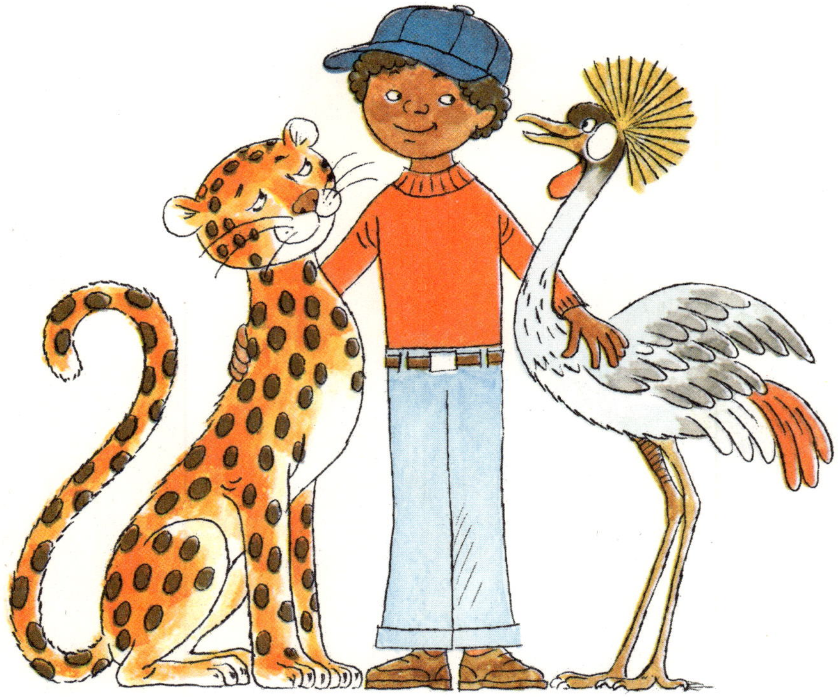

Mammals (including humans) and birds are warm-blooded. Their body temperature doesn't change with the weather.

Our **BODY TEMPERATURE,** in good health, is about 98.6 degrees on the Fahrenheit thermometer. It varies a little bit during the day, but only a degree or so.

We create heat in our bodies by the action of our muscles and organs, and by burning food. The body's temperature is affected by two things—how much heat the body is making, and what the temperature of its surroundings is. If the body is getting too cold, it has ways of warming itself. If it is getting too hot, it has ways of cooling itself.

In a cold place, the body will lose a lot of its heat to its surroundings. To keep the body from getting too cold, the blood vessels near the skin's surface automatically contract (close up a little) to keep most of the warm blood deep inside the body, and away from the skin, where it would give off its warmth to the colder air around it. Also, if the body is getting too cold, the muscles automatically begin to shiver—through their actions the muscles are trying to create more heat for the body.

In a hot place, the body might overheat if it didn't have ways to get rid of some of its heat. The blood vessels in the skin dilate (open wider) to allow more blood to come to the body's surface, where it can get rid of some of its heat. To lose more heat, we perspire. The sweat glands bring perspiration, which is mostly water, out of the

There is very little change in body temperature even if the air temperature goes up to 100 degrees . . .

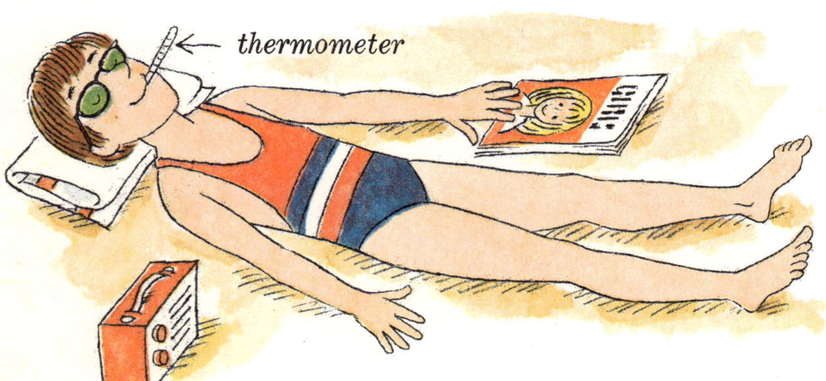

. . . or down to zero!

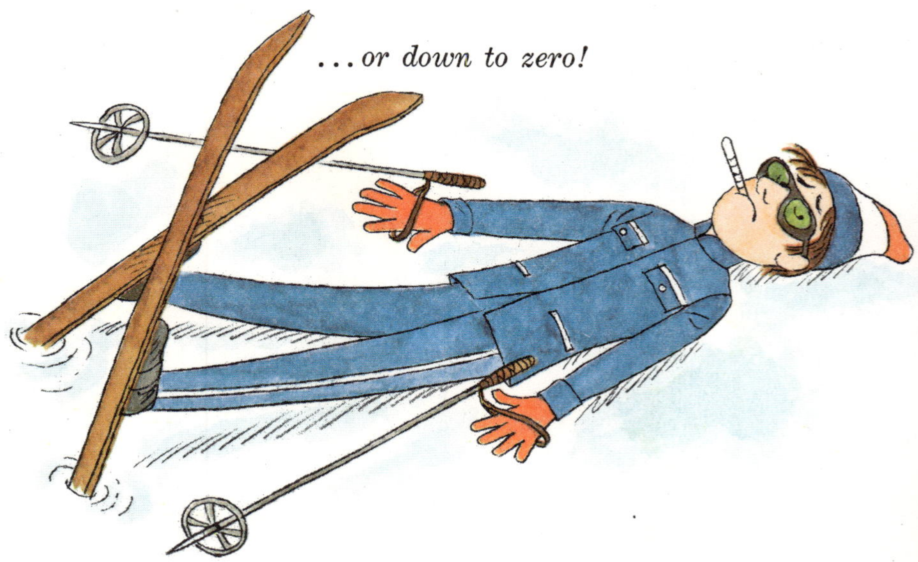

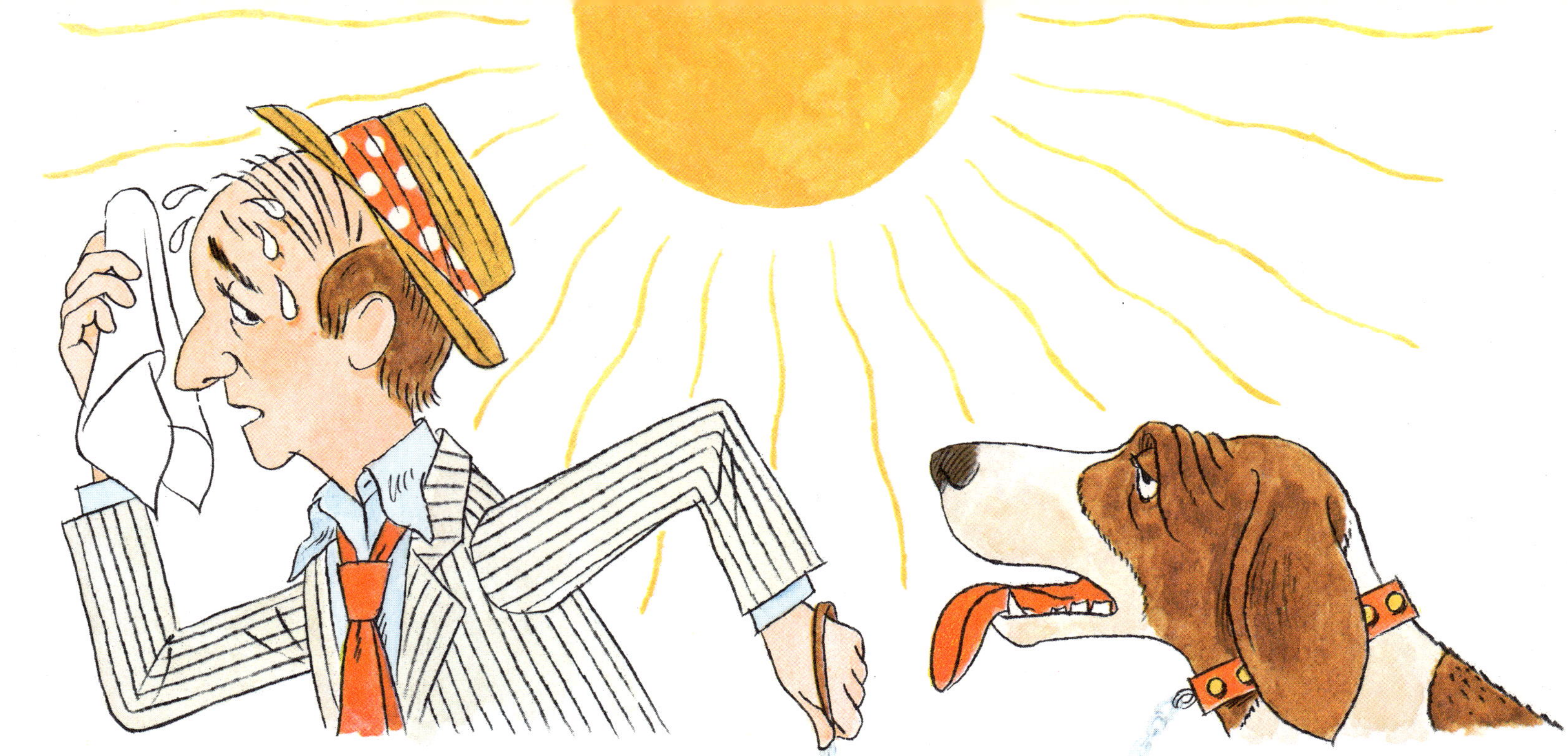

When hot, we perspire. As the perspiration evaporates, it cools the skin. This helps to cool the rest of the body.

A dog can't perspire—he has hardly any sweat glands. To get cool, he pants, and water evaporates from his tongue.

blood and force it to the skin's surface through the pores. As this perspiration evaporates into the air, heat is withdrawn from the outer tissues of the body.

On a hot humid day, we are very uncomfortable for two reasons. The air may be close to body temperature and will not draw away much heat from the blood. And, since humid air already has a lot of moisture in it, not much perspiration can evaporate into it. With both cooling mechanisms slowed down, no wonder we feel hot and sticky.

Of course, choosing the right clothes is another thing we humans can do to help control our body temperature. Our heating system is not good enough to protect us from severe cold without some warm clothes to help. And our cooling system couldn't do its job very well if we wore tight or heavy clothes on a hot day.

Like humans, other warm-blooded animals can vary their body temperatures from inside. But the body temperature of cold-blooded animals such as snakes, frogs, turtles, and salamanders depends only on their surroundings. For example, if a snake stayed in the hot sun, its body would get hotter and hotter. So it has to hide in the ground or in the shade to keep cool. If it is driven out it wriggles as fast as it can to another shady spot; otherwise the heat might kill it.

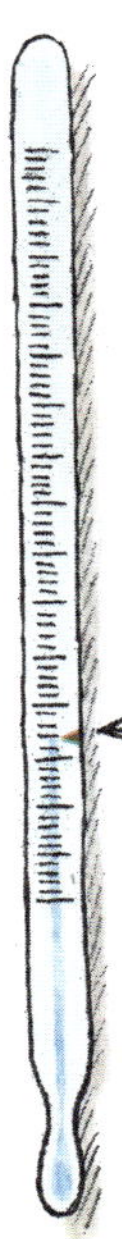

This is 98.6 degrees on a Fahrenheit thermometer, normal temperature for people.

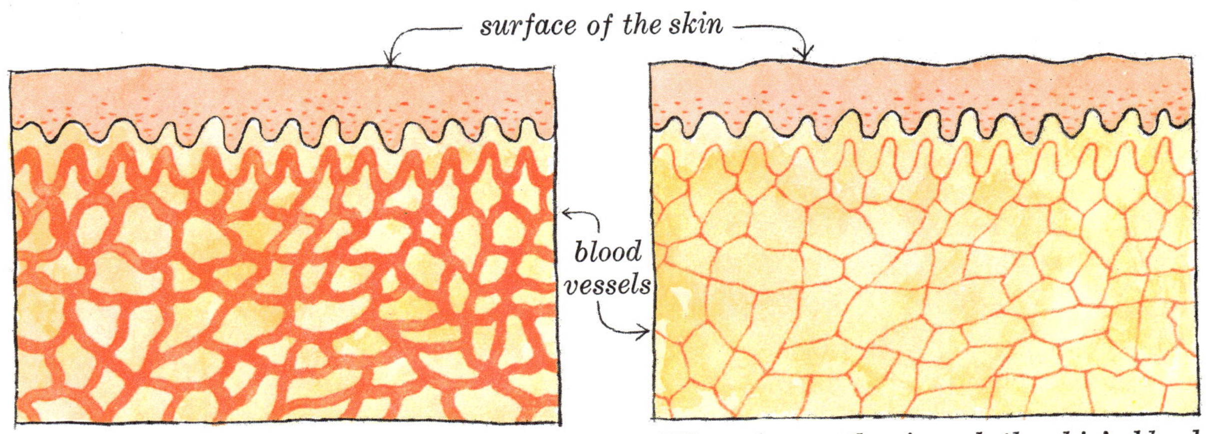

When the weather is hot, the skin's blood vessels open wider. More blood comes to the surface to lose its heat to the air.

When the weather is cool, the skin's blood vessels contract. More blood stays to the inside of the body, keeping warmth in.

SICKNESS means that some part of your body is not working well. It is under attack. Usually, harmful bacteria or virus germs are causing the trouble. When your body is healthy you stand a good chance of resisting the attack, but when you haven't been taking good care of yourself, when you haven't been eating the kind of food you should and getting as much rest as you need, you are likely to get sick. These are some of the more common sicknesses:

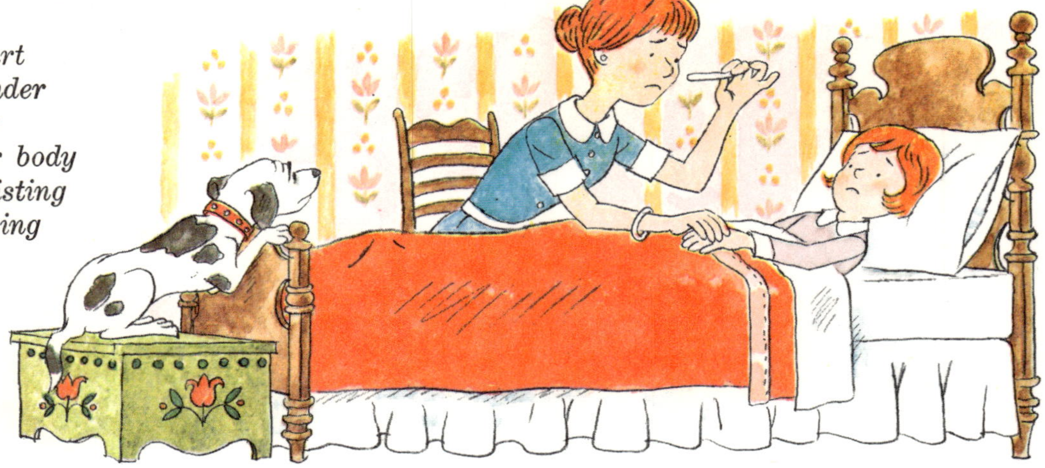

A COLD is caused by a virus so tiny that we can see it only with the most powerful electron microscope. The virus infects the lining of the nasal passages and spreads easily from person to person through sneezes and coughs. It seems that being too tired makes you less able to fight a cold that you may come in contact with. Once a cold infects the nasal passages, it often spreads to the throat. The cold makes the little blood vessels in your nose swell up, and mucous seeps out, blocking the nose and making it hard to breathe. You cough and may have a fever. It's all very uncomfortable. But fortunately it's not serious. Most colds last about a week or so. Plenty of rest and liquids are recommended.

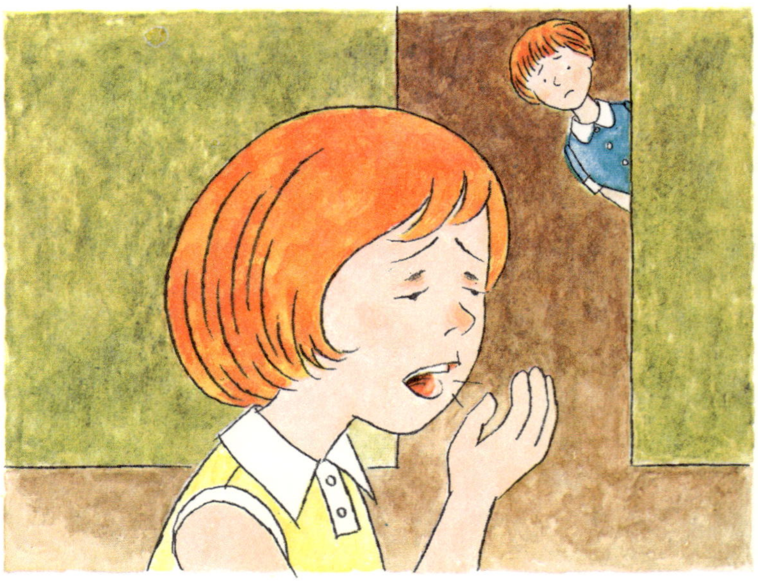

A FEVER means the body temperature is higher than normal (98.6° F.), although normal varies during the day by about one degree—usually being highest late in the afternoon and lowest early in the morning. Fever is not a sickness itself, but it means the body is fighting an infection of some kind, trying to stay well. When the brain gets a message that harmful bacteria are in the body, it sends signals to close the sweat glands and contract the surface blood vessels. The body temperature goes up, which kills many kinds of bacteria. More blood is kept deep in the body where white cells can fight the infection. It is wise to see a doctor about a fever, for help in fighting the infection causing it.

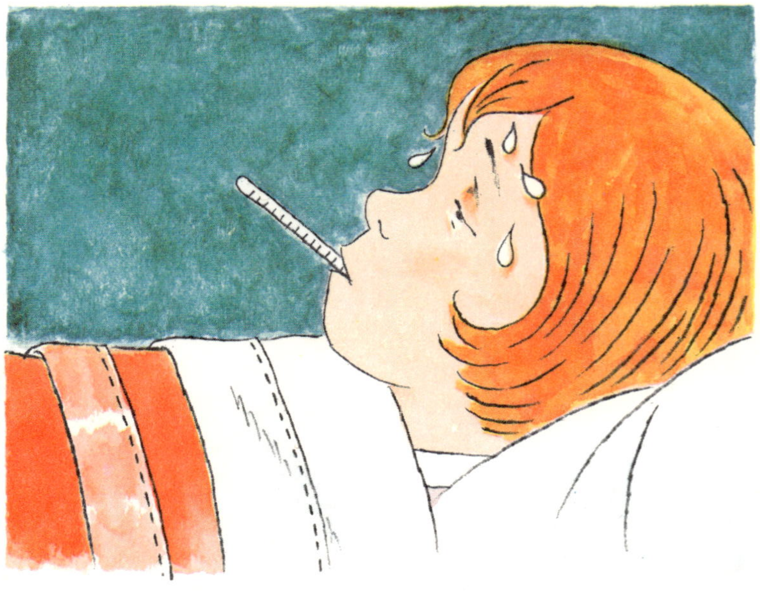

An EARACHE can have different causes. If the pain is in the outer ear it might be caused by too much ear wax, or something in the ear that doesn't belong there. Most often the earache is caused by an infection in the middle ear. A tube connects the middle ear to the back of the throat. It helps keep the air pressure in the middle ear the same as the outside air pressure. But harmful bacteria can sometimes pass along the tube from the throat to the middle ear, causing an infection. Bacteria might be forced up the tube into the middle ear if you have a cold and blow your nose too hard. Either kind of earache could become serious if not promptly cared for by a doctor.

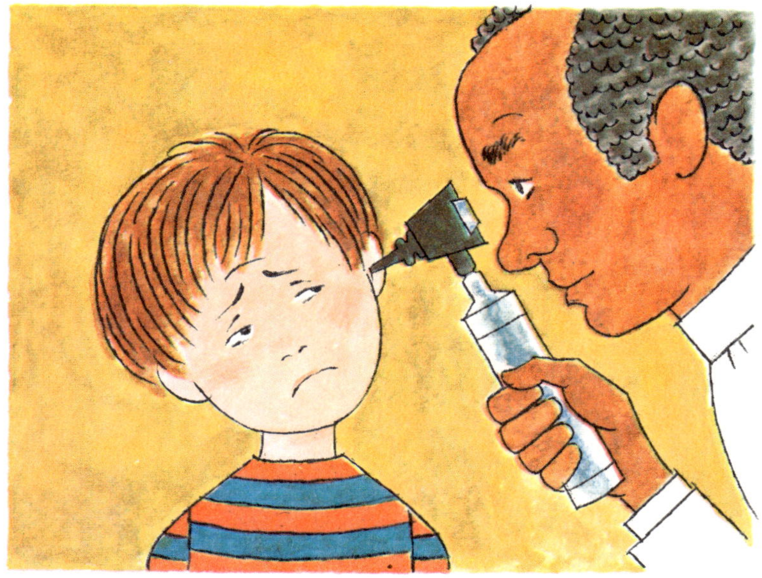

A RASH can break out for many reasons. Any serious irritation to the skin may cause it, and what irritates one person's skin may not have any effect on another's. Some people have skin allergies. Food is a common one. Some people's skin reacts violently after they have eaten strawberries; other people are sensitive to fish, nuts, or other food. Some skins are allergic to certain fabrics—wool is often an irritant. Plants can mean trouble—most people will get a severe rash if they touch poison ivy. A rash is also a sign of some diseases, such as measles. The doctor must determine what, among so many possibilities, caused the rash before it can be successfully treated.

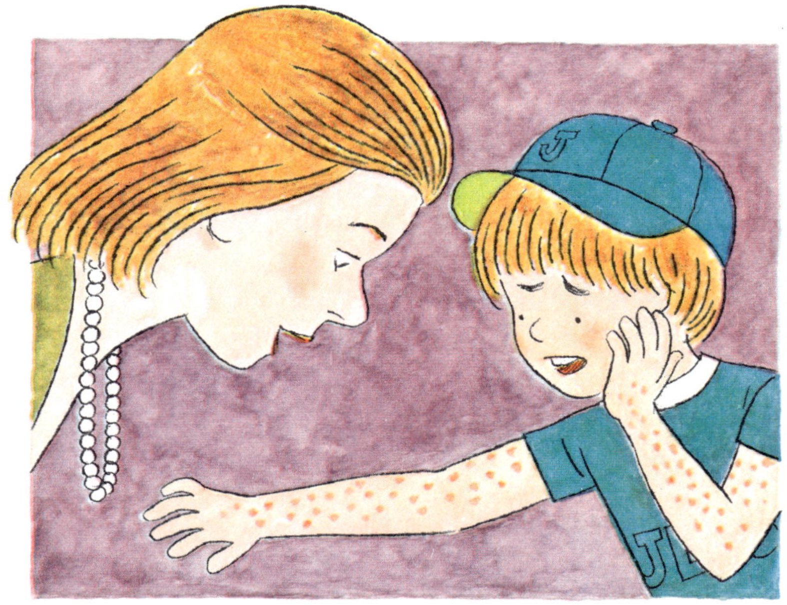

A TOOTHACHE probably won't happen if you see your dentist regularly. Most often a toothache starts when a tooth is so decayed that the pulp of the tooth is exposed to infection. If you visit your dentist regularly cavities can be discovered and filled long before they are deep enough to reach the pulp, where the nerve is. The larger and deeper the decay, the more intense a toothache may be. Sometimes the first indication of a deep cavity is a sudden, sharp pain while eating something hot, cold, or very sweet. Of course, if you break a tooth and expose the pulp, that, too, will cause a toothache. A dentist should treat the tooth as soon as possible, to keep it from becoming infected.

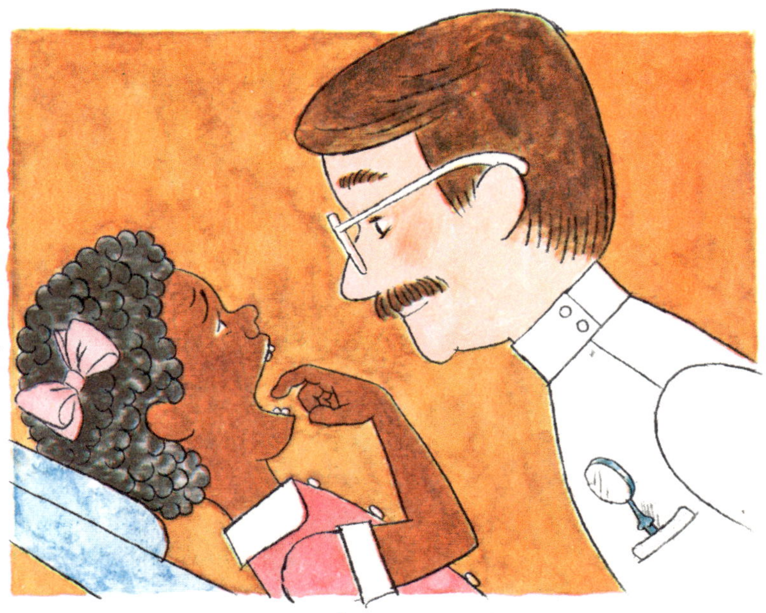

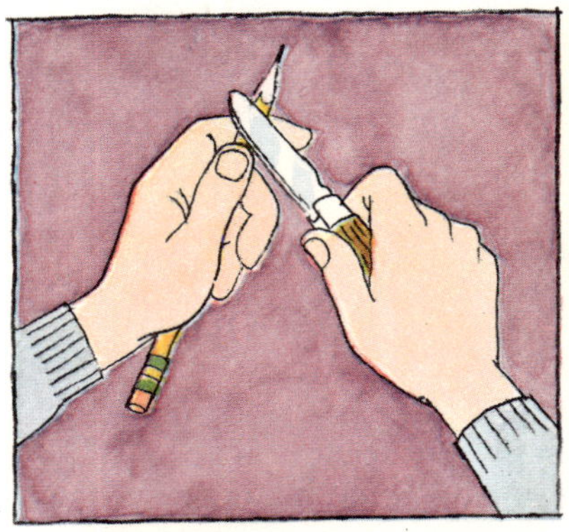

You're sharpening a pencil. Whoops—the knife slips!

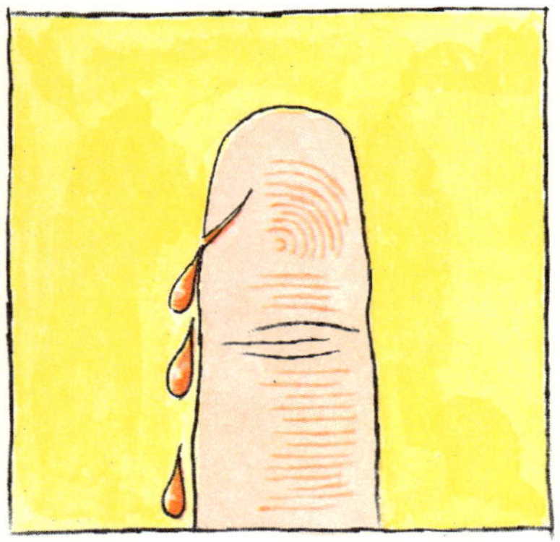

You have a cut—harmful bacteria get into the wound.

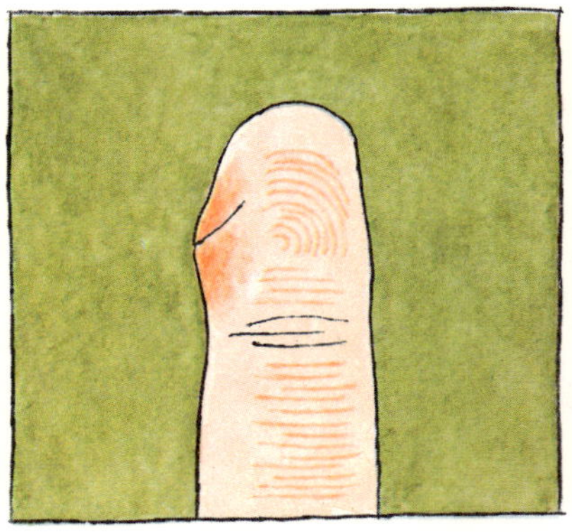

The wounded area gets red. It swells—it's painful.

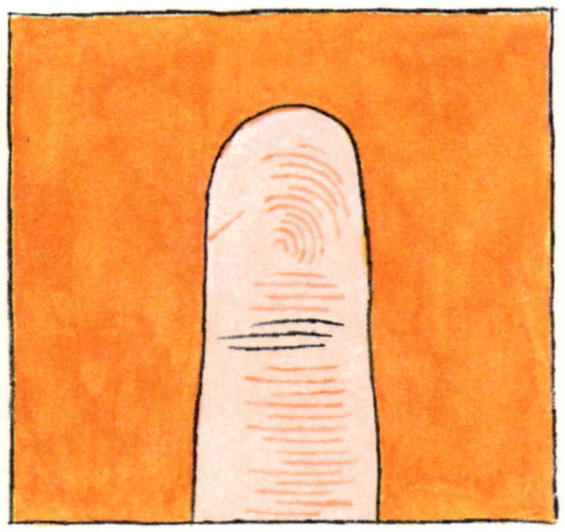

Your body overcomes the infection—the wound heals.

HEALING of an infected cut begins after the body's protective system has won its battle with the invading bacteria.

The skin is the body's natural armor against harmful bacteria. But when it has been cut by something that had bacteria on it, an infection might start. An infection might also start from bacteria getting into the cut from anything nearby. The body then calls on its inner protective forces to destroy the invader.

The area around the bacteria-infected cut becomes red, swollen, and painful. *Red,* because blood vessels react to injury by enlarging so that more blood comes to the area; *swollen,* because the swollen blood vessels leak fluid from the blood into the injured areas; and *painful,* because the injured tissue releases special chemicals which irritate nerve endings, causing pain (so you'll know you've cut yourself).

The extra blood flow brings an army of white blood cells to the infection. The white cells work their way out of the blood vessels and into the infected tissue, and the fight is on. The first thing the white-blood-cell army does is surround the enemy to keep them from spreading any farther—the white cells form a wall with their own bodies around the bacteria. Inside the wall other white cells attack the trapped bacteria to destroy them. Some of the bacteria may sometimes be carried away by the lymph vessels to the lymph nodes to be destroyed there by other white cells. Meanwhile the bacteria keep multiplying, so that the fighting is furious and many white blood cells die before the battle is won. Their dead bodies and those of the dead bacteria are gathered up in the infected area and form the white matter called pus, which is eventually drained away. The battle is over and the cut heals.

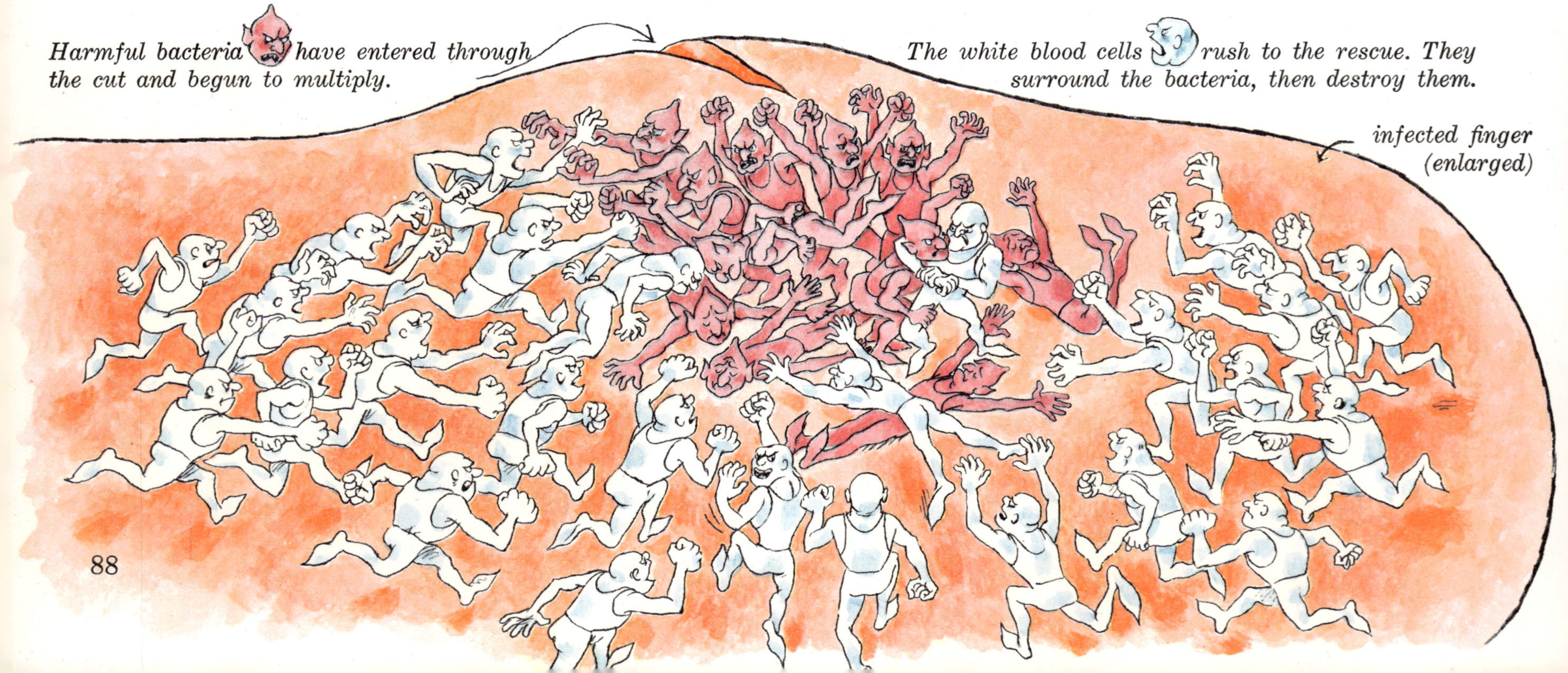
Harmful bacteria have entered through the cut and begun to multiply.
The white blood cells rush to the rescue. They surround the bacteria, then destroy them.
infected finger (enlarged)

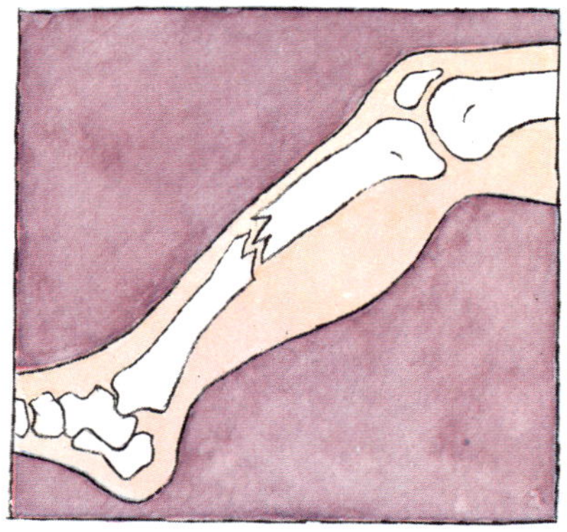

There's been a serious fall— the shinbone is broken!

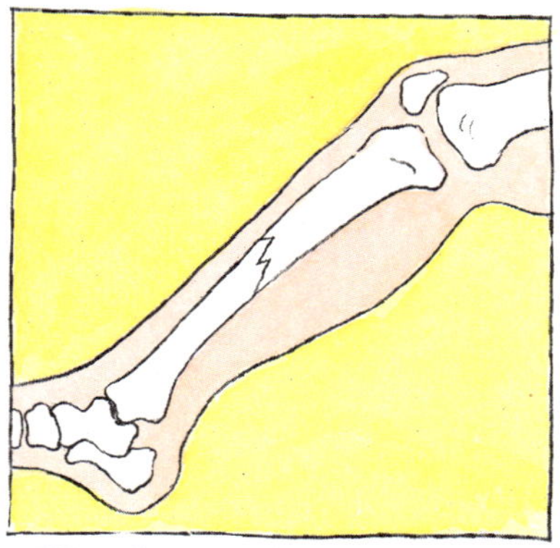

The doctor fits the bone's edges together carefully.

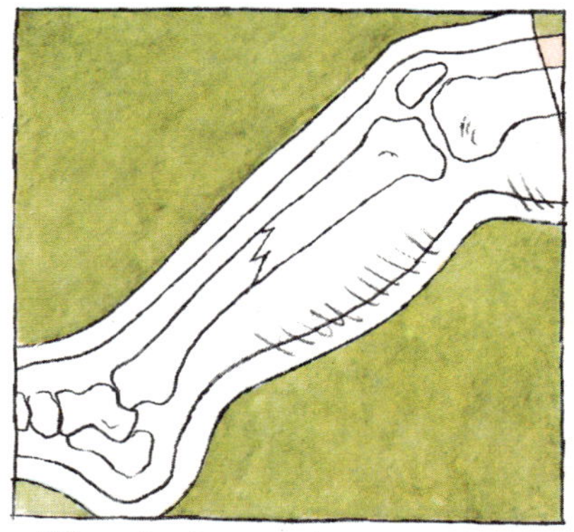

The doctor puts a cast on to hold the bone in place.

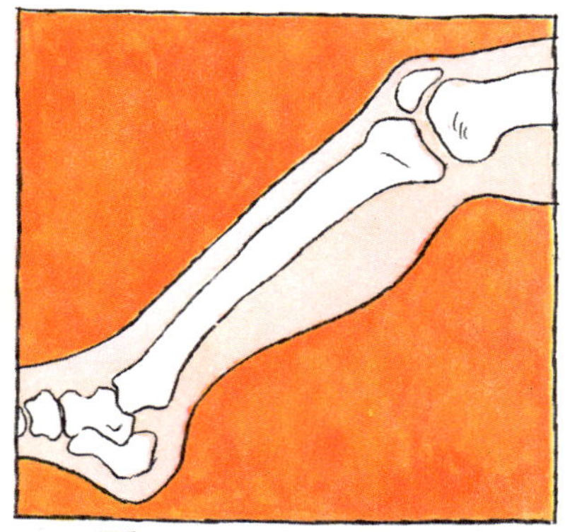

The cast is removed when the bone is healed.

HEALING of a broken bone takes place best if the broken ends are put back together and held firmly until they grow together. If this is not done, the bone may not heal properly. It might be crooked, too long or short, or weak.

An X ray (a picture of the inside of the body) shows the doctor how the bone is broken. After matching the broken ends and making sure the bone is straight, the doctor usually applies a cast to hold it in that position until it heals. A cast is made with bandage that has plaster in it. The doctor wets the bandage and wraps it around and around the broken arm or leg (casts are used mostly for arms and legs). The plaster bandage dries quickly, becomes hard, and keeps the healing bone from moving out of place. Sometimes the doctor won't use a cast. You couldn't breathe if you had a tight plaster cast around your chest for a broken rib, so the doctor uses adhesive tape to hold the rib in place. For a broken finger the doctor often uses a splint, a piece of plastic or metal taped to the finger to keep it from bending while the finger bone is healing.

Once the doctor's work is finished, and the broken bone is kept from moving, nature takes over and the healing begins. First, blood from the broken blood vessels near the break begins to clot. The clotting seals the torn vessels and stops any more blood flow. Nearby vessels take over the broken vessels' job until they heal. Then each broken bone end begins to grow new bone cells. The new cells grow toward each other, touch, then start to knit together. This goes on until there is more bone material at that spot than there was before the break. This bulge is called a callus—because the bone is thicker there, it is even stronger than it was before it was broken!

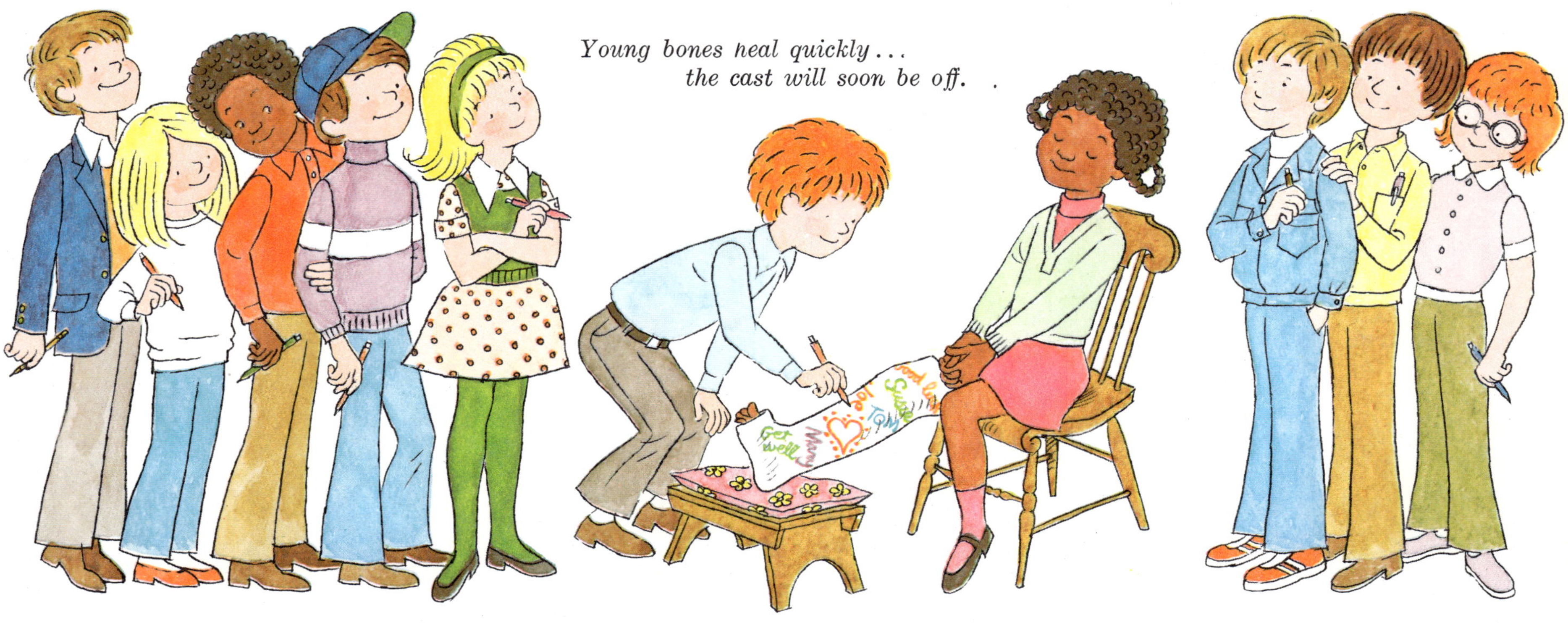

Young bones heal quickly . . . the cast will soon be off.

DISCOVERIES about the body have a long history. Sickness used to be blamed on evil spirits. Primitive people tried to frighten away these spirits with masks and dances. Then came a search for natural causes of disease. Leaves and bark of certain trees were early medicines. Egypt, Greece, and Rome had many doctors. Romans knew how important it was to keep clean and drink clean water. They built public baths and water supply systems. After that, for a thousand years, little was learned about the body or sickness. When plagues came and millions died, doctors were helpless. Then, in 1543, Vesalius

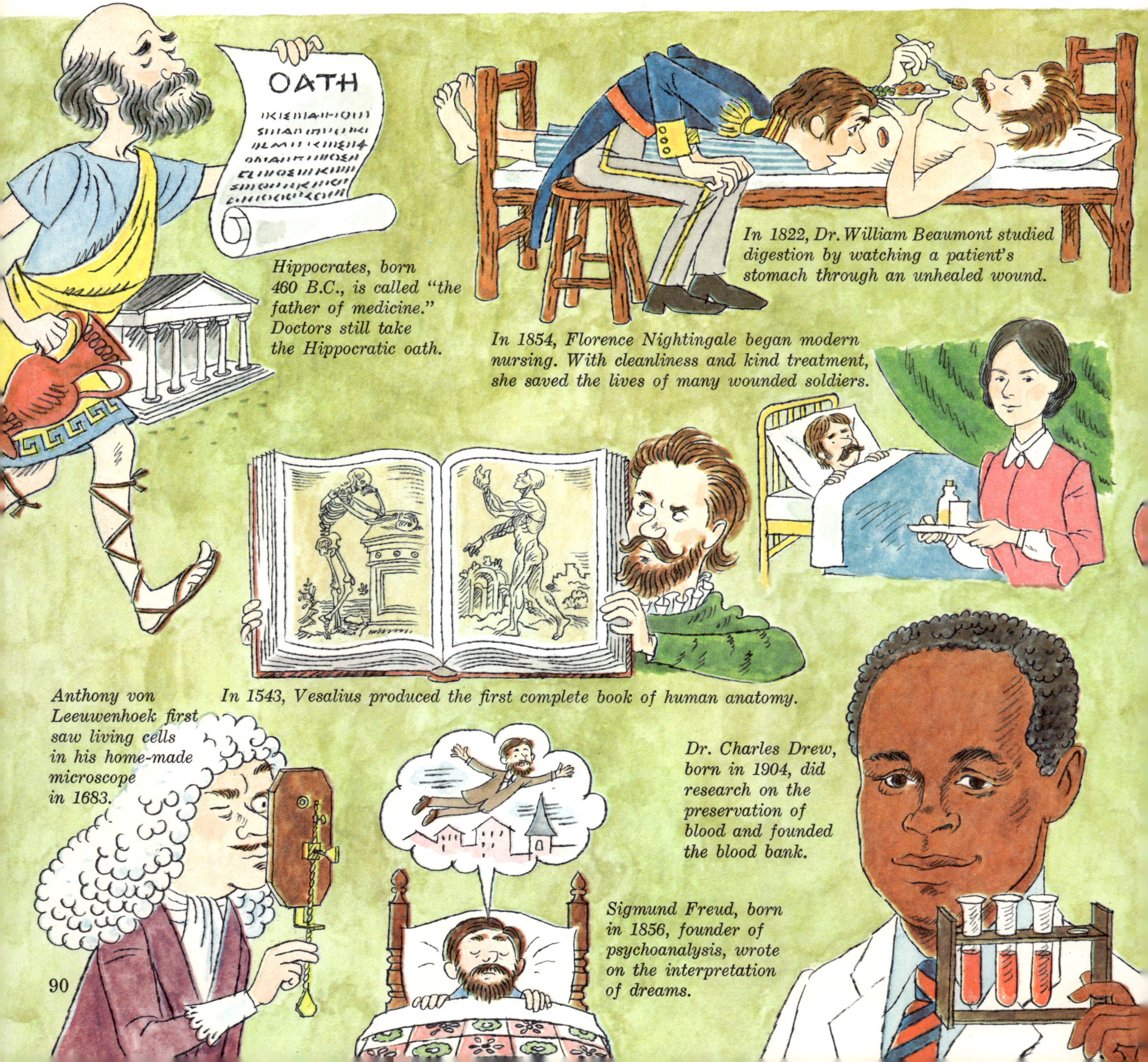

Hippocrates, born 460 B.C., is called "the father of medicine." Doctors still take the Hippocratic oath.

In 1822, Dr. William Beaumont studied digestion by watching a patient's stomach through an unhealed wound.

In 1854, Florence Nightingale began modern nursing. With cleanliness and kind treatment, she saved the lives of many wounded soldiers.

In 1543, Vesalius produced the first complete book of human anatomy.

Anthony von Leeuwenhoek first saw living cells in his home-made microscope in 1683.

Dr. Charles Drew, born in 1904, did research on the preservation of blood and founded the blood bank.

Sigmund Freud, born in 1856, founder of psychoanalysis, wrote on the interpretation of dreams.

published the first book that described the body pretty accurately. Harvey, in 1628, showed that the heart pumps the blood through the body in a continuous, returning stream. Leeuwenhoek (LAY-ven-hook) saw germs in his microscope, but 170 years passed before Pasteur and others proved that germs cause disease and that sterilization can kill germs. This made surgery safer. Roentgen's X rays let doctors see inside the body. Miracle drugs were developed. Today, researchers all over the world continue to make exciting discoveries about how the body works and how illnesses can be treated.

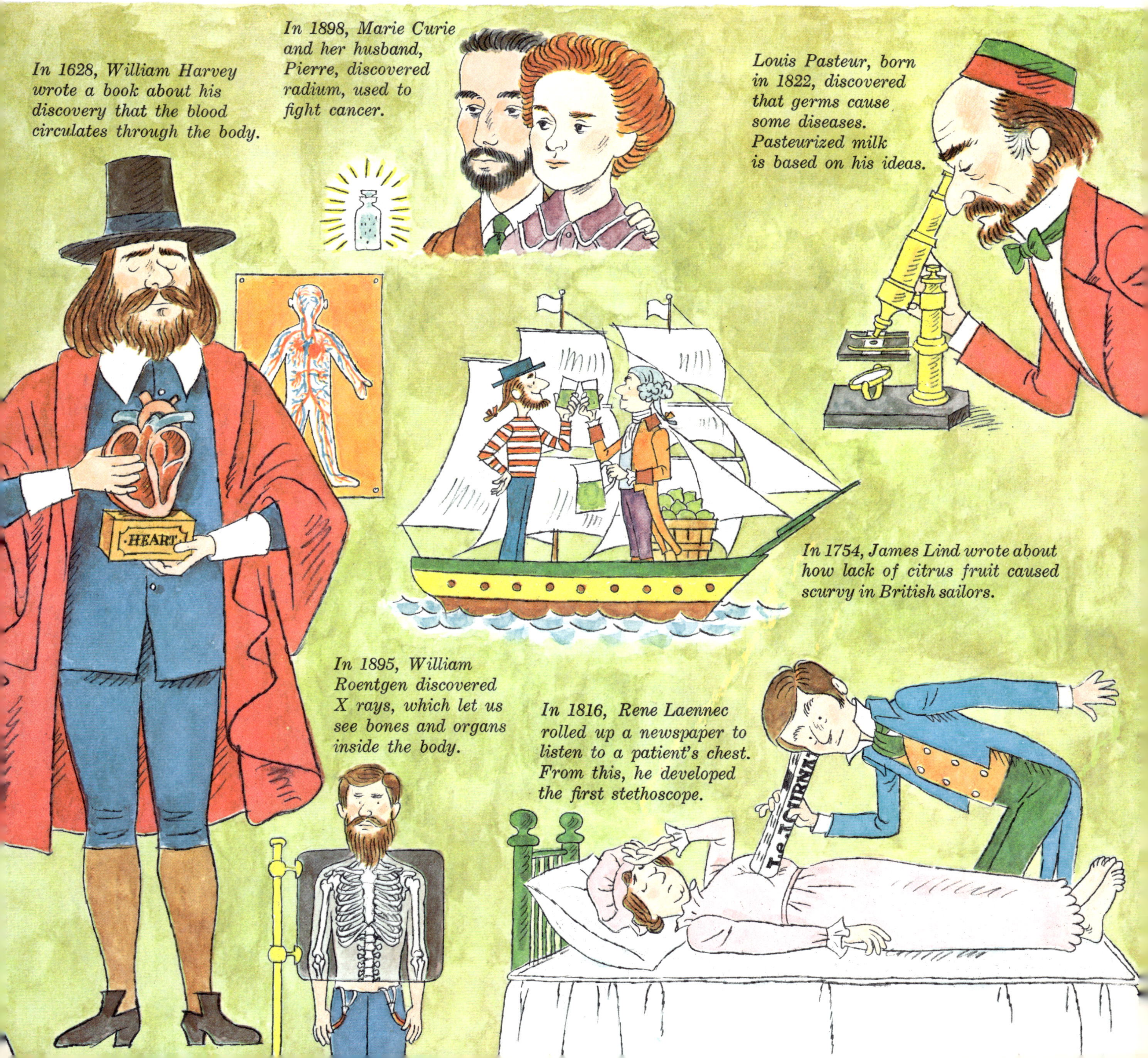

In 1628, William Harvey wrote a book about his discovery that the blood circulates through the body.

In 1898, Marie Curie and her husband, Pierre, discovered radium, used to fight cancer.

Louis Pasteur, born in 1822, discovered that germs cause some diseases. Pasteurized milk is based on his ideas.

In 1754, James Lind wrote about how lack of citrus fruit caused scurvy in British sailors.

In 1895, William Roentgen discovered X rays, which let us see bones and organs inside the body.

In 1816, Rene Laennec rolled up a newspaper to listen to a patient's chest. From this, he developed the first stethoscope.

Will we be **BORN**
more mature?

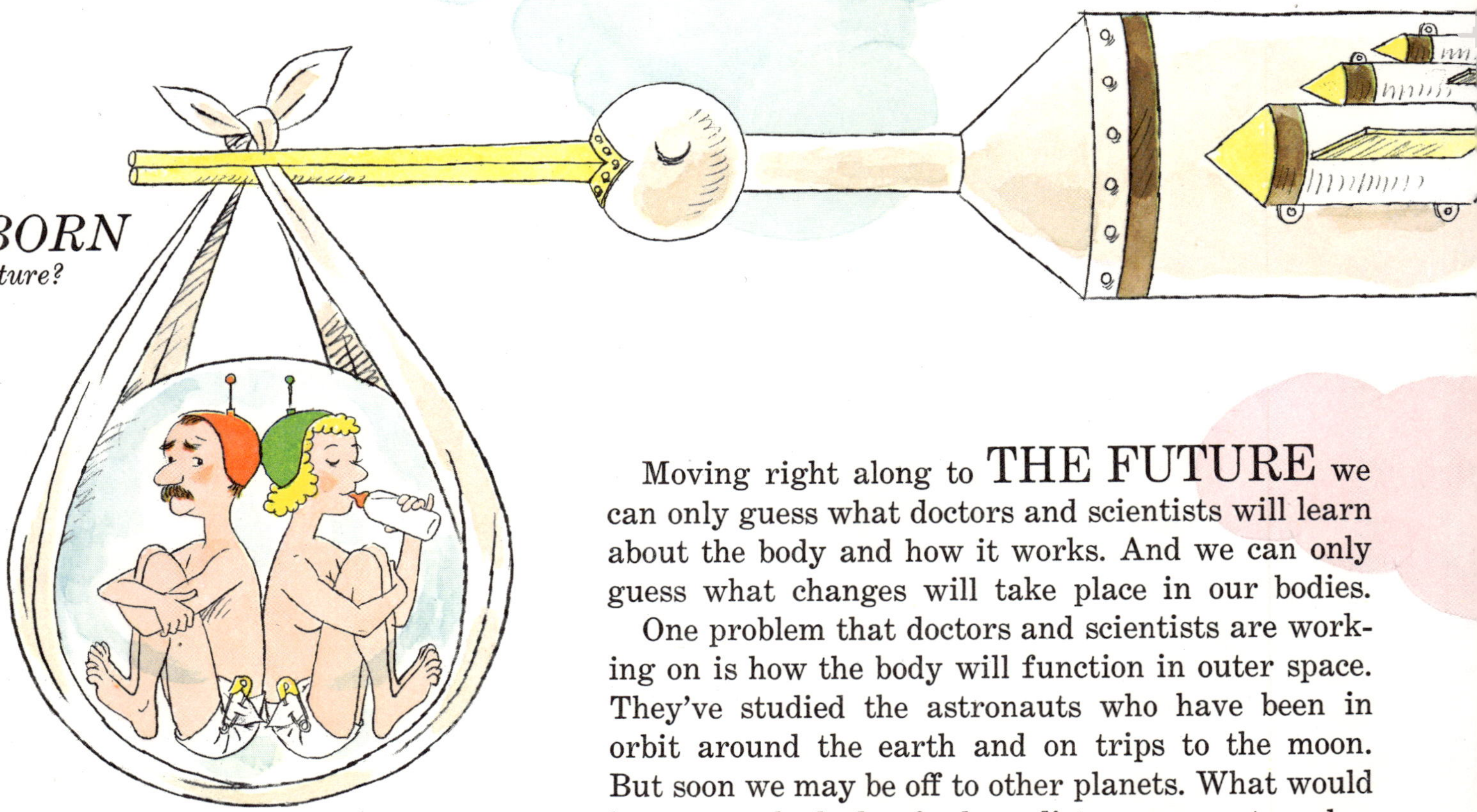

Moving right along to THE FUTURE we can only guess what doctors and scientists will learn about the body and how it works. And we can only guess what changes will take place in our bodies.

One problem that doctors and scientists are working on is how the body will function in outer space. They've studied the astronauts who have been in orbit around the earth and on trips to the moon. But soon we may be off to other planets. What would happen to the body of a long-distance space traveler, floating around weightless for a year or two? What would happen to the heart, the lungs, and the digestive system? Would the muscles lose their strength, and would the bones get weak?

And what about future changes in our bodies? Most likely we will change in size. If you look at suits of armor in a museum, you can see that the people who wore them were much smaller than people

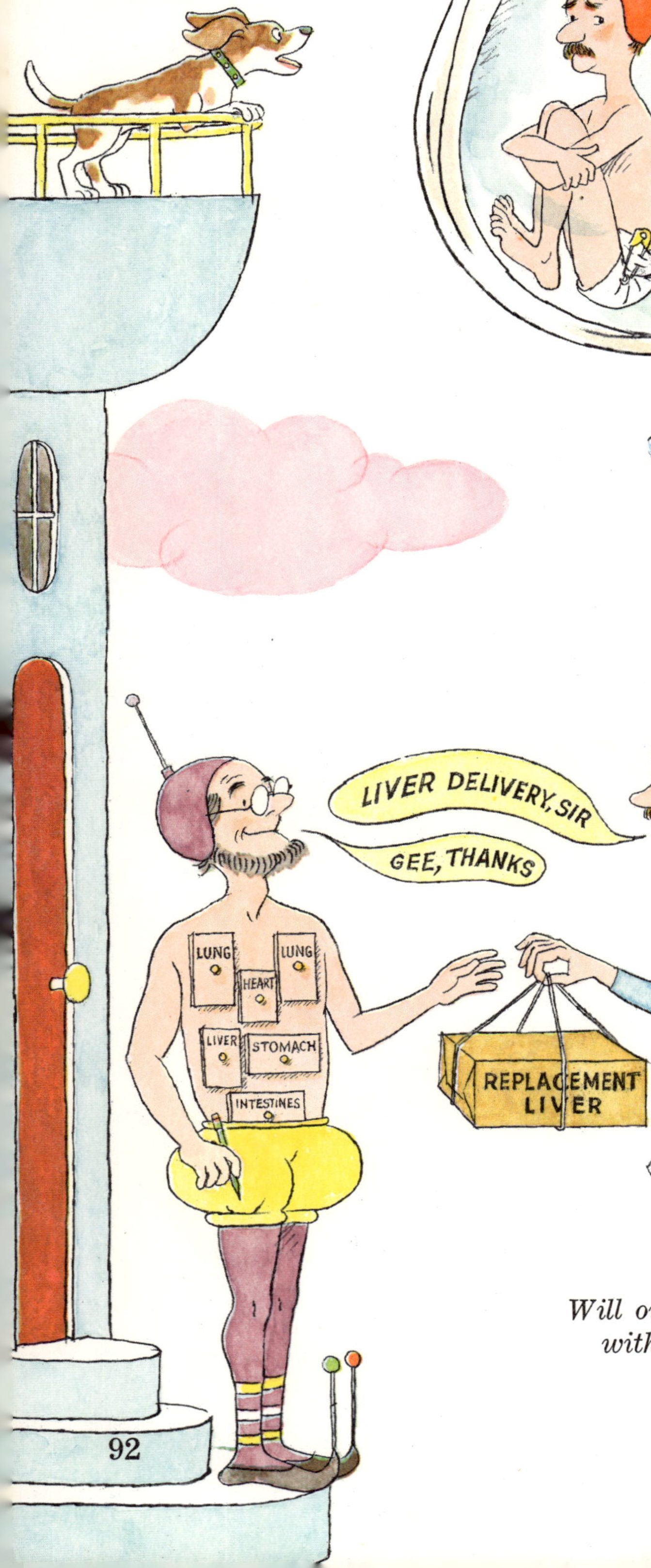

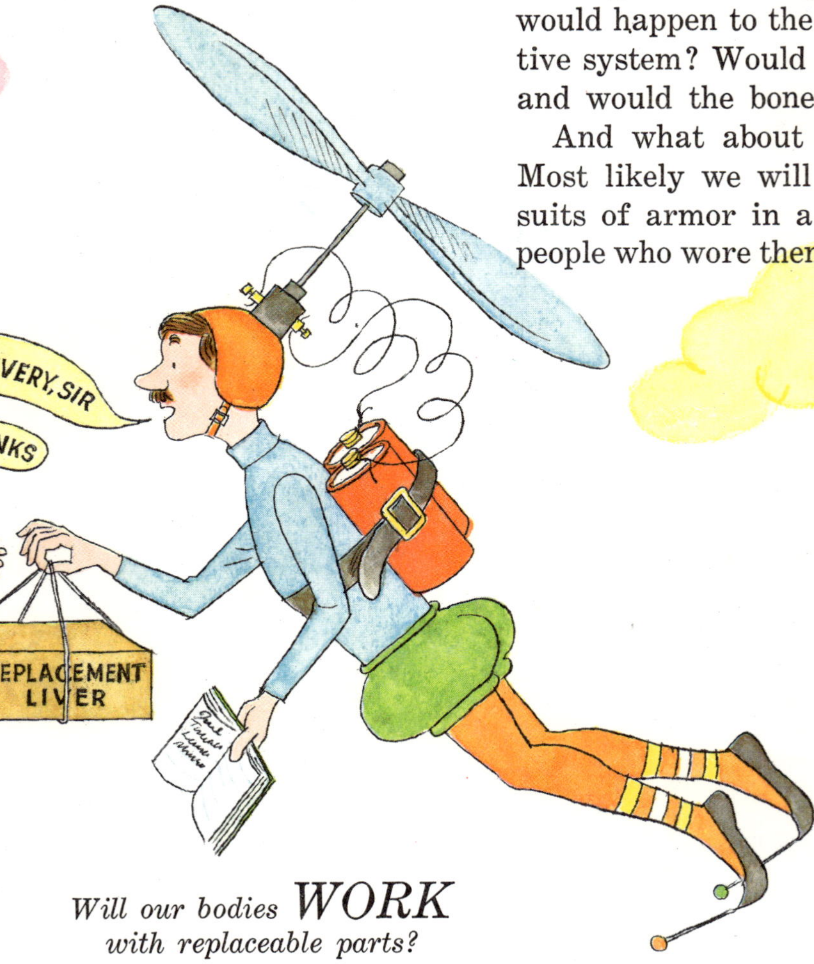

Will our bodies **WORK**
with replaceable parts?

Will we **LEARN** *everything*
while we are asleep?

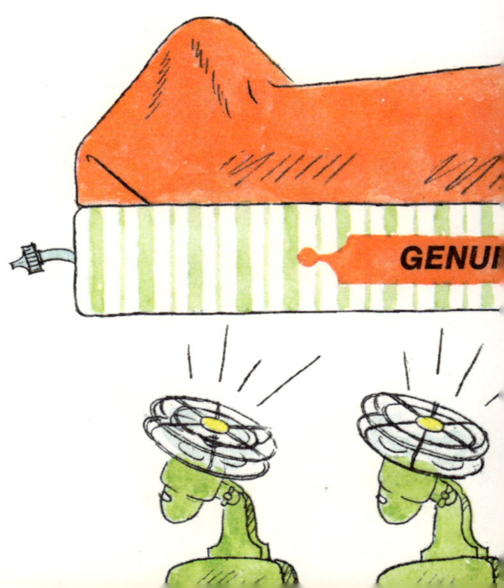

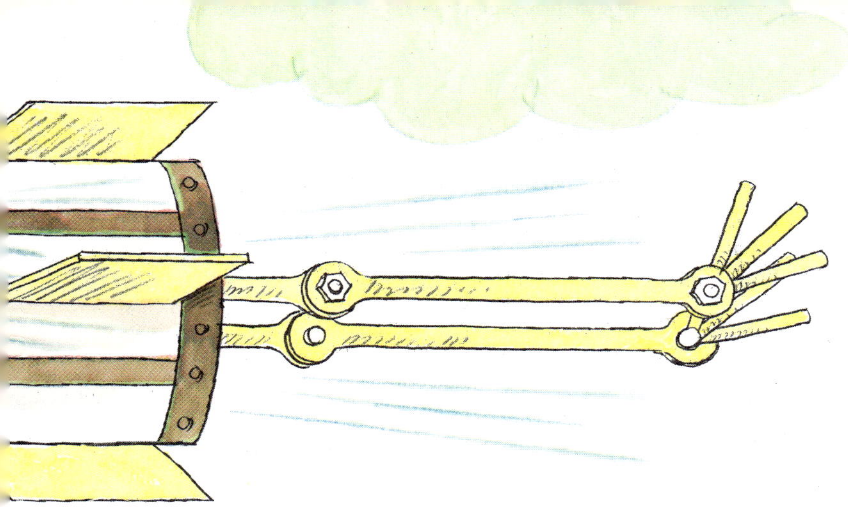

are today. In the future, people seven feet tall might be just average, and basketball players might be eight feet and taller!

Will man-made mechanical hearts and other organs be perfected to replace seriously damaged natural ones? Lots of work is being done in this area right now.

But even without replacements for worn-out parts of the body, people seem to be living longer and longer. In the future, 150-year-olds might be quite common. It would then be possible for a baby to have 25-year-old parents, 50-year-old grandparents, 75-year-old great-grandparents, 100-year-old great-great-grandparents, 125-year-old great-great-great-grandparents, and 150-year-old great-great-great-great-grandparents.

Who knows how different a future book about the human body might be from this one?

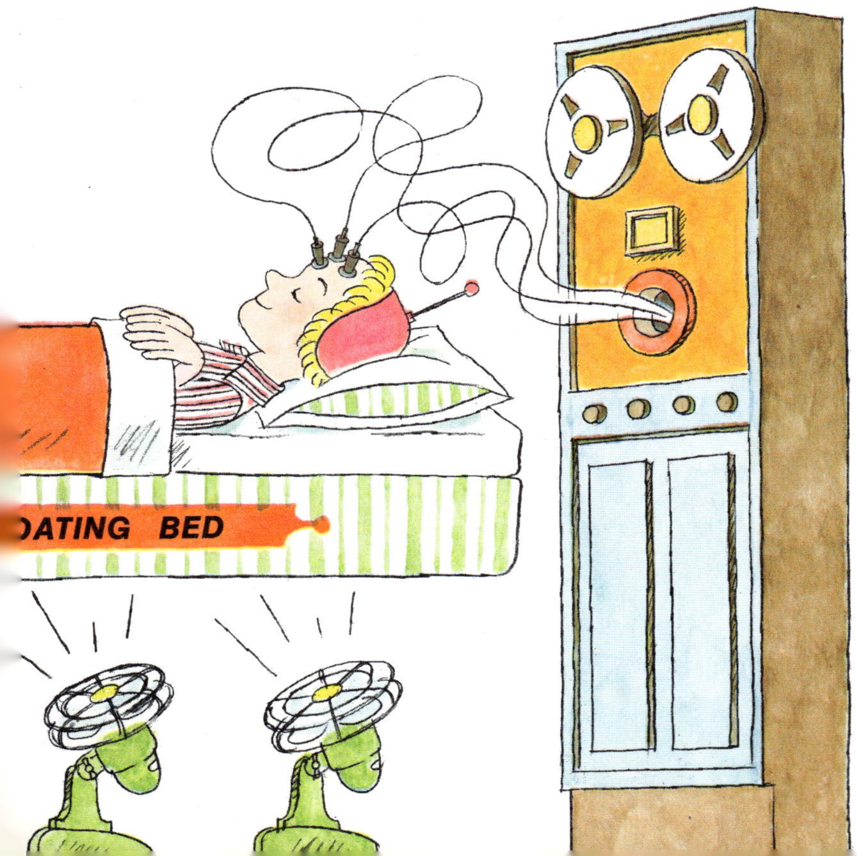

Will every generation **GROW** *taller and still taller?*

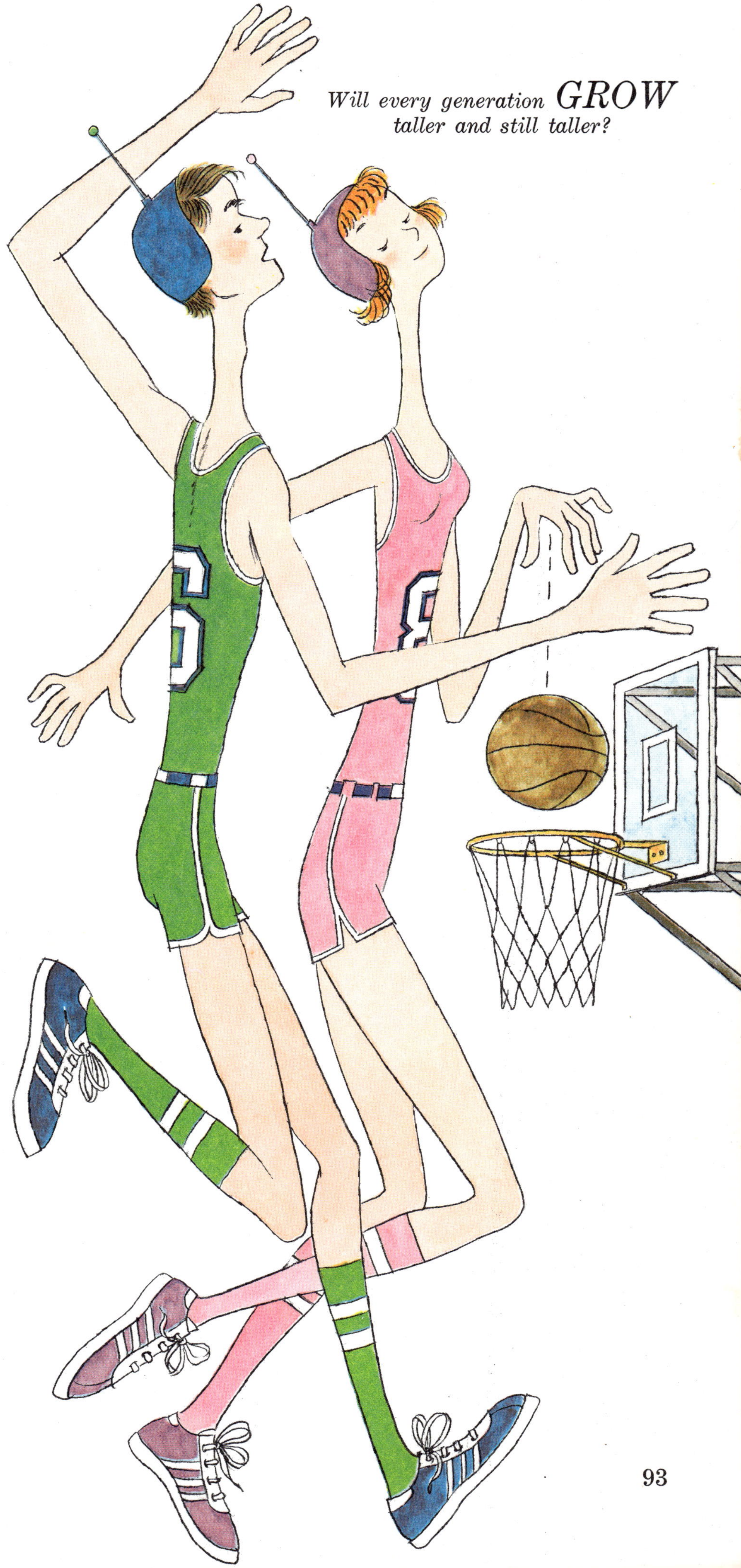

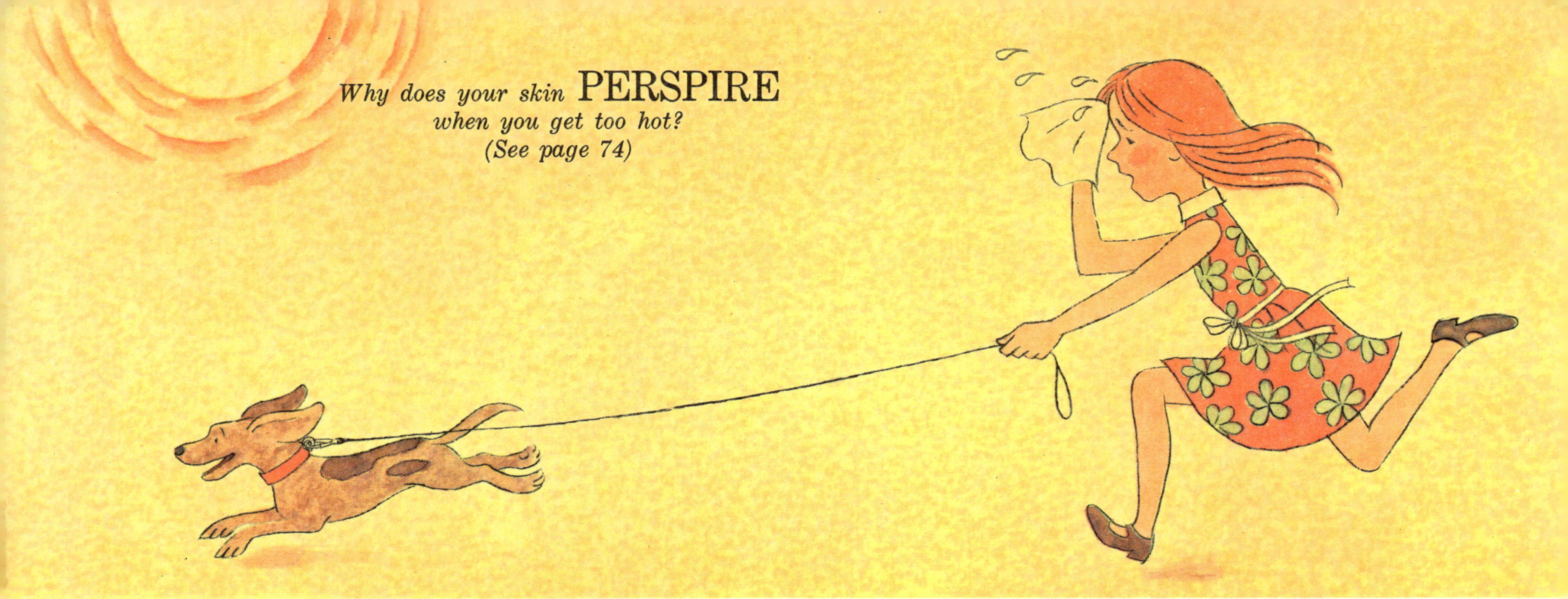

Why does your skin PERSPIRE
when you get too hot?
(See page 74)

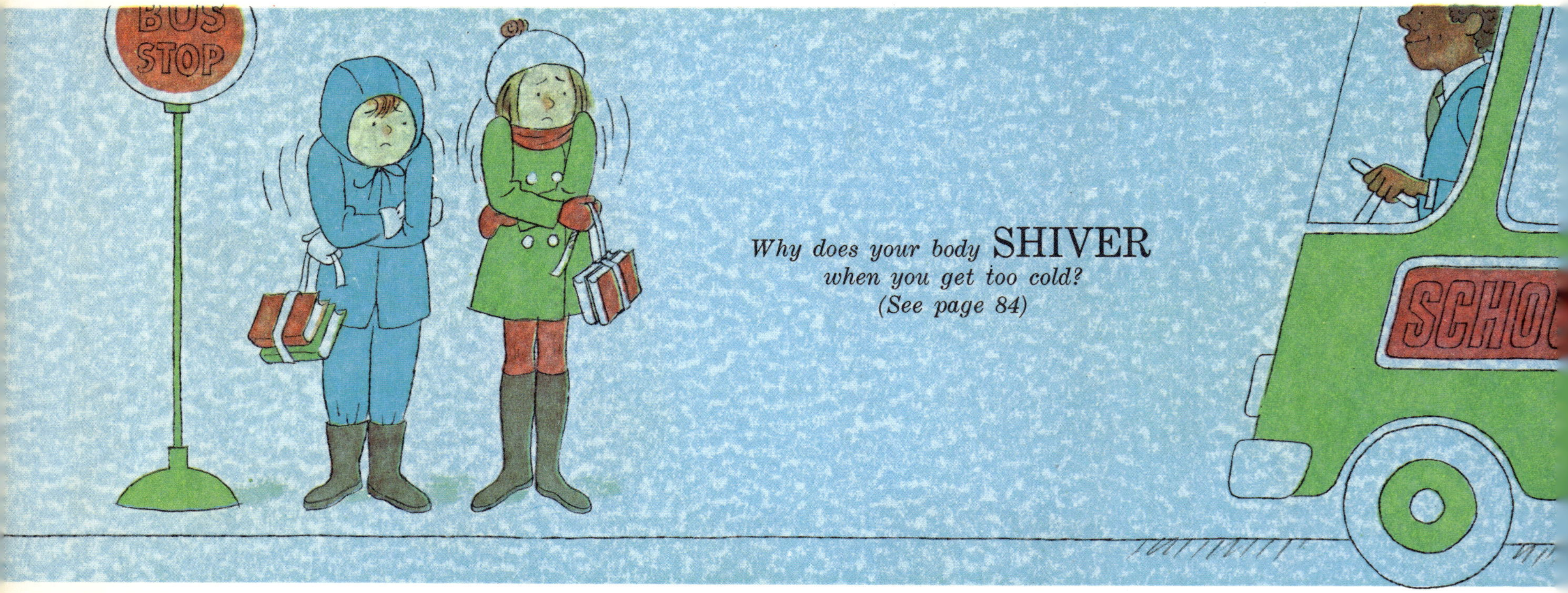

Why does your body SHIVER
when you get too cold?
(See page 84)

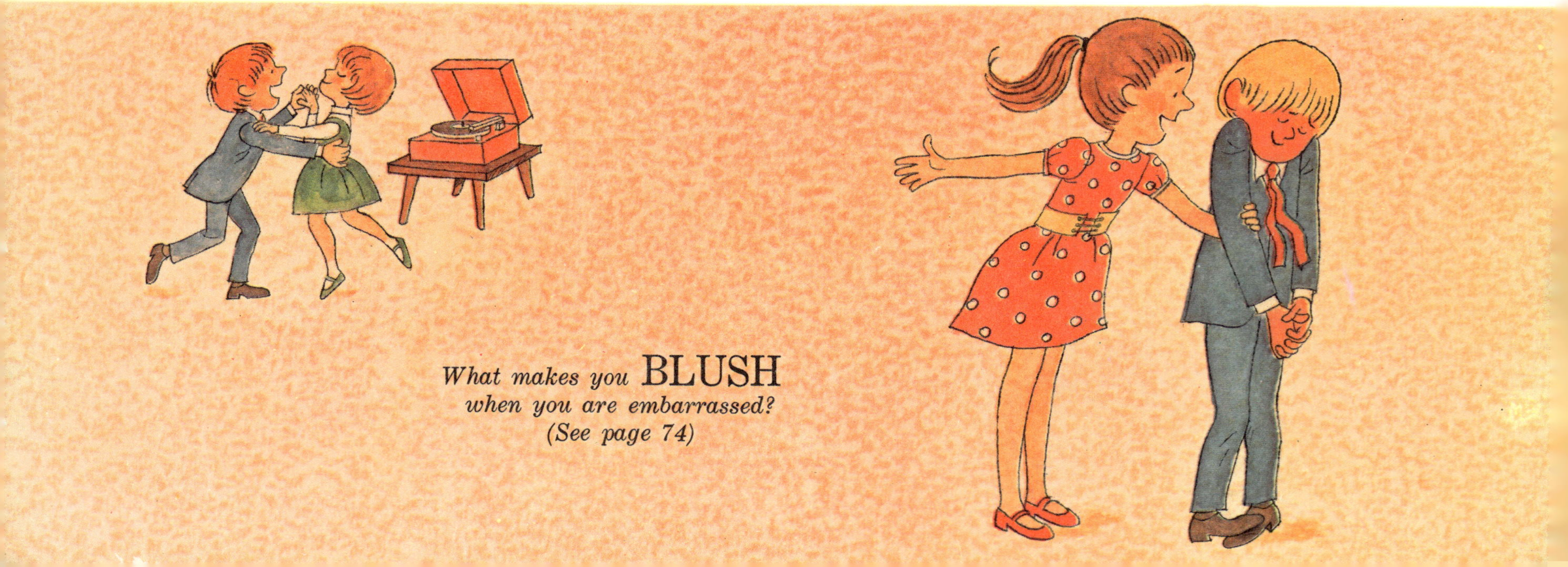

What makes you BLUSH
when you are embarrassed?
(See page 74)